Pain Management

Editor

JOHANN (HANS) COETZEE

VETERINARY CLINICS OF NORTH AMERICA: FOOD ANIMAL PRACTICE

www.vetfood.theclinics.com

Consulting Editor
ROBERT A. SMITH

March 2013 • Volume 29 • Number 1

ELSEVIER

1600 John F. Kennedy Boulevard ● Suite 1800 ● Philadelphia, Pennsylvania, 19103-2899

http://www.theclinics.com

VETERINARY CLINICS OF NORTH AMERICA: FOOD ANIMAL PRACTICE Volume 29, Number 1
March 2013 ISSN 0749-0720, ISBN-13: 978-1-4557-7349-7

Editor: John Vassallo; j.vassallo@elsevier.com
Developmental Editor: Teia Stone

Veterinary Clinics of North America: Food Animal Practice (ISSN 0749-0720) is published in March, July, and November by Elsevier Inc., 360 Park Avenue South, New York, NY 10010-1710. Subscription prices are $224.00 per year (domestic individuals), $308.00 per year (domestic institutions), $104.00 per year (domestic students/residents), $253.00 per year (Canadian individuals), $402.00 per year (Canadian institutions), $319.00 per year (international individuals), $402.00 per year (international institutions), and $159.00 per year (international and Canadian students/residents). To receive student/resident rate, orders must be accompanied by name of affiliated institution, date of term, and the signature of program/residency coordinator on institution letterhead. Clinics subscription prices. All prices are subject to change without notice. POSTMASTER: Send address changes to Veterinary Clinics of North America: Food Animal Practice, Elsevier Health Sciences Division, Subscription Customer Service, 3251 Riverport Lane, Maryland Heights, MO 63043. Customer Service (orders, claims, online, change of address): Elsevier Health Sciences Division, Subscription Customer Service, 3251 Riverport Lane, Maryland Heights, MO 63043. Tel: 1-800-654-2452 (U.S. and Canada); 314-447-8871 (ouside U.S. and Canada). Fax: 314-447-8029. E-mail: journalscustomerservice-usa@elsevier.com (for print support); journalsonlinesupport-usa@elsevier.com (for online support).

Reprints. For copies of 100 or more, of articles in this publication, please contact the Commercial Reprints Department, Elsevier Inc., 360 Park Avenue South, New York, NY 10010-1710. Tel.: 212-633-3812; Fax: 212-462-1935; E-mail: reprints@elsevier.com.

Veterinary Clinics of North America: Food Animal Practice is covered in Current Contents/Agriculture, Biology and Environmental Sciences, MEDLINE/PubMed (Index Medicus), and Excerpta Medica.

Printed and bound by CPI Group (UK) Ltd, Croydon, CR0 4YY

Transferred to digital print 2012

Contributors

CONSULTING EDITOR

ROBERT A. SMITH, DVM, MS
Diplomate, American Board of Veterinary Practitioners; Veterinary Research and
Consulting Services, LLC, Greeley, Colorado

EDITOR

JOHANN (HANS) COETZEE, BVSc, Cert CHP, PhD
Diplomate, American College of Veterinary Clinical Pharmacology; Associate
Professor, Department of Biomedical Science; Department of Veterinary Diagnostic
and Production Animal Medicine, College of Veterinary Medicine, Iowa State University,
Ames, Iowa

AUTHORS

ERIC J. ABRAHAMSEN, DVM
Diplomate, American College of Veterinary Anesthesiologists; Kalamazoo, Michigan

DAVID E. AMRINE, DVM
Department of Diagnostic Medicine and Pathobiology, College of Veterinary Medicine,
Kansas State University, Manhattan, Kansas

DAVID E. ANDERSON, DVM, MS
Diplomate, American College of Veterinary Surgeons; Professor and Head, Large Animal
Clinical Sciences, College of Veterinary Medicine, University of Tennessee, Knoxville,
Tennessee

SARAH L. BALDRIDGE, DVM, MS
Department of Clinical Sciences, College of Veterinary Medicine, Kansas State University,
Manhattan, Kansas

JOHANN F. COETZEE, BVSc, Cert CHP, PhD
Diplomate, American College of Veterinary Clinical Pharmacology; Associate
Professor, Department of Biomedical Science; Department of Veterinary Diagnostic
and Production Animal Medicine, College of Veterinary Medicine, Iowa State University,
Ames, Iowa

MISTY A. EDMONDSON, DVM, MS
Diplomate, American College of Theriogenology; Assistant Professor, Department of
Clinical Sciences, College of Veterinary Medicine, Auburn University, Auburn, Alabama

DEE GRIFFIN, DVM, MS
Great Plains Veterinary Educational Center, University of Nebraska-Lincoln, Clay Center,
Nebraska

SUZANNE T. MILLMAN, BSc(Agr), PhD
Associate Professor of Animal Welfare, Departments of Veterinary Diagnostic & Production Animal Medicine and Biomedical Sciences, Lloyd Veterinary Medical Center, Iowa State University, Ames, Iowa

SANJA MODRIC, DVM, PhD
FDA Center for Veterinary Medicine, Office of New Animal Drug Evaluation, Rockville, Maryland

HEATHER P. NEWTON, BS
DVM Candidate, Department of Veterinary Diagnostic and Production Animal Medicine, College of Veterinary Medicine, Iowa State University, Ames, Iowa

ANNETTE M. O'CONNOR, BVSc, MVSc, DVSc, FACVSc (Epidemiology)
Veterinary Epidemiologist; Professor, Department of Veterinary Diagnostic and Production Animal Medicine, College of Veterinary Medicine, Iowa State University, Ames, Iowa

PAUL J. PLUMMER, DVM, PhD
Diplomate, American College of Veterinary Internal Medicine (Large Animal Internal Medicine); Assistant Professor, Veterinary Diagnostic and Production Animal Medicine, Lloyd Veterinary Medical Center, College of Veterinary Medicine, Iowa State University, Ames, Iowa

JENNIFER A. SCHLEINING, DVM, MS
Diplomate, American College of Veterinary Surgeons (Large Animal); Veterinary Diagnostic and Production Animal Medicine, Lloyd Veterinary Medical Center, College of Veterinary Medicine, Iowa State University, Ames, Iowa

JAN K. SHEARER, DVM, MS
Diplomate, American College of Animal Welfare; Professor and Dairy Extension Specialist, Dairy Production Medicine, Lameness, Animal Welfare, Iowa State University, Ames, Iowa

EMILY R. SMITH, DVM
FDA Center for Veterinary Medicine, Office of New Animal Drug Evaluation, Rockville, Maryland

GEOF SMITH, DVM, MS, PhD
Diplomate, American College of Veterinary Internal Medicine; Associate Professor, Department of Population Health & Pathobiology, North Carolina State University, Raleigh, North Carolina

MATTHEW L. STOCK, VMD
Diplomate, American Board of Veterinary Practitioners (Food Animal); Department of Veterinary Diagnostic and Production Animal Medicine; Department of Biomedical Sciences, College of Veterinary Medicine, Iowa State University, Ames, Iowa

MILES E. THEURER, BS
Department of Diagnostic Medicine and Pathobiology, College of Veterinary Medicine, Kansas State University, Manhattan, Kansas

SAREL R. VAN AMSTEL, BVSc, Dip Med Vet, M MED VET
Diplomate, American College of Veterinary Internal Medicine; Diplomate, American Board of Veterinary Practitioners; Professor, Department of Large Animal Clinical Sciences, College of Veterinary Medicine, The University of Tennessee, Knoxville, Tennessee

BRAD J. WHITE, DVM, MS
Associate Professor, Department of Clinical Sciences, College of Veterinary Medicine, Kansas State University, Manhattan, Kansas

Contents

of diagnosis and treatment of bovine pain. In this review, attitudes of citizens, producers, and veterinarians are explored regarding pain and its associations with animal welfare and husbandry procedures. Behavior used to quantify pain in cattle is identified in terms of pain-specific behaviors and general behavioral responses that can be observed during painful procedures or convalescence. Finally, nociception and cognitive tests used for reporting pain in human patients are investigated for application to bovine patients.

Cattle behavior is frequently monitored to determine the health of the animal. This article describes potential benefits and challenges of remotely monitoring cattle behavior with available methodologies. The behavior of interest, labor required, and monitoring expenses must be considered before deciding which remote behavioral monitoring device is appropriate. Monitoring the feeding behavior of an animal over time allows establishment of a baseline against which deviations can be evaluated. Interpretation of multiple behavioral responses as an aggregate indicator of animal wellness status instead of as individual outcomes may be a more accurate measure of true state of pain or wellness.

Validated pain assessment tools are needed to support approval of analgesic compounds to alleviate pain associated with castration. Accelerometers, videography, heart rate variability, electroencephalography, thermography, and plasma neuropeptide measurement to assess behavioral, physiologic, and neuroendocrine changes associated with castration are discussed. Preemptive local and systemic analgesia are also reviewed. Previous studies found that preemptive administration of nonsteroidal antiinflammatory drug (NSAID) and local anesthesia significantly decreased peak serum cortisol concentration after castration. Local anesthesia alone tended to decrease peak cortisol concentrations more than NSAIDs, whereas NSAIDs alone tended to decrease the area under the cortisol-time curve more than local anesthesia alone.

Dehorning or disbudding in cattle is performed for a variety of reasons using various methods. Pain associated with this procedure has been mostly evaluated through behavioral, physiologic, and neuroendocrine changes following dehorning. Analgesics, including local nerve blockades, anti-inflammatories, and opioids have demonstrated an effective attenuation of the cortisol response. The administration of sedatives with analgesic properties has been indicated in the attenuation of the acute phase of pain associated with dehorning. Following a literature review, this article recommends a multimodal approach to analgesia for dehorning procedures, including the use of a local anesthetic and anti-inflammatory and, when possible, a sedative-analgesic.

ruminant triple drip, provide a more stable plane of injectable anesthesia than bolus administration techniques.

Using castration and dehorning as the test base, this article evaluates whether pain management is associated with increased production and whether this motivates producers. The literature supporting increased production parameters is limited. Studies have evaluated short periods and often use few animals. Few studies are repeated and the potential for publication bias is high. There is little evidence that pain management is associated with increased production. This is a concern because survey data suggest producers are partly motivated based on economic factors. The unanswered question is whether economic incentive programs would be greater motivators than increased production.

VETERINARY CLINICS OF NORTH AMERICA: FOOD ANIMAL PRACTICE

THE CLINICS ARE NOW AVAILABLE ONLINE!
Access your subscription at:
www.theclinics.com

Preface

Pain Management

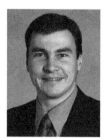

Johann (Hans) Coetzee BVSc, Cert CHP, PhD, DACVCP
Editor

It is an honor for me to serve as the guest editor for this, the first issue of *Veterinary Clinics of North America: Food Animal Practice* dedicated to pain management. The provision of analgesia is considered an essential part of overall patient care in human medicine, creating an expectation that veterinarians should also be able to recognize and manage pain in animals effectively. This, combined with increased public awareness of pain associated with routine livestock management practices, has resulted in calls for the development of procedures that alleviate pain and suffering in production animals. Surveys suggest that 81% of consumers believe that animals and humans have the same ability to feel pain, with 76% stating that animal welfare considerations are more important than product price. One example of the impact that this has had on livestock production practices is a recent European Commission Directive requiring that surgical castration of pigs after 1 January 2012 be performed with prolonged analgesia and/or anesthesia. Current information about pain assessment and management in livestock, as contained in this collection of review articles, is therefore critical for food animal veterinarians to address these emerging issues effectively.

The desire for veterinarians to be at the forefront of advocating pain management in animals is not new. The first Veterinarian's Oath adopted by the American Veterinary Medical Association (AVMA) House of Delegates in 1954 contained a specific pledge that veterinarians will "temper pain with anesthesia where indicated." Subsequent amendments to the Oath removed this phrase and replaced it with a commitment that veterinarians will use their "scientific knowledge and skills for the benefit of society through the protection of animal health and welfare, and the prevention and relief of animal suffering." In spite of this, surveys of food animal veterinarians in the United States and Canada reported that less than 20% of respondents routinely use analgesics at the time of dehorning and castration. The reason for the low prevalence of analgesic use can be attributed to several challenges and misconceptions encountered by food animal veterinarians when implementing analgesic regimens on a routine basis. These include that (1) pain recognition is difficult in stoic species such as cattle, sheep, and

Vet Clin Food Anim 29 (2013) xi–xii
http://dx.doi.org/10.1016/j.cvfa.2012.11.013
0749-0720/13/$ – see front matter © 2013 Published by Elsevier Inc.

vetfood.theclinics.com

goats; (2) there are no analgesic compounds specifically approved by the Food and Drug Administration for analgesic use in livestock in the United States; (3) analgesic use constitutes extra label drug use (ELDU), which is regulated by Animal Medicinal Drug Use Clarification Act (AMDUCA) and which effectively places the responsibility for determining an appropriate meat and milk withhold period on the veterinarian; (4) there is often a delay between drug administration and onset of analgesic activity; (5) analgesic drug administration often involves inconvenient routes of drug administration, which may require additional training; (6) most analgesic compounds have short plasma elimination half-lives, necessitating repeated drug administration; and (7) it is unclear if analgesic administration is associated with health and performance benefits that could help offset the cost of treatment.

The talented contributors to this issue were selected across disciplines to provide the latest expert information that would assist veterinarians in addressing these challenges. The first 3 articles introduce the analgesic compounds that are available for use in cattle and the regulatory considerations with respect to the drug approval process and the establishment of withdrawal periods needed for ELDU. The fourth and fifth articles are devoted to the assessment of pain through either the direct or the indirect assessment of changes in animal behavior in response to pain. Articles 6 through 9 are devoted specifically to the assessment and management of pain associated with castration, dehorning, lameness, and surgery. The focus of the 10th article is specifically on the analgesic needs of small ruminants and camelids, and the 11th article describes protocols for field anesthesia and chemical restraint in ruminants. The final article is a systematic review of the published literature evaluating the economics of pain management administered at the time of dehorning and castration. Taken together, this issue provides readers with practical, science-based information regarding management of painful conditions routinely encountered in food animal practice as well as addressing broader issues related to the drug approval process and the economics of providing analgesia. Ultimately, the success of this endeavor will be judged by how many copies find their way from the bookshelf into the vet truck. My hope is that most of the pages will be well worn!

I am indebted to all the authors for accepting the invitation to contribute to this issue and for accommodating a tight timetable in meeting deadlines in the midst of their extraordinarily busy schedules. Acknowledgements are also due to the editors of the series, Dr Robert A. Smith and Mr John Vassallo, for their support and guidance during the editorial process. Last, but certainly not least, I am especially grateful for all the miracles in my life, especially my wife, Tiffany, for her unwavering support throughout the process of preparing and assembling these articles.

Johann (Hans) Coetzee, BVSc, Cert CHP, PhD, DACVCP
Diplomate of the American College of Veterinary Clinical Pharmacology
Department of Veterinary Diagnostic
and Production Animal Medicine
College of Veterinary Medicine
Iowa State University
1600 South 16th Street
Ames, IA 50011, USA

E-mail address:
hcoetzee@iastate.edu

Regulatory Considerations for the Approval of Analgesic Drugs for Cattle in the United States

Emily R. Smith, DVM*, Sanja Modric, DVM, PhD

KEYWORDS

- Analgesics • Nonsteroidal anti-inflammatory drugs • Cattle • Pain • Regulatory

KEY POINTS

- The Food and Drug Administration's Center for Veterinary Medicine (CVM) ensures that safe and effective approved animal drugs are available for use in the United States.
- Although no drugs are currently approved for analgesic use in cattle, CVM supports the ethical treatment and management of cattle and aims to improve the availability of safe and effective drugs for the control of pain.
- CVM encourages drug companies to use innovative approaches to demonstrate the effectiveness of drugs for analgesic use in cattle.
- There is an obvious need for continued research into the development of adequate behavioral and physiologic measures that can be used to reliably demonstrate the effectiveness of new animal drugs for the control of pain in cattle.

INTRODUCTION

Animal drugs intended for use in the United States are regulated by the US Food and Drug Administration (FDA) Center for Veterinary Medicine (CVM). CVM is a consumer-protection organization with a mission to protect human and animal health. The authority to carry out CVM's public health mission comes from the Federal Food, Drug, and Cosmetic Act (FFDCA). The United States Congress passed the animal drug amendments to the FFDCA in 1968 because they recognized the need for the use of animal drugs to meet the therapeutic and production needs of animals. FDA interprets the FFDCA and publishes regulations in the Code of Federal Regulations (CFR). Chapter 21 of the CFR addresses new animal drugs. As mandated by the FFDCA, a new animal drug may not be introduced into interstate commerce unless it is: the subject of an approved new animal drug application (NADA); the subject of an abbreviated NADA (ANADA); the subject of a conditional approval (CNADA)

FDA Center for Veterinary Medicine, Office of New Animal Drug Evaluation, 7500 Standish Place, Rockville, MD 20855, USA
* Corresponding author.
E-mail address: emily.smith2@fda.hhs.gov

Vet Clin Food Anim 29 (2013) 1–10
http://dx.doi.org/10.1016/j.cvfa.2012.11.009
0749-0720/13/$ – see front matter Published by Elsevier Inc.

pursuant to 21 U.S.C. §360 ccc; or there is an index listing in effect pursuant to 21 U.S.C. §360 ccc-1 (21 U.S.C. §§331(a) and 360b(a)). Under section 512(j) of the Act, new animal drugs may be exempt from the approval requirements of the Act if they are intended solely for investigational use to evaluate the safety and effectiveness of the drug.

To approve and sustain a new animal drug for commercial use, 4 critical requirements must be met: (1) the animal drug product must be safe for the target animal, safe for the humans consuming food derived from treated animals, safe for the user or the person administering the drug, and safe for the environment; (2) the animal drug must be effective for its intended uses as stated in labeling of the product; (3) the animal drug must be a quality manufactured product, being the result of a validated manufacturing process; and (4) the product must be properly labeled to inform the user of the product how to use it and to provide safety information, withdrawal times, and storage and handling instructions. Once in the market place, the FDA continues to monitor the animal drug to ensure that these characteristics are sustained. The post-approval evaluation includes monitoring the drug's safety and effectiveness, manufacturing processes, and labeling through surveillance and the submission of proposed changes by the sponsor.

The development and marketing of a new animal drug in the United States is a complex undertaking. Meeting the rigorous standards for safety and effectiveness and sustaining a quality manufactured product is a challenge. However, CVM believes that its public health mission is achieved when a safe, effective, quality manufactured, properly labeled new animal drug is put in the hands of the user. For food-producing animals, CVM wants to ensure that the use of therapeutic animal drugs will serve to improve animal health and welfare. Therefore, the approval of safe and effective analgesic drugs for cattle is an important part of the public health mission of CVM.

NEW ANIMAL DRUG APPROVAL PROCESS IN THE UNITED STATES

The new animal drug approval process often involves many years of research on the part of the drug sponsor and significant collaboration with CVM to provide appropriate and adequate data supporting the safety, effectiveness, and manufacture of the drug. For approval of any new animal drug, drug sponsors are encouraged to have early discussions with CVM to create a development plan based on the drug, species, and intended use of the product.

To assist sponsors with the drug approval process, CVM provides Guidance for Industry (GFI) documents, which represent the Agency's current thinking on various topics related to the drug approval process. These documents are not legally binding, but are helpful in designing pivotal studies in support of NADAs. Drug sponsors should consider the information contained in guidance documents as recommendations unless specific regulatory requirements are discussed. Drug sponsors may use alternative approaches if the approach satisfies the requirements of the applicable statues and regulations. In such cases, CVM encourages sponsors to discuss their ideas with CVM. Published literature can be used to demonstrate safety and effectiveness of a new animal drug. Important factors to consider when using published literature include the use of appropriate and objective end points that are not dependent on investigator's subjective judgment; a high level of detail in the published report; and robust analyses and conclusions based on protocol-specified parameters. In general, literature can be relied on to a greater degree if there are multiple studies conducted by independent investigators with adequate study designs; properly documented operating procedures, and a history of implementing such procedures effectively, as well as consistent findings between investigators. When literature is used in support of the safety and effectiveness of a new animal drug, it is important to provide a balanced discussion of the published studies that raise questions relating to the safety and effectiveness of the new animal drug, as well as the published studies that support a finding of safety and effectiveness.

There are 7 components (referred to as technical sections) that must be addressed for approval of a new animal drug in food animals: Effectiveness, Target Animal Safety (TAS), Chemistry, Manufacturing, and Controls (CMC), Human Food Safety (HFS), Environmental Impact, Labeling, and All Other Information (AOI). Each technical section is briefly discussed here. (For more detail on the NADA regulatory requirements, see 21 CFR 514.)

Effectiveness

The Effectiveness technical section must contain full reports of all studies that show whether the new animal drug is effective for its intended use [21 CFR §514.1(b)(8)(i)]. To demonstrate effectiveness, the sponsor must show by substantial evidence that the new animal drug will have the effect it purports or is represented to have under the conditions of use prescribed, recommended, or suggested in the proposed labeling. One part of the Effectiveness technical section is the characterization of the dosage (dose, frequency, and duration of administration). For the purpose of dosage characterization, the sponsor may submit information (such as a dose titration study, a pilot effectiveness study, in vitro studies, scientific literature, or assessments based on pharmacokinetic and pharmacodynamic modeling) to explain the dose selection. Substantial evidence may be demonstrated through 1 or more adequate and well-controlled studies that include the measurement of appropriate parameters that reflect the effectiveness of the drug and provide repeatable results with inferential value. Studies such as those conducted in the target species or laboratory animals, a field study, a bioequivalence study, or an in vitro study may fulfill the substantial evidence of effectiveness requirements. Pharmacokinetic and pharmacodynamic studies may augment and further document the nature of the drug's effectiveness. Depending on the type of drug (eg, antimicrobial, anthelmintic, nonsteroidal anti-inflammatory, and so forth) and the proposed indication(s), different studies may be necessary, such as a validated animal model study, a dose-confirmation study, and a field-effectiveness study.

CVM encourages sponsors to submit and obtain CVM concurrence on all study protocols before conducting pivotal studies to ensure that the study design and success criteria are acceptable to support the intended indication(s) and use. All pivotal studies are designed based on the proposed indications, dosage, and target population for which the new animal drug is intended.

Target Animal Safety

The TAS technical section must contain full reports of all studies that show whether the new animal drug is safe to the target species [21 CFR §514.1(b)(8)(i)]. The specific TAS information needed for approval depends on factors such as the type of drug, species and class of animals, route of administration, indications, dosage, and available scientific knowledge about the pharmacology and toxicology of the drug. For new animal drugs, TAS may be demonstrated in a margin of safety study, such as a 0, 1×, 3×, and 5× dose study (1× = highest recommended dose level), with the drug administered for a period of time in excess of the recommended maximum duration of use. CVM also encourages sponsors to consider other study designs or approaches to evaluate the safety of the drug for the target animal, where appropriate. TAS is established by demonstrating an acceptable margin of safety and, where possible, identifying the toxic syndrome. Additional studies such as reproductive safety, safety in neonates, or application/injection site studies may also be required, depending on the intended use of the new animal drug. GFI #185 entitled *Target Animal Safety for Veterinary Pharmaceutical Products, VICH GL43*,[1] is available on the CVM Web site, and was written to assist sponsors in the development of their target animal safety assessment.

Chemistry, Manufacturing, and Controls

The CMC technical section must contain complete information regarding the manufacture of the new animal drug active ingredient and the new animal drug product [21 CFR §514.1(b)(4)&(5)]. The CMC section includes information on the new drug's identity, strength, components and composition, quality, purity, potency, manufacturing sites and process, specifications such as assays, expiry dating, and stability, and the container closure system. The regulations set forth in 21 CFR Parts 210 through 226 contain the minimum current Good Manufacturing Practice (cGMP) requirements for methods used, and the facilities or controls to be used for the manufacture, processing, packaging, or holding of a drug.

Human Food Safety

For drugs intended for use in food-producing animals, sponsors must demonstrate that residues in edible tissues derived from treated animals are safe for human consumption. Edible tissues are defined as muscle, injection-site muscle, muscle underlying a pour-on site, muscle with skin in natural proportions (fish), liver, kidney, fat, skin with fat in natural proportions, eggs, milk, and honey (21 CFR §556.1). To complete the HFS technical section, sponsors must submit a description of practicable methods for determining the quantity, if any, of the new animal drug in or on food, and any substance formed in or on food because of its use, and the proposed tolerance or withdrawal period or other use restrictions to ensure that the proposed use of the drug will be safe [21 CFR §514.1(b)(7)].

The HFS technical section may include, but is not limited to, information on the following: short-term and long-term toxicology, total residue and metabolism, analytical method validation, tissue residue depletion, and, if the drug has antimicrobial properties, microbial food safety. First, toxicology information is used to determine the toxicologic acceptable daily intake (tADI) of a chemical. The tADI represents residues that may be consumed daily in the human diet for a lifetime without appreciable risk to the health of the consumer. If the drug is antimicrobial in nature or exhibits antimicrobial properties, sponsors must demonstrate that the use of the drug does not cause bacteria in or on treated animals to become resistant, and that any resistance will not affect public health. In addition, following an evaluation of an antimicrobial or compound with antimicrobial activity, a microbiological ADI (mADI) may be assigned. CVM will select the most appropriate of the calculated ADIs, either the tADI or, if applicable, the mADI, as the final ADI for the drug. Using this ADI, CVM establishes safe concentrations for total residues of the drug in each of the edible tissues. Once the safe concentrations are established, a target tissue and a marker residue are identified. A tolerance for the marker residue, which is the maximum legally permitted concentration for residues in or on a food, is determined in the target tissue using the official regulatory method. Tolerances are established for the target tissue and, where applicable, for milk and eggs. Information on residue depletion is collected under conditions of use to establish the withdrawal period and, where applicable, a milk discard time, based on the respective tolerances. The withdrawal period/milk discard time is the interval between the last administration of a sponsored compound and when the animal can be safely harvested for food or the milk safely consumed. If the withdrawal time is followed, food products derived from treated animals are considered safe for people to eat.

Environmental Impact

The Environmental Impact technical section must contain either an environmental assessment (EA) under 21 CFR §25.40, or a request for categorical exclusion under 21 CFR §25.33 [21 CFR §514.1(b)(14)]. Environmental information is submitted to comply with the National Environmental Policy Act. Before approving a new animal drug, the agency must consider potential effects on the environment. In many cases, including those for many intended uses for minor species, a categorical exclusion from the need to provide an EA can be granted. In other cases, such as new chemical entities, some type of EA will be necessary to support a "finding of no significant impact" or FONSI. The EA may include information on the introduction of the drug into the environment through manufacture, use, and disposal, the fate of the drug in the environment, and the effects of the drug in the environment.

Labeling

The labeling includes the immediate container label, package insert, outer packaging (box, carton), and shipper (multiple container) labeling. Label statements are data driven and should not be promotional in tone nor false or misleading, and should ensure the new animal drug product is used in a proper, safe, and effective manner.

Sponsors should provide labeling language with each technical section submitted for review to reflect information from that particular section. For example, the indication, dose, administration information, and adverse reactions seen in field studies should accompany the Effectiveness technical section. Results from target animal safety studies and appropriate warnings and contraindication statements should be submitted with the TAS technical section. Withdrawal times for edible tissues may be part of the HFS technical section. Storage conditions and formulation information should be submitted with the CMC technical section.

The proprietary (trade) name of the product is also subject to review by CVM to ensure the name is not promotional, nor false or misleading. CVM ensures the adherence to 21 CFR 201.10, as well as sections 201 and 502 of the FFDCA.

All Other Information

The AOI technical section includes all information pertinent to the review of safety and effectiveness received or otherwise obtained by the applicant from any source [21 CFR §514.1(b)(8)(iv)]. For the AOI section, the sponsor submits all other available information on the new animal drug that has not been previously submitted to any of the other technical sections. It should contain information from any investigations, foreign marketing and scientific literature, and any other data that were not already submitted by the sponsor as part of a major technical section (Effectiveness, TAS, CMC, HFS, and Environmental Impact).

FREEDOM OF INFORMATION SUMMARY

A Freedom of Information (FOI) Summary is made public at the time that a drug is approved or conditionally approved, and includes general information about the product and a summary of the information the agency relied on to demonstrate that the Effectiveness, TAS, and HFS technical sections were complete. FOI Summaries for approved and conditionally approved products are available on the FDA Web site searchable by NADA or CNADA number, drug name, or trade name.

IDENTIFICATION OF APPROVED VERSUS UNAPPROVED DRUGS

When veterinarians buy FDA-approved drugs, they are choosing the only marketed products shown to be safe and effective. In addition, if the drugs are for food animals and are used according to the label, veterinarians can have confidence that food made from treated animals is safe for people to eat. Also, by choosing FDA-approved drugs, veterinarians are assured that they are using the only marketed products manufactured to meet the agency's strict standards for quality, purity, and potency.

There are several ways by which veterinarians can confirm if a drug is FDA approved. All FDA-approved new animal drugs have a 6-digit NADA number, which is usually on the drug's label. Generic animal drugs will have an Abbreviated New Animal Drug Application (ANADA) number and conditionally approved drugs will have a Conditional New Animal Drug Application (CNADA) number. FDA-approved drugs are codified in the CFR Part 500.[2] In addition, most FDA-approved drugs are listed in "Animal Drugs @ FDA," a searchable database available through the FDA Web site. The presence of a National Drug Code (NDC) number or the statement "caution: Federal law restricts this drug to use by or on the order of a licensed veterinarian" does not mean that the drug is FDA approved. Finally, simply because a product has the same established name (nonproprietary name) as an FDA-approved drug does not mean that it is approved.

Unapproved drugs fall into two categories: illegally marketed unapproved animal drugs and legally marketed indexed drugs. Indexed animal drugs are drugs on the FDA's Index of Legally Marketed Unapproved New Animal Drugs for Minor Species. A drug on the index can be legally marketed for a specific use in non–food-producing minor species, such as pet birds, hamsters, and ornamental fish; and early life stages of a food-producing minor species, such as oyster spat (immature oysters). Illegally marketed unapproved animal drugs are a serious concern to FDA. These drugs are not reviewed by FDA and may not meet FDA's strict standards for safety and effectiveness. Illegally marketed unapproved animal drugs also may not be labeled or advertised appropriately or truthfully.

SPECIFIC ISSUES RELATED TO THE APPROVAL OF ANALGESIC DRUGS IN CATTLE

Although a variety of drugs are approved by FDA for analgesic use in companion animals (nonsteroidal anti-inflammatory drugs [NSAIDs], opioids, and α2-agonists), there are currently no drugs approved for analgesic use in cattle in the United States. Of all the analgesic classes used in veterinary medicine, only one NSAID, flunixin meglumine (Banamine), is approved in cattle. However, it is indicated for the control of pyrexia and inflammation, not for the control of pain.

To help sponsors in the development of new NSAIDs for use in veterinary species, CVM issued GFI #123 entitled *Development of Target Animal Safety and Effectiveness Data to Support Approval of Nonsteroidal Anti-Inflammatory Drugs (NSAIDS) for Use in Animals*.[3] The document provides guidance on the approval of NSAIDs that reduce the production of prostaglandins by inhibiting the cyclooxygenase (COX) pathway, by outlining the types of studies and requirements for demonstration of drug effectiveness and safety in the target species. However, many of the principles outlined in this guidance document are applicable to other types of analgesics as well. The FDA also collaborates with regulatory agencies outside the United States in an effort to harmonize and promote the continued development of appropriate and efficient methods for the evaluation of analgesic drugs for cattle.

For the evaluation of the TAS of analgesics, CVM recommends that the studies include specific tests or examinations as defined by the pharmacologic and toxicologic characteristics of the drug or drug class. For example, TAS studies for NSAIDs should include tests to detect NSAID-specific toxicity such as gastrointestinal toxicity, renal toxicity, or effects on platelet aggregation.

Studies on the evaluation of effectiveness of analgesic drugs for cattle should be designed with the intended indication in mind. If pain is present in a disease condition, CVM generally recommends that sponsors pursue an indication for control of pain associated with that specific disease condition. The emphasis is on the control of pain because NSAIDs ameliorate pathophysiologic responses (including pain) rather than cure the underlying disease. In general, indications do not include the concurrent use of another drug. When the analgesic efficacy is evaluated with the concurrent use of another drug, it is difficult to separate the effect of each drug on the pathophysiologic process associated with the disease condition. However, there may be cases whereby such concurrent use is appropriate and may be adequately incorporated into the design of studies to support such an indication.

There are multiple ways to show substantial evidence of effectiveness for the control of pain in cattle. A validated model study may be used to show the physiologic effect of the drug, and a field study may be conducted using clinically relevant end points to confirm the results of the model study. Alternatively, clinically relevant end points may be measured in a field study under conditions of actual use. The types of studies necessary will depend on the pharmacologic characteristics of the drug being investigated and the end points measured to demonstrate effectiveness.

For a model study to be used in support of effectiveness, the model needs to be validated by confirmation of its reliability and relevance. More specifically, the end points (eg, biomarkers) selected to demonstrate the treatment efficacy need to be physiologically and clinically relevant, and previously qualified (validated as suitable biomarkers). The pathophysiologic processes evaluated in the model study should be representative of the clinical conditions for which the drug is intended (type of inflammatory response and or pain, clinical presentation, severity). Finally, the results need to be reproducible by different investigators and in different clinical settings using the same model and methods.

Cattle present specific challenges with regard to designing studies that reliably evaluate and measure pain. Although researchers have proposed several subjective and objective methods to evaluate pain in cattle, there are currently no validated pain-assessment tools available. The subjective methods of evaluating pain in cattle rely on the observation and scoring of visible physical signs of pain shown by cattle, which may be masked because of their status as prey animals. Typical signs of pain in cattle are either characterized by abnormal behaviors, such as excessive vocalization (grunting and bellowing), postural changes (rigid posture, holding a head low, and so forth), tail swishing, limping, kicking or stamping of feet, grinding of teeth, excessive licking of a localized area of pain, and depression; or a reduction in normal behaviors, such as reluctance to move or lay down, decreased interest in the animal's surroundings, and inappetence.[4–7]

Many of the subjective signs are nonspecific, difficult to quantify, and subject to observer bias; therefore, researchers have focused their attention on the identification of robust biomarkers and assessment tools for the objective measurement of pain in cattle. Validated and practical objective assessment tools are critical for assessing pain and, thus, the effectiveness of any pain-control measures. Various quantifiable methods have been evaluated in pain studies including accelerometers, electroen-cephalography, pressure algometers, infrared thermography, pressure mats, vocali-zation measurements, chute exit speeds, and average daily gain in weight.[7–11] Although some of these methods are potentially promising for providing specific, objective, and quantifiable measures of animal behavior and physiologic responses to pain, more research is needed to validate them for use in cattle and other food animal species. Other physiologic responses to painful stimuli, such as changes in respiration, heart rate, body temperature, and pupil size, can be objectively measured. Although potentially useful, these quantifiable physiologic responses to pain may be caused by stress and influenced by other endogenous and exogenous factors, and are thus not specific to the assessment of pain.

Several research groups have identified and evaluated potential biomarkers for use in the evaluation of drugs for the control of pain and distress in cattle, such as substance P, cortisol, acute-phase proteins, and interferon-γ.[12–15] Microarray-based gene expression profiling also shows promise in the search for biomarkers associated with pain.[16] Further research is needed to validate these biomarkers for use in the evaluation of pain control.

CVM encourages continued research to validate pain-assessment tools for cattle and the use of innovative approaches, using a combination of different methods, to evaluate the effectiveness of drugs for analgesic use in cattle.

EXTRALABEL USE OF APPROVED DRUGS TO CONTROL PAIN IN CATTLE

The Animal Medicinal Drug Use Clarification Act of 1994 (AMDUCA) allows veterinar-ians to prescribe extralabel use of certain approved animal drugs and approved human drugs for animals under certain conditions. Extralabel drug use refers to the use of an approved drug in a manner that is not in accordance with the approved label directions; this includes, but is not limited to, use in species not listed in the labeling, use for indications (disease and other conditions) not listed in the labeling, and use at dosage levels, frequencies, or routes of administration other than those stated in the labeling.

The key constraints of AMDUCA are that any extralabel use must be by or on the order of a licensed veterinarian within the context of a veterinarian-client-patient rela-tionship, must not result in violative residues in food animals, and the use must conform with the regulations published in 21 CFR Part 530. A list of drugs specifically prohibited from extralabel use appears in 21 CFR 530.41.

Although there are currently no drugs approved for analgesic use in cattle, the use of analgesics for routine pain-eliciting procedures in cattle such as castration and dehorning is recommended and taught in veterinary schools and at various continuing education venues for veterinary practitioners. The American Veterinary Medical Asso-ciation (AVMA), in its policy on castration and dehorning,[17] recommends the use of procedures and practices that reduce or eliminate pain in cattle, "including the use of approved or AMDUCA-permissible clinically effective medications whenever possible." AVMA also published an article on the welfare implications of castration in cattle,[18] in which different types of local and systemic anesthetics and analgesics were reviewed. The AVMA suggests that the use of multimodal analgesic regimens (eg, NSAID and a local anesthetic) may be more effective than the use of a single drug at mitigating pain and distress associated with castration.

It should be emphasized that the extralabel use of approved drugs for the control of pain in cattle has not been rigorously evaluated in pivotal effectiveness and safety studies. Therefore, the availability of approved drugs for analgesic use in cattle will serve to improve animal health and welfare, and is thus an important part of the public health mission of CVM.

SUMMARY

The approval of safe and effective new animal drugs for analgesic use is an important part of the mission of CVM to protect human and animal health. The new animal drug approval process ensures that an approved new animal drug is safe and effective for its intended use; the manufacturing process is adequate to preserve the drug's identity, strength, quality, and purity; and the labeling is appropriate, truthful, and not misleading. CVM encourages drug sponsors and researchers to use all available information to develop new and innovative approaches to address the specific challenges of analgesic evaluation and approval in food animals. Continued collaboration between academia, the pharmaceutical industry, FDA, and regulatory agencies around the world is needed to develop such innovative approaches, thereby to demonstrate the effectiveness of new animal drugs for the control of pain in cattle.

REFERENCES

1. CVM. Guidance for Industry #185, target animal safety for veterinary pharmaceutical products (VICH GL43). 2009. Available at: http://www.fda.gov/downloads/AnimalVeterinary/GuidanceComplianceEnforcement/GuidanceforIndustry/UCM052464.pdf. Accessed November 30, 2012.
2. Electronic Code of Federal Regulations, Title 21, Chapter I: Food and Drug Administration, Department of Health and Human Services, Subchapter E—animal drugs, feeds, and related products. Available at: http://www.ecfr.gov/cgi-bin/text-idx?SID=604894779bddf665ad1580a629d4c66f&tpl=/ecfrbrowse/Title21/21tab_02.tpl. Accessed November 30, 2012.
3. CVM. Guidance for Industry #123, development of target animal safety and effectiveness data to support approval of non-steroidal anti-inflammatory drugs (NSAIDS) for use in animals. 2006. Available at: http://www.fda.gov/downloads/AnimalVeterinary/GuidanceComplianceEnforcement/GuidanceforIndustry/UCM052663.pdf. Accessed November 30, 2012.
4. Underwood WJ. Pain and distress in agricultural animals. J Am Vet Med Assoc 2002;221:208–11.
5. Chapinal N, de Passillé AM, Rushen J, et al. Effect of analgesia during hoof trimming on gait, weight distribution, and activity of dairy cattle. J Dairy Sci 2010;93:3039–46.
6. Hudson C, Whay H, Huxley J. Recognition and management of pain in cattle. In Practice 2008;30:126–34.
7. Robert BD, White BJ, Renter DJ, et al. Determination of lying behavior patterns in healthy beef cattle by use of wireless accelerometers. Am J Vet Res 2011;72:467–73.
8. Heinrich A, Duffield TF, Lissemore KD, et al. The effect of meloxicam on behavior and pain sensitivity of dairy calves following cautery dehorning with a local anesthetic. J Dairy Sci 2010;93:2450–7.
9. Stewart M, Verkerk GA, Stafford KJ, et al. Noninvasive assessment of autonomic activity for evaluation of pain in calves, using surgical castration as a model. J Dairy Sci 2010;93:3602–9.
10. Bergamasco L, Coetzee JF, Gehring R, et al. Effect of intravenous sodium salicylate administration prior to castration on plasma cortisol and electroencephalography parameters in calves. J Vet Pharmacol Ther 2011;34:565–76.

11. Theurer ME, White BJ, Coetzee JF, et al. Assessment of behavioral changes associated with oral meloxicam administration at time of dehorning in calves using a remote triangulation device and accelerometers. BMC Vet Res 2012;8:48.
12. Pang WY, Earley B, Sweeney T, et al. Effect of carprofen administration during banding or burdizzo castration of bulls on plasma cortisol, in vitro interferon-γ production, acute-phase proteins, feed intake, and growth. J Anim Sci 2006; 84:351–9.
13. Coetzee JF, Lubbers BV, Toerber SE, et al. Plasma concentrations of substance P and cortisol in beef calves after castration or simulated castration. Am J Vet Res 2008;69(6):751–62.
14. Baldridge SL, Coetzee JF, Dritz SS, et al. Pharmacokinetics and physiologic effects of intramuscularly administered xylazine hydrochloride-ketamine hydrochloride-butorphanol tartrate alone or in combination with orally administered sodium salicylate on biomarkers of pain in Holstein calves following castration and dehorning. Am J Vet Res 2011;72:1305–17.
15. Whitlock BK, Coffman EA, Coetzee JF, et al. Electroejaculation increased vocalization and plasma concentrations of cortisol and progesterone, but not substance P, in beef bulls. Theriogenology 2012;78(4):737–46.
16. Almeida PE, Weber PS, Burton JL, et al. Gene expression profiling of peripheral mononuclear cells in lame dairy cows with foot lesions. Vet Immunol Immunopathol 2007;120:234–45.
17. AVMA. AVMA policy on castration and dehorning in cattle. 2012. Available at: https://www.avma.org/KB/Policies/Pages/Castration-and-Dehorning-of-Cattle.aspx. Accessed November 30, 2012.
18. AVMA. Welfare implications of castration in cattle. 2012. Available at: https://www.avma.org/KB/Resources/Backgrounders/Documents/castration_cattle_bgnd.pdf. Accessed November 30, 2012.

A Review of Analgesic Compounds Used in Food Animals in the United States

Johann F. Coetzee, BVSc, Cert CHP, PhD

KEYWORDS

- Local anesthetics • Nonsteroidal antiinflammatory drugs (NSAIDs) • Opioids
- α2-Agonists • N-Methyl-D-aspartate receptor antagonists • Gabapentin

KEY POINTS

- Extralabel drug use for pain relief in the United States is regulated under the Animal Medicinal Drug Use Clarification Act.
- Agents that may provide analgesia in livestock include local anesthetics, nonsteroidal antiinflammatory drugs, opioids, α2-agonists, and N-methyl-D-aspartate receptor antagonists.
- The addition of sodium bicarbonate in a 1:10 ratio with lidocaine may decrease pain associated with drug administration and increase the speed of onset of local anesthesia.
- Oral meloxicam tablets provide an effective and convenient means of providing long-lasting analgesia to ruminant cattle.
- The pharmacokinetic profile of oral gabapentin supports clinical evaluation of this compound for management of neuropathic pain associated with lameness in cattle.

INTRODUCTION

Societal concern about the moral and ethical treatment of animals is increasing.[1] In particular, negative public perception of pain associated with routine animal management practices such as dehorning and castration is mounting, with increasing call for the development of practices to relieve pain and suffering in livestock.[2] Preemptive analgesia can be applied in advance of the painful stimulus, thereby reducing sensitization of the nervous system to subsequent stimuli that could amplify pain. Agents that

Dr Coetzee is supported by Agriculture and Food Research Initiative Competitive grants #2008-35204-19238 and #2009-65120-05729 from the USDA National Institute of Food and Agriculture.
Conflict of interest statement: Dr Coetzee has been a consultant for Intervet-Schering Plough Animal Health, Norbrook Laboratories Ltd, and Boehringer Ingelheim Vetmedica.
Department of Veterinary Diagnostic and Production Animal Medicine, College of Veterinary Medicine, Iowa State University, Ames, IA 50011, USA
E-mail address: hcoetzee@iastate.edu

could be used to provide preemptive analgesia include local anesthetics, nonsteroidal antiinflammatory drugs (NSAIDs), opioids, α2-agonists, and N-methyl-D-aspartate (NMDA) receptor antagonists.[3] However, less that 20% of US veterinarians currently report using analgesia routinely at the time of dehorning and castration.[4]

The capacity to experience pain is considered to have a protective role by eliciting behavioral responses that reduce further tissue damage and enhance wound healing.[5] However, persistent pain syndromes offer no biological advantage and are associated with suffering and distress.[5] Pathologic pain states in cattle occur as a result of tissue damage, nerve damage, and inflammation and are frequently associated with pain hypersensitivity.[6] Pain hypersensitivity manifests as hyperalgesia (exaggerated responses to painful stimuli) and allodynia (pain resulting from normally innocuous stimuli).

Hyperalgesia has been reported to persist in dairy cattle and lame sheep for at least 28 days after the causal lesion has resolved.[7,8] As a result, chronic pain associated with lameness is considered one of the most significant welfare concerns in dairy cows.[9] Inflammatory pain associated with lameness responds modestly to treatment with NSAIDs[10,11] but neuropathic pain (caused by nerve damage or neuronal dysfunction) is considered refractory to the effects of NSAIDs and many opioid analgesics.[5] Therefore, there is a need to identify novel drugs and drug targets for alleviating chronic pain of neuropathic origin in animals.[6]

This article reviews the challenges associated with providing analgesia in food animals in the United States and the salient pharmacokinetic and pharmacodynamic features of the analgesic compounds that are commonly used in livestock. The use of novel agents such as bicarbonate, magnesium, ethanol, gabapentin, and vitamin B complex to augment analgesia is also discussed.

CHALLENGES ASSOCIATED WITH PROVIDING ANALGESIA IN FOOD ANIMALS

There are several challenges associated with providing effective analgesia in food animals in the United States. First, there are currently no analgesic drugs specifically approved for the alleviation of pain in livestock.[12] Therefore, use of any drug for pain relief constitutes extralabel drug use (ELDU).[13] Under the Animal Medicinal Drug Use Clarification Act (AMDUCA) of 1994,[14] ELDU is permitted for relief of suffering in cattle provided specific conditions are met. These conditions include that (1) ELDU is allowed only by or under the supervision of a veterinarian, (2) ELDU is allowed only for US Food and Drug Administration (FDA)–approved animal and human drugs; (3) ELDU is only permitted when the health of the animal is threatened and not for production purposes; (4) ELDU in feed is prohibited, and (5) ELDU is not permitted if it results in a violative drug residue in food intended for human consumption. Therefore, use of an analgesic to alleviate pain associated with castration in calves in the United States would be required by law to comply with these regulations.

A second challenge to providing effective analgesia in cattle is that there is often a delay between the time of drug administration and the onset of analgesic activity. For example, local anesthetics require 2 to 5 minutes before a maximal effect is achieved,[15,16] which may slow animal processing because producers must wait for local anesthesia to take effect. This delay may serve as a disincentive for them to provide routine preemptive analgesia. Furthermore, the requirement for large numbers of animals to be processed quickly may result in procedures being initiated before optimal analgesia is achieved. A third challenge is that the route or method of analgesic drug administration may require specialized training and expertise or may be hazardous to the operator. For example, the NSAID flunixin meglumine is only approved for intravenous (IV) administration in the United States.[13] Therefore, administration requires the animal to be adequately restrained and the operator to be proficient in IV administration. Similar issues are encountered with epidural analgesic drug administration and administration of local anesthesia into the scrotum. The latter procedure is also considered especially hazardous by many livestock handlers. In addition, most analgesic drugs that are available in the United States have a short elimination half-life necessitating frequent administration to be effective.[13] This increases the stress on the individual animal and increases labor and drug costs.

In addition to the regulatory considerations discussed previously, certain drug classes such as the opioid and NMDA-receptor antagonists are designated as schedule 3 drugs and are subject to regulation by the US Drug Enforcement Administration (DEA).[17] Therefore, administration of these compounds to provide preemptive analgesia is restricted to use by licensed veterinarians. In addition, the cost associated with providing preemptive analgesia contributes to the reluctance of producers to adopt these measures, especially because there is no perceived economic benefit for doing so. It may also be difficult for producers and veterinarians to determine whether analgesic compounds are effective because cattle may not show overt signs of pain and distress. Thus determining the need for analgesia and the dose, route, duration, and frequency of drug administration in cattle can be especially challenging.

ANALGESIC COMPOUNDS AND THEIR EFFECT IN CATTLE

Pain perception involves the transduction of chemical signals into electrical energy at the site of injury (**Fig. 1**). This transduction is followed by transmission of the electrical signal via nerve fibers up the spinothalamic tracts where modulation may occur in the dorsal horn.[18] The impulse is then projected to the brain where pain perception

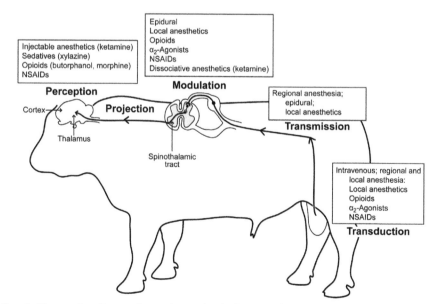

Fig. 1. The nociceptive pathway in cattle, indicating the anatomic location of target receptors for analgesic drug activity. (*Courtesy of* Mal Hoover, CMI, Manhattan, KS.)

occurs.[19] The initial response to a noxious stimulus is typically brief, well localized, and proportional to the intensity of the insult. The second phase of the response is prolonged, diffuse, and often associated with hypersensitivity around the point where the initial stimulus was applied.[19] This effect may lead to persistent postinjury changes in the central nervous system (CNS) resulting in pain hypersensitivity or central sensitization (so called wind-up).[19,20] These effects lead to hyperalgesia (increased pain from previously painful stimuli) and allodynia (a previously nonpainful stimulus now produces pain).[21]

Surgery-induced pain and central sensitization consist of 2 phases: an immediate incisional phase and a prolonged inflammatory phase that arises primarily from tissue damage.[20] The goal of administering analgesic compounds before castration is to mitigate both the incisional and inflammatory phases of the pain response. Effective analgesia therefore requires a multimodal approach using compounds that act on different receptor targets along the nociceptive pathway (see **Fig. 1**).[18] This approach can be achieved through a combination of local anesthesia, NSAIDs, and sedative-analgesic combinations of opioids, α2-agonists, and NMDA-receptor antagonists.

LOCAL ANESTHESIA

Local anesthetics are the most commonly prescribed preemptive analgesic drugs used in food animal practice.[22] These compounds produce reversible loss of sensation in a localized area without causing loss of consciousness. Local anesthetics enter and block open sodium channels of nerve cells and prevent generation and propagation of nerve impulses.[23] Nerve cells that are repeatedly stimulated are therefore more susceptible to the effects of local anesthetics. Furthermore, unmyelinated nerve fibers that transmit pain signals are preferentially blocked by local anesthetics compared with myelinated fibers that are responsible for pressure sensation and motor activity. The quality of local anesthesia in an acidic environment, such as infected tissues, is often poor because these compounds are weak bases that must dissociate in an alkaline environment to exert their effect. Lidocaine has a rapid onset of activity (2–5 minutes) and an intermediate duration of action (90 minutes). Local anesthetic administration into the epidural space has also been shown to provide regional analgesia of the perineal region commencing 5 minutes after administration of 0.2 mg/kg lidocaine and lasting 10 to 115 minutes.[22]

COMPOUNDS THAT POTENTIATE LOCAL ANESTHESIA
Magnesium Sulfate

Magnesium sulfate has been combined with lidocaine to potentiate the local anesthetic effects.[24] Magnesium competitively antagonizes NMDA receptors and their associated ion channels in the same manner as ketamine, thus reducing central sensitization caused by peripheral nociceptive stimulation.[25,26] It was recently reported that the combination of lidocaine with magnesium sulfate produced epidural analgesia of longer duration than lidocaine with distilled water.[24] Local anesthesia with 2% lidocaine solution administered at 0.22 mg/kg was potentiated with 1 mL of 10% magnesium sulfate solution.[24] Magnesium also reportedly has antinociceptive effects in animals and humans after systemic administration.[27] These effects are considered to be associated with the inhibition of calcium influx into the cell and antagonism of NMDA receptors. Further studies with respect to the safety and efficacy of magnesium augmentation of local anesthesia are needed before this technique can be recommended.

Sodium Bicarbonate

Commercial preparations of lidocaine are prepared as acidic solutions to promote solubility and stability.[28] The addition of sodium bicarbonate before administration significantly reduces pain produced by infiltration of lidocaine in humans probably because of the reduced acidity of the commercial formulation.[28] The addition of sodium bicarbonate to lidocaine has also been found to reduce the time taken for the nerve block to take effect and enhance analgesia in humans.[29,30] However, the addition of bicarbonate may decrease the duration of the block.[30] A 10:1 ratio of 2% lidocaine with 8.4% sodium bicarbonate is recommended for optimal buffering of lidocaine. Thus 1 mL of commercially available 8.4% sodium bicarbonate solution can be added to 10 mL of 2% lidocaine immediately before administration to buffer the acidic effects of the formulation.

ALTERNATIVES TO LOCAL ANESTHESIA

Ethanol injection demyelinates nerves fibers and may be a promising long-acting local anesthetic for use at the time of disbudding.[31] When ethanol was administered as a corneal nerve block before disbudding, calves failed to display increased pain sensitivity in response to pressure algometry relative to their baseline values.[31] Furthermore, ethanol-treated calves differed significantly from calves treated with the local anesthetic lidocaine at 1-hour after disbudding, when the lidocaine is assumed to be wearing off. Ethanol blocks seemed to desensitize the site of cautery dehorning for longer than 83 hours, at which time the experiment concluded.[31] In this experiment, 2 mL of 100% ethanol were injected at the site of the corneal nerve block. However, more than half the calves subjected to ethanol anesthesia required a second injection to achieve complete loss of sensation in 1 or both horns.[31] Further studies with respect to the safety and efficacy of ethanol blocks for local anesthesia are needed before this technique can be recommended.

NSAIDS

NSAIDs produce analgesia and antiinflammatory effects by reducing prostaglandin (PG) synthesis through inhibition of the enzyme cyclooxygenase (COX) in the peripheral tissues and CNS.[21] COX exists in 2 isoforms. COX-1 is constitutively expressed in both the peripheral nervous system and CNS, although expression is enhanced by pain and inflammatory mediators. COX-2 is ubiquitous in the CNS but only becomes the major enzyme for PG synthesis after induction by factors released during cell damage and death.[32] It takes 2 to 8 hours for maximal COX-2 mRNA expression to occur in the peripheral tissues, therefore initial release of PG is primarily caused by COX-1.[33] PG in the peripheral tissues lowers the activation threshold of sensory neurons and may initiate nociceptive activity. PG also works in concert with substance P, histamine, calcitonin gene–related peptide (CGRP), and bradykinin to lower the firing threshold of sensory nerves and produce inflammation. Therefore, NSAIDs that inhibit COX-1 may have a more immediate impact on pain by inhibiting PG production in the periphery than COX-2 selective compounds.[21] However, NSAIDs that inhibit COX-1 may be associated with increased risk for adverse gastrointestinal and renal effects.

Spinal PG, notably PGE_2, is responsible for increased excitability of the dorsal root ganglia leading to centrally mediated hyperalgesia. Given that COX-2 is constitutively expressed in the CNS, inhibition of spinal PGE_2 production by NSAIDs that inhibit COX-2 may be an important mechanism in preventing the establishment of hyperalgesia.[21,33] The effect of NSAIDs on both central and peripheral PG synthesis suggests that these compounds have an important role in multimodal analgesic protocols.

The dose and pharmacokinetic parameters of the commonly used NSAIDs in the United States are summarized in **Table 1**.

FLUNIXIN MEGLUMINE

Flunixin is a highly substituted derivative of nicotinic acid. Flunixin meglumine is currently the only NSAID approved for use in cattle in the United States.[13] The plasma elimination half-life of flunixin is reported to be 3 to 8 hours.[34] Following a single IV dose of 2.2 mg/kg of body weight, plasma concentrations decreased from 16.16 ± 5.28 µg/mL to 1.22 ± 0.16 µg/mL in 2 hours, and reached 0.5 ± 0.02 µg/mL by 30 hours.[35] A peak concentration (C_{max}) of 0.9 ± 0.05 mcg/mL occurred at 3.5 ± 1.0 hours (T_{max}) after a single oral dose of 2.2 mg/kg with an estimated half-life of 6.2 hours and bioavailability of 60%.[35,36] Therefore, once-daily administration is likely required to maintain effective plasma drug concentrations. Although this drug class is recognized as having analgesic properties, flunixin is only indicated for control of fever associated with respiratory disease or mastitis and fever and inflammation associated with endotoxemia, rather than for control of pain. Studies showing the analgesic effects of flunixin administered alone at the approved dose of 2.2 mg/kg are deficient in the published literature. Use of flunixin meglumine is further complicated by the requirement for IV administration, which is more stressful on the animal and involves more skill and training on the part of the operator. Several reports have suggested that the intramuscular (IM) administration of flunixin may result in significant myonecrosis and tissue residues.[13]

PHENYLBUTAZONE

Phenylbutazone is not approved for use in cattle in the United States, although it has been used in veterinary medicine for more than 50 years.[37,38] The pharmacokinetics of phenylbutazone is characterized by a slow clearance and longer terminal half-life compared with other NSAIDs.[39] The oral bioavailability of phenylbutazone ranges from 54% to 69%, with peak plasma concentrations achieved in 8.9 to 10.5 hours.[39]

Phenylbutazone has been associated with rare but fatal blood dyscrasias, including aplastic anemia, leukopenia, agranulocytosis, thrombocytopenia, and deaths in humans.[40] The risk for developing these lethal adverse effects in humans is not dose dependent. The human mortality following aplastic anemia induced by phenylbutazone and oxyphenbutazone is reported to be 94% and 71%, respectively. The risk of mortality from oxyphenbutazone is estimated to be 3.8/100,000 exposures and, from phenylbutazone, the rates varied from less than 1 death/100,000 for men aged 65 years to 6/100,000 for women aged 65 years and older.[41] No particular indication for treatment seemed to carry a higher risk. The primary concern was the use of these two drugs in elderly patients.[41] Hypersensitivity reactions of the serum-sickness type have also been reported. In addition, phenylbutazone is recognized as a carcinogen by the FDA.[40]

In light of these potential adverse effects associated with exposure to phenylbutazone, the FDA has issued an order prohibiting the extralabel use of phenylbutazone animal and human drugs in female dairy cattle 20 months of age or older.[40] There is also a zero tolerance for phenylbutazone residues in edible tissues from any class of animal.[40] Use of phenylbutazone as an analgesic in food animals is therefore strongly discouraged.[13]

Table 1
Nonsteroidal antiinflammatory compounds available for use in cattle

Drug	Approved Species	Indications	Dose (mg/kg)	Half-life	Withhold Period
Flunixin meglumine	Cattle, horses, and pigs	NSAID: antipyretic, antiinflammatory	2.2; IV only	3–8 h	Meat: 4 d Milk: 36 h
Phenylbutazone	Horses and dogs	NSAID: antiinflammatory	4; IV only 4.4 in horses 8 in dogs 10 loading dose in cattle followed by 5 mg/kg every 48 h	40–55 h	Not approved in cattle in the United States
Ketoprofen	Horses and dogs	NSAID: antiinflammatory	3 IV, IM	0.42 h	Not approved in cattle in the United States
Aspirin	No FDA approval Horses and cattle	NSAID: reduction of fever Relief of minor muscle aches and joint pain	50–100 by mouth Oral F < 20%	0.5 h (IV salicylate)	No formal FDA approval Not for use in lactating cattle
Carprofen	EU approval in cattle Dogs	NSAID: adjunctive therapy for acute respiratory disease and mastitis	1.4 IV or SC	Age dependent <10 wk: 49.7 ± 3.9 h (R−) and 37.4 ± 2.4 h (S+) Adult cows, 30.7 ± 2.3 h	Not approved in cattle in the United States
Meloxicam	EU and Canadian approval in cattle Dogs and cats	NSAID: adjunctive therapy for acute respiratory disease; diarrhea, and acute mastitis (Europe)	0.5 IV, SC 0.5–1 by mouth	27 h (range 19.97–43.29 h)	Not approved in cattle in the United States

Abbreviations: EU, European Union; IM, intramuscular; SC, subcutaneous.

KETOPROFEN

Ketoprofen is a member of the propionic acid class of NSAIDs.[42] Ketoprofen has a short plasma elimination half-life of 0.42 hours in adult cattle, making it less attractive for use as a preemptive analgesic.[43] Although it has been shown that concentrations of ketoprofen are higher in inflammatory exudates than plasma, 80% of a parenteral dose is reportedly eliminated in the urine within 24 hours of administration.[42] Therefore, multiple doses of ketoprofen are likely required to maintain adequate analgesic concentrations.

Ketoprofen exists in 2 enantiomeric forms: R(−) and S(+).[42] Commercial formulations contain a 50:50 mixture of the 2 enantiomers; however, it is estimated that 31% of the R(−) enantiomer is converted to the S(+) enantiomer in calves after IV administration. The extent of chiral inversion may vary depending on the age and production class of the animal. The S(+) enantiomer is thought to be 250 times more potent than the R(−) enantiomer in inhibiting PGE_2 production.[44] The duration of PgE_2 inhibition in a tissue cage model in sheep was 4 times longer with S(+)-ketoprofen compared with R(−)-ketoprofen.[45] The clinical significance of chirality in term of analgesic effects in cattle requires further investigation. The development and production of enantiomer-specific formulations could provide superior analgesia to current racemic mixtures in cattle in the future.

Ketoprofen is approved in the European Union and Canada for the alleviation of inflammation and pain associated with arthritis and traumatic musculoskeletal injuries and as an adjunctive therapy for the alleviation of fever, pain, and inflammation associated with acute clinical mastitis.[42] The recommended dose is 3 mg/kg of body weight by IM or IV injection, every 24 hours for up to 3 days. Ketoprofen is commonly used in small animal and equine medicine in the United States; however; there are currently no approved formulations for use in livestock.[13]

SALICYLIC ACID DERIVATIVES

Salicylic acid derivatives, including aspirin (acetylsalicylic acid) and sodium salicylate, were the first NSAIDs to be used in modern medicine and are still widely used for their analgesic, antipyretic, and antiinflammatory properties.[46] Although the veterinary forms of aspirin are extensively marketed with label indications for the treatment of fever, inflammation, and pain relief, these have never been approved by the FDA Center for Veterinary Medicine for these indications.[47] Therefore, the legality of using salicylic acid derivatives in cattle is questionable because these are technically compounded products.

Aspirin is a weak acid with a pK_a of 3.5. In the alkaline environment of the rumen (pH 5.5–7.0), approximately 1000 times as much aspirin is in the ionized form compared with the more diffusible nonionized form,[47] which results in a slow absorption rate in cattle. It is estimated that the oral bioavailability of aspirin in cattle may only be 20%.[48] Aspirin is also highly protein bound (70%–90%), a characteristic shared by all NSAIDs discussed in this article. Administration of 2 NSAIDs at one time, or an NSAID in conjunction with another highly protein-bound drug, may result in higher concentrations of free drug in the plasma because of competition for binding sites.

Aspirin elimination half-lives after oral administration range from approximately 4 hours after oral administration in cattle to approximately 38 hours in cats.[47] The slow absorption rate after oral administration shown in adult dairy cows is evident in the difference between elimination half-times for IV sodium salicylate (0.54 ± 0.04 hours)[49] and oral acetylsalicylic acid (3.70 ± 0.44 hours).[50] The elimination half-life is longer after oral administration of aspirin because the rumen acts as a slow-release reservoir for aspirin absorption. The low volume of distribution (0.24 ± 0.02 L/kg) indicates limited distribution to tissues. Salicylic acid derivatives are not associated with clotting deficits in cattle.[46]

In previous bovine castration studies, plasma concentrations of sodium salicylate of more than 25 µg/mL have coincided with decreased peak cortisol concentrations compared with castration with no analgesia.[48] In one study, an oral dose of 100 mg/kg (70 grains/100 lbs) maintained serum concentrations in excess of 30 µg/mL between approximately 1 hour and 5 hours after administration.[50] The mean peak serum concentration was close to 50 µg/mL. An oral dose of 50 mg/kg failed to reach serum concentrations of 30 µg/mL. Gingerich and colleagues[50] used 30 µg/mL as the minimum concentration for pain relief, based on the human serum concentrations required for relief of headaches, aches, and pains. Serum concentrations near 100 µg/mL are necessary in humans to relieve severe arthritis pain. The investigators noted clinical improvement in 2 cows with nonsuppurative tarsitis at 100 mg/kg orally, but noted no improvement at this dose in a bull with suppurative tarsitis.[50] They recommended 100 mg/kg every 12 hours to maintain serum concentrations at more than 30 µg/mL.

CARPROFEN

Carprofen is a member of the propionic acid class of NSAIDs.[51] The relative antiinflammatory, analgesic, and antipyretic activity of carprofen is reported to be greater than phenylbutazone or aspirin.[52] Carprofen exists in 2 enantiomeric forms: R(−) and S(+). In vitro studies in canine plasma suggest that the S(+) enantiomer is 100 times more active against COX-2 than the R(−) enantiomer.[53] Carprofen also shows age-dependent pharmacokinetics. The reported half-life of the R(−) and S(+) enantiomer in calves less than 10 weeks of age is 49.7 ± 3.9 hours and 37.4 ± 2.4 hours respectively.[51,52] In adult cows after subcutaneous (SC) administration, the half-life of the racemic mixture is 30.7 ± 2.3 hours.[51] Carprofen is approved in the European Union as an adjunct to antimicrobial therapy to reduce clinical signs in acute infectious respiratory disease and acute mastitis in cattle. The recommended dose for SC or IV administration is 1.4 mg/kg bodyweight. Carprofen is commonly used in small animal medicine in the United States; however; there are currently no approved formulations for use in livestock.[13]

MELOXICAM

Meloxicam is an NSAID of the oxicam class that is approved in the European Union for adjunctive therapy for acute respiratory disease, diarrhea, and acute mastitis when administered at 0.5 mg/kg IM or SC.[54] Heinrich and colleagues[55] showed that 0.5 mg/kg meloxicam IM combined with a cornual nerve block reduced serum cortisol response for longer compared with calves receiving only local anesthesia before cautery dehorning. Furthermore, calves receiving meloxicam had lower heart rates and respiratory rates than placebo-treated control calves in the 24 hours after dehorning. Stewart and colleagues[56] found that meloxicam at 0.5 mg/kg IV mitigated the onset of pain responses as measured by heart rate variability and eye temperature, compared with administration of a cornual nerve block alone. Coetzee and colleagues[57] observed that meloxicam administered at 0.5 mg/kg IV before dehorning in 16-week-old calves reduced plasma substance P concentrations and improved weight gain over 10 days compared with untreated controls. These reports show that administration of meloxicam before dehorning at 0.5 mg/kg IV or IM may be effective at alleviating pain and distress associated with painful procedures in cattle.

The pharmacokinetic-pharmacodynamic relationship and dose response to meloxicam in horses with induced carpal arthritis has been reported.[58] Based on this work, the reported median effective concentration (EC_{50}) for meloxicam in the plasma of lame horses is approximately 0.2 µg/mL. The pharmacokinetics of meloxicam after oral and IV administration have recently been described.[59] A mean plasma C_{max} of 3.10 µg/mL (range 2.64–3.79 µg/mL) was recorded at 11.64 hours (range 10–12 hours) with an elimination half-life (T 1/2 λz) of 27.54 hours (range 19.97–43.29 hours) after oral meloxicam administration. The bioavailability (F) of oral meloxicam corrected for dose was 1.00 (range 0.64–1.66).[59] These findings indicate that oral meloxicam administration could be an effective and convenient means of providing long-lasting analgesia to ruminant calves.

Meloxicam (20 mg/mL) is approved for use in cattle in several European countries, with a 15-day meat withdrawal time and a 5-day milk withdrawal time following administration of 0.5 mg/kg IM or SC.[54] An oral meloxicam suspension (1.5 mg/mL) and injectable formulation (5 mg/mL) are approved in the United States for the control of pain and inflammation associated with osteoarthritis in dogs. Furthermore, an injectable formulation (5 mg/mL) is approved for the control of postoperative pain and inflammation in cats. Several inexpensive generic tablet formulations containing meloxicam (7.5 and 15 mg) have recently been approved for relief of signs and symptoms of osteoarthritis in human medicine. In the absence of FDA-approved analgesic compounds in food animals, use of oral meloxicam tablets for alleviation of pain in cattle could be considered under AMDUCA.[14]

SEDATIVE-ANALGESIC DRUGS

Opioids, α2-agonists, and NMDA-receptor antagonists are the most commonly used sedative-analgesic compounds in veterinary medicine. These compounds may act synergistically and are therefore increasingly coadministered. A recent survey of Canadian veterinarians found that respondents who did use an analgesic at the time of castration used xylazine (>50% of respondents) more frequently than lidocaine (<30% of respondents).[60] Administration of local anesthetics into the testicles is considered by some to be dangerous and time consuming with unpredictable efficacy, especially when circumstances do not allow sufficient time for maximal anesthesia to take effect.[60] Sedative-analgesic compounds may replace the need for intratesticular anesthetic injection and thus enhance animal well-being and operator safety. A subanesthetic combination of xylazine, administered at 0.02 to 0.05 mg/kg and ketamine at 0.04 to 0.1 mg/kg given IV or IM (so-called ketamine stun) is reported to provide mild sedation without recumbency in cattle.[61,62] Butorphanol (0.01 mg/kg) or morphine (0.05 mg/kg) may be included for enhanced analgesic effects.[61]

OPIOID ANALGESICS

The analgesic effect of opioids are associated with binding to spinal and supraspinal µ, κ and δ receptors.[63] Drug binding decreases propagation of the nociceptive signal by activating receptor-linked potassium channels and inhibiting voltage-gated calcium channels. In addition to producing analgesia, µ-receptor activation is associated with respiratory depression, decreased gastrointestinal motility, increased appetite, sedation, euphoria, and nausea. Therefore, partial and mixed receptor opioids have been developed with fewer adverse effects and, in some cases, a lower abuse potential than pure µ agonists. There are currently no narcotic analgesics approved for use in cattle in the United States. Opioids are designated as schedule 3 drugs in the United States and are subject to regulation by the DEA.[17]

Butorphanol is a κ-opioid–receptor agonist and either a partial μ agonist or antagonist. The potency of butorphanol is reported to be 5 to 7 times that of morphine, although some investigators dispute this.[63] The efficacy of butorphanol is limited to mild and moderate pain but it is one of the most common narcotic analgesics used in veterinary medicine. The half-life of butorphanol in dairy cows administered 0.25 mg/kg IV was 82 minutes.[64] Baldridge and colleagues[65] reported a peak plasma concentration for butorphanol of 7.07 ± 0.55 ng/mL at 9.5 ± 0.50 minutes after coadministration of 0.025 mg/kg butorphanol, 0.05 mg/kg xylazine, and 0.1 mg/kg ketamine IM immediately before dehorning and castration with a plasma elimination half-life of 71.28 ± 7.64 minutes. In dogs, a plasma concentration of 45 ng/mL is considered an effective analgesic concentration, but this has not been confirmed in cattle.[63]

Nalbuphine is a synthetic opioid that is a κ-receptor agonist and a μ-receptor antagonist with similar pharmacologic effects to butorphanol. Nalbuphine has analgesic potency similar to morphine on a milligram basis.[63] The onset of activity of nalbuphine reportedly occurs within 2 to 3 minutes after IV administration in humans with a plasma elimination half-life of 5 hours. Duration of activity of 3 to 6 hours has been reported after nalbuphine administration in human clinical studies.[63]

Nalbuphine injection may be associated with fewer adverse effects than morphine because κ agonists cause less respiratory depression compared with μ-receptor agonists. Furthermore, κ agonists carry a significantly lower risk of dependency because opioid addiction is mediated primarily through activation of the μ receptor. As a result, nalbuphine is presently not scheduled as a controlled substance in most parts of the United States in accordance with the Controlled Substances Act (21 U.S.C. § 812) based on the exclusion detailed in 21 C.F.R. § 1308.12.[17] Therefore, special storage and record keeping is not necessary. The potential for fewer adverse effects and reduced regulatory restrictions may make nalbuphine an attractive narcotic analgesic option for use in cattle if clinical efficacy were shown.

α2-ADRENERGIC AGONISTS

α2-Adrenergic agonists produce profound sedation, chemical restraint, and analgesia in cattle. Activation of α2-adrenergic receptors inhibits the positive feedback mechanism for the release of norepinephrine from the presynaptic nerve endings by reducing calcium conductance.[66] Attenuation of norepinephrine release causes dose-dependent sedation and inhibits the afferent pain pathway.[66] In addition, α2-adrenergic agonists decrease cardiac output, cause a centrally mediated reduction in respiratory rate, produce muscle relaxation, and depress gastrointestinal motility. Epidural administration of α2-agonists can produce analgesia with minimal sedative and cardiovascular effects compared with IV administration.

Xylazine is the most commonly used α2-adrenergic agonist used in cattle and is approved in the European Union for IM administration at 0.05 to 0.3 mg/kg. Administration of the lower dose is characterized by a slight decrease in muscle tone but the ability to stand is maintained. Higher doses cause recumbency, very deep sedation, and a degree of analgesia. It is recommended that cattle are starved before systemic administration of higher doses of xylazine to reduce the risk of rumen tympany and aspiration of rumen contents.

Xylazine epidural has been shown to produce greater perineal analgesia than xylazine given intramuscularly.[67] Xylazine epidural has been proposed as a method of providing sedation and analgesia to facilitate castration in mature bulls.[68] Grubb and colleagues[69] compared the time of onset and duration of analgesia produced by lidocaine and xylazine alone and in combination. The onset of analgesia following administration of xylazine alone was significantly longer (11.7 ± 1 minute) than the combination of xylazine and lidocaine (5.1 ± 0.9 minutes) and lidocaine alone (4.8 ± 1.0 minutes). The combination of lidocaine and xylazine produced analgesia of significantly longer duration (302.8 ± 11.0 minutes) than xylazine alone (252.9 ± 18.9 minutes) or lidocaine alone (81.8 ± 11.8 minutes). Xylazine induced mild to moderate sedation and ataxia. Ataxia was also noted in cattle receiving lidocaine alone.

Grant and Upton[70] (2004) reported that 0.05 mg/kg xylazine IV in sheep produced analgesia lasting 25 minutes with only 3 out of 7 animals showing signs of mild sedation. Garcia-Villar and colleagues[71] (1981) reported that an IV dose of 0.2 mg/kg xylazine in cattle was associated with a peak plasma concentration of 1.050 μg/mL, a plasma elimination half-life of 36 minutes, and a total body clearance of 42 mL/min/kg. Baldridge and colleagues[65] (2010) reported a peak plasma concentration for xylazine of 20.95 ± 1.68 ng/mL at 9.5 ± 0.50 minutes after coadministration of 0.025 mg/kg butorphanol, 0.05 mg/kg xylazine, 0.1 mg/kg ketamine IM immediately before dehorning and castration in calves. The plasma elimination half-life of xylazine was 96.40 ± 20.33 minutes.

NMDA-RECEPTOR ANTAGONISTS

Ketamine is an NMDA-receptor antagonist that produces analgesia and dissociative anesthetic effects when administered to calves at a dose of 2 to 4 mg/kg IV.[66] Ketamine and its active metabolite, norketamine, also bind μ-opioid and κ-opioid receptors producing analgesia.[72] Data from rats suggest that norketamine contributes to the analgesic effect of ketamine, with a potency that is one-third that of the parent drug.[73]

Subanesthetic ketamine administered at 0.1 to 1 mg/kg as an IV bolus is effective in managing acute postoperative pain in human medicine.[74] In humans, plasma ketamine concentrations more than 4 to 5 μmol/L (1000 ng/mL) are required to produce anesthetic effects, whereas analgesic effects are associated with plasma concentrations less than 1 μmol/L (275 ng/mL) or one-tenth to one-fifth of the anesthetic dose.[75] Grant and colleagues[76] reported that plasma ketamine concentrations ranging from 40 to 150 ng/mL were associated with analgesia in humans. Our group previously showed that mean plasma ketamine and norketamine concentrations in cattle decreased to less than 40 ng/mL and 10 ng/mL after 30 and 60 minutes respectively after administration of a subanesthetic combination of xylazine (0.05 mg/kg) and ketamine (0.1 mg/kg).[77] NMDA-receptor antagonists are designated as schedule 3 drugs and are subject to regulation by the DEA.[17]

FUTURE PROSPECTS FOR TREATING CHRONIC PAIN AND CENTRAL SENSITIZATION IN CATTLE
Gabapentin

Gabapentin, or 1-(aminomethyl) cyclohexane acetic acid, is a γ-aminobutyric acid (GABA) analogue originally developed for the treatment of spastic disorders and epilepsy.[78] Studies have reported that gabapentin is also effective for the management of chronic pain of inflammatory of neuropathic origin.[79] Although the mechanism of action of gabapentin is poorly understood, it is thought to bind to the α2-δ subunit of voltage-gated calcium channels acting presynaptically to decrease the release of excitatory neurotransmitters.[80] Efficacy of gabapentin in humans is associated with 2 μg/mL plasma drug concentrations.[81] It has also been reported that gabapentin can interact synergistically with NSAIDs to produce antihyperalgesic effects.[79,82] In a recent study, we reported a mean plasma gabapentin C_{max} of 3.40 µg/mL (range 1.70–4.60 µg/mL) at 7.20 hours (range 6–10 hours) after oral gabapentin administration at 15 mg/kg. A T 1/2 λz of 7.9 hours (range 6.9–12.4 hours) was recorded.[83] Oral administration of gabapentin at 15 mg/kg may be associated with plasma concentrations of greater than 2 µg/mL for up to 15 hours. The pharmacokinetics of gabapentin suggest that this compound may be useful in mitigating chronic neuropathic and inflammatory pain in ruminant cattle.

Vitamin B Complex Injections

B vitamins have been found to produce antinociceptive and antiinflammatory effects in the rat tail pressure test,[84] and are able to significantly decrease the responses evoked in spinal dorsal horn nociceptive neurons in the cat.[85] An SC injection of a combination of vitamin $B_1:B_6:B_{12}$ at 20:20:0.2 mg/kg has been proposed. Several studies have documented that lower NSAID doses are needed for pain relief when combined with B vitamins.[85,86] Cocktails of B vitamins have also been shown to ameliorate allodynia and formalin-evoked hyperalgesia in diabetic rats, suggesting that the use of such a cocktail may prove to be a potentially inexpensive and safe long-term approach for treating neuropathies such as lameness.[87] However, in the absence of controlled studies, further research is needed to determine whether this would be effective in cattle. Further studies with respect to the safety and efficacy of vitamin B augmentation of NSAID analgesia are needed before this technique can be recommended.

ACKNOWLEDGMENTS

The author acknowledges the assistance of Mal Hoover at Kansas State University in preparing this article for publication.

REFERENCES

1. Rollin BE. Annual meeting keynote address: animal agriculture and emerging social ethics for animals. J Anim Sci 2004;82:955–64.
2. Weary DM, Fraser D. Rethinking painful management practices. In: Benson GJ, Rollin BE, Ames IA, editors. The well-being of farm animals: challenges and solutions. 1st edition. Ames, IA: Blackwell Publishing; 2004. p. 325–38.
3. Thurmon JC, Tranquilli WJ, Benson GJ. Preanesthetics and anesthetic adjuncts. In: Lumb and Jones veterinary anesthesia. 3rd edition. Baltimore (MD): Lippincott Williams & Wilkins; 1996. p. 183–209.
4. Coetzee JF, Nutsch A, Barbur LA, et al. A survey of castration methods and associated livestock management practices performed by bovine veterinarians in the United States. BMC Vet Res 2010;6:12. http://dx.doi.org/10.1186/1746-6148-6-12.
5. Woolf CJ, Mannion RJ. Neuropathic pain: aetiology, symptoms, mechanisms, and management. Lancet 1999;353:1959–64.
6. Viñuela-Fernández I, Jones E, Welsh EM, et al. Pain mechanisms and their implication for the management of pain in farm and companion animals. Vet J 2007; 147:227–39.
7. Ley SJ, Waterman AE, Livingston A. Measurement of mechanical thresholds, plasma cortisol and catecholamines in control and lame cattle: a preliminary study. Res Vet Sci 1996;61:172–3.

8. Whay HR, Waterman AE, Webster AJ, et al. The influence of lesion type on the duration of hyperalgesia associated with hindlimb lameness in dairy cattle. Vet J 1998;156:23–9.

9. Whay HR, Main DC, Green LE, et al. Assessment of the welfare of dairy cattle using animal-based measurements: direct observations and investigation of farm records. Vet Rec 2003;153:197–202.

10. Whay HR, Webster AJ, Waterman-Pearson AE. Role of ketoprofen in the modulation of hyperalgesia associated with lameness in dairy cattle. Vet Rec 2005;157: 729–33.

11. Flower FC, Sedlbauer M, Carter E, et al. Analgesics improve the gait of lame dairy cattle. J Dairy Sci 2008;91:3010–4.

12. Bayley AJ, editor. Compendium of veterinary products. 13th edition. Port Huron (MI): North American Compendiums; 2010. p. 1159.

13. Smith GW, Davis JL, Tell LA, et al. Extralabel use of nonsteroidal anti-inflammatory drugs in cattle. J Am Vet Med Assoc 2008;232(5):697–701.

14. Animal Medicinal Drug Use Clarification Act of 1994 (AMDUCA). US Food and Drug Administration website. Available at: http://www.fda.gov/RegulatoryInformation/Legislation/FederalFoodDrugandCosmeticActFDCAct/SignificantAmendmentsto theFDCAct/AnimalMedicinalDrugUseClarificationActAMDUCAof1994/default. htm. Accessed March 18, 2011.

15. Spoormakers TJ, Donker SH, Ensink JM. Diagnostic anaesthesia of the equine lower limb: a comparison of lidocaine and lidocaine with epinephrine. Tijdschr Diergeneeskd 2004;129(17):548–51.

16. Lemke KA, Dawson SD. Local and regional anesthesia. Vet Clin North Am Small Anim Pract 2000;30(4):839–57.

17. DEA. Drug Scheduling. US Drug Enforcement Administration. Available at: http://www.justice.gov/dea/pubs/scheduling.html. Accessed March 18, 2011.

18. Muir WW, Woolf CL. Mechanisms of pain and their therapeutic implications. J Am Vet Med Assoc 2001;219(10):1346–56.

19. Gottschalk A, Smith DS. New concepts in acute pain therapy: preemptive analgesia. Am Fam Physician 2001;63(10):1979–84.

20. Kissin I. Preemptive analgesia. Anesthesiology 2000;93:1138–43.

21. Ochroch EA, Mardini IA, Gottschalk A. What is the role of NSAIDs in pre emptive analgesia. Drugs 2003;63(24):2709–23.

22. Muir WW, Hubbell JA, Skarda R, et al. Local anesthesia in cattle, sheep, goats, and pigs. In: Muir WM, Hubbell JA, Skarda R, et al, editors. Handbook of veterinary anesthesia. 2nd edition. St Louis (MO): Mosby; 1995. p. 53–77.

23. Webb AI, Pablo LS. Injectable anaesthetic agents. In: Riviere JE, Papich MG, editors. Veterinary pharmacology and therapeutics. 9th edition. Ames (IA): Wiley-Blackwell; 2009. p. 383.

24. Dehghani SN, Bigham AS. Comparison of caudal epidural anesthesia by use of lidocaine versus a lidocaine–magnesium sulfate combination in cattle. Am J Vet Res 2009;70:194–7.

25. Liu HT, Hollman MW, Liu WH, et al. Modulation of NMDA receptor function by ketamine and magnesium: part I. Anesth Analg 2001;92:1173–81.

26. Schulz-Stübner S, Wettmann G, Reyle-Hahn SM, et al. Magnesium as part of balanced general anaesthesia with propofol, remifentanil and mivacurium: a double-blind, randomized prospective study in 50 patients. Eur J Anaesthesiol 2001;18:723–9.

27. Kara H, Sahin N, Ulusan V, et al. Magnesium infusion reduces perioperative pain. Eur J Anaesthesiol 2002;19:52–6.

28. McKay W, Morris R, Mushlin MD. Sodium bicarbonate attenuates pain on skin infiltration with lidocaine, with or without epinephrine. Anesth Analg 1987;66(6): 572–4.
29. Curatolo M, Petersen-Felix S, Arendt-Nielsen L, et al. Adding sodium bicarbonate to lidocaine enhances the depth of epidural blockade. Anesth Analg 1998;86(2): 341–7.
30. Sinnott CJ, Garfield JM, Thalhammer JG, et al. Addition of sodium bicarbonate to lidocaine decreases the duration of peripheral nerve block in the rat. Anesthesiology 2000;93(4):1045–52.
31. Tapper KR, Goff JP, Leuschen BL, et al. Novel techniques for anesthesia during disbudding of calves. J Anim Sci 2011;8(E-Suppl 1):413 J Dairy Sci 94(E-Suppl 1).
32. Smith WL, Langenbach R. Why there are two cyclooxygenase isozymes. J Clin Invest 2001;107(12):1491–5.
33. Svensson CI, Yaksh TL. The spinal phospholipase-cyclooxygenase-prostanoid cascade in nociceptive processing. Annu Rev Pharmacol Toxicol 2002;42:553–83.
34. Anderson KL, Neff-Davis CA, Davis LE, et al. Pharmacokinetics of flunixin meglumine in lactating cattle after single and multiple intramuscular and intravenous administrations. Am J Vet Res 1990;51(9):1464–7.
35. USP veterinary pharmaceutical information monographs – anti-inflammatories. Flunixin. J Vet Pharmacol Ther 2004;27(1):70–5.
36. Odensvik K. Pharmacokinetics of flunixin and its effect on prostaglandin F2 alpha metabolite concentrations after oral and intravenous administration in heifers. J Vet Pharmacol Ther 1995;18(4):254–9.
37. Arifah AK, Lees P. Pharmacodynamics and pharmacokinetics of phenylbutazone in calves. J Vet Pharmacol Ther 2002;25(4):299–309.
38. USP veterinary pharmaceutical information monographs – anti-inflammatories. Phenylbutazone. J Vet Pharmacol Ther 2004;27(1):92–100.
39. Lees P, Ayliffe T, Maitho TE, et al. Pharmacokinetics, metabolism and excretion of phenylbutazone in cattle following intravenous, intramuscular and oral administration. Res Vet Sci 1988;44:57–67.
40. FDA-CVM. US Food and Drug Administration, FDA order prohibits extralabel use of phenylbutazone in certain dairy cattle. Available at: http://www.fda.gov/AnimalVeterinary/NewsEvents/CVMUpdates/ucm124078.htm. Accessed March 18, 2011.
41. Inman WH. Study of fatal bone marrow depression with special reference to phenylbutazone and oxyphenylbutazone. Br Med J 1977;1(11):1500–5.
42. USP veterinary pharmaceutical information monographs – anti-inflammatories. Ketoprofen. J Vet Pharmacol Ther 2004;27(1):75–85.
43. Landoni MF, Cunningham FM, Lees P. Pharmacokinetics and pharmacodynamics of ketoprofen in calves applying PK/PD modeling. J Vet Pharmacol Ther 1995;18: 315–24.
44. Aberg G, Ciofalo VB, Pendleton RG, et al. Inversion of (R)- to (S)-ketoprofen in eight animal species. Chirality 1995;7(5):383–7.
45. Landoni MF, Comas W, Mucci N, et al. Enantiospecific pharmacokinetics and pharmacodynamics of ketoprofen in sheep. J Vet Pharmacol Ther 1999;22(6): 349–59.
46. Langston VC. Therapeutic management of inflammation. In: Howard JL, Smith RA, editors. Current veterinary therapy 4: food animal practice. Philadelphia: WB Saunders; 2003. p. 7–12.
47. USP veterinary pharmaceutical information monographs – anti-inflammatories. Aspirin. J Vet Pharmacol Ther 2004;27(1):4–14.

48. Coetzee JF, Gehring R, Bettenhausen AC, et al. Mitigation of plasma cortisol response in bulls following intravenous sodium salicylate administration prior to castration. J Vet Pharmacol Ther 2007;30:305–13.

49. Kotschwar JL, Coetzee JF, Anderson DE, et al. Analgesic efficacy of sodium salicylate in an amphotericin B induced bovine synovitis-arthritis model. J Dairy Sci 2009;92(8):3731–43.

50. Gingerich DA, Baggot JD, Yeary RA. Pharmacokinetics and dosage of aspirin in cattle. J Am Vet Med Assoc 1975;167:945–8.

51. USP veterinary pharmaceutical information monographs – anti-inflammatories. Carprofen. J Vet Pharmacol Ther 2004;27(1):15–25.

52. Delatour P, Foot R, Foster AP, et al. Pharmacodynamics and chiral pharmacokinetics of carprofen in calves. Br Vet J 1996;152(2):183–98.

53. Ricketts AP, Lundy KM, Seibel SB. Evaluation of selective inhibition of canine cyclooxygenase 1 and 2 by carprofen and other nonsteroidal anti-inflammatory drugs. Am J Vet Res 1998;59(11):1441–2.

54. EMEA. European Agency for the Evaluation of Medicinal Products (EMEA) Web site: Committee for Veterinary Medicinal Products. Meloxicam. Maximum Residue Limit (MRL) Summary Report (2). Available at: http://www.emea.europa.eu/pdfs/vet/mrls/057199en.pdf. Accessed March 18, 2011.

55. Heinrich A, Duffield TF, Lissemore KD, et al. The impact of meloxicam on postsurgical stress associated with cautery dehorning. J Dairy Sci 2009;92(2):540–7.

56. Stewart M, Stookey JM, Stafford KJ, et al. Effects of local anesthetic and nonsteroidal anti-inflammatory drug on pain responses of dairy calves to hot-iron dehorning. J Dairy Sci 2009;92(4):1512–9.

57. Coetzee JF, Mosher RA, KuKanich B, et al. Pharmacokinetics and effect of intravenous meloxicam in weaned Holstein calves following scoop dehorning without local anesthesia. BMC Vet Res 2012;8:153.

58. Toutain PL, Cester CC. Pharmacokinetic-pharmacodynamic relationships and dose response to meloxicam in horses with induced arthritis in the right carpal joint. Am J Vet Res 2004;65:1533–41.

59. Coetzee JF, KuKanich B, Mosher R, et al. Pharmacokinetics of intravenous and oral meloxicam in ruminant calves. Vet Ther 2009;10(4):E1–8.

60. Hewson CJ, Dohoo IR, Lemke KA, et al. Canadian veterinarians' use of analgesics in cattle, pigs, and horses in 2004 and 2005. Can Vet J 2007;48(2):155–64.

61. Abrahamsen EJ. Chemical restraint in ruminants. In: Anderson DE, Rings DM, editors. Current veterinary therapy food animal practice. 5th edition. St Louis (MO): Saunders Elsevier; 2009. p. 546–9.

62. Coetzee JF, Gehring R, Anderson DE, et al. Effect of sub-anaesthetic xylazine and ketamine ("ketamine stun") administered to calves prior to castration. Vet Anaesth Analg 2010;37(6):566–78.

63. KuKanich B, Papich M. Opioid analgesics. In: Riviere JE, Papich MG, editors. Veterinary pharmacology and therapeutics. 9th edition. Ames (IA): Wiley-Blackwell; 2009. p. 301–35.

64. Court MH, Dodman NH, Levine HD, et al. Pharmacokinetics and milk residues of butorphanol in dairy cows after single intravenous administration. J Vet Pharmacol Ther 1992;15(1):28–35.

65. Baldridge SL, Coetzee JF, Dritz SS, et al. Pharmacokinetics and physiologic effects of xylazine-ketamine-butorphanol administered intramuscularly alone or in combination with orally administered sodium salicylate on biomarkers of pain in Holstein calves following concurrent castration and dehorning. Am J Vet Res 2010;72(10):1305–17.

66. Postner LP, Burns P. Injectable anaesthetic agents. In: Riviere JE, Papich MG, editors. Veterinary pharmacology and therapeutics. 9th edition. Ames (IA): Wiley-Blackwell; 2009. p. 283.
67. Caron JP, LeBlanc PH. Caudal epidural analgesia in cattle using xylazine. Can J Vet Res 1989;53(4):486–9.
68. Caulkett NA, MacDonald DG, Janzen ED, et al. Xylazine hydrochloride epidural analgesia: A method of providing sedation and analgesia to facilitate castration of mature bulls. Compend Contin Educ Pract Vet 1993;15:1155–9.
69. Grubb TL, Riebold TW, Crisman RO, et al. Comparison of lidocaine, xylazine, and lidocaine-xylazine for caudal epidural analgesia in cattle. Vet Anaesth Analg 2002;29(2):64–8.
70. Grant C, Upton RN. Comparison of the analgesic effects of xylazine in sheep via three different administration routes. Aust Vet J 2004;82:304–7.
71. Garcia-Villar R, Toutain PL, Alvinerie M, et al. The pharmacokinetics of xylazine hydrochloride: an interspecific study. J Vet Pharmacol Ther 1981;4:87–92.
72. Annetta MG, Iemma D, Garisto C, et al. Ketamine: new indications for an old drug. Curr Drug Targets 2005;6:789–94.
73. Leung LY, Baillie TA. Comparative pharmacology in the rat of ketamine and its two principal metabolites, norketamine and (Z)-6-hydroxynorketamine. J Med Chem 1986;29:2396–9.
74. Schmid RL, Sandler AN, Katz J. Use and efficacy of low-dose ketamine in the management of acute postoperative pain: a review of current techniques and outcomes. Pain 1999;82:111–25.
75. Eide PK. Clinical trials of NMDA-receptor antagonists as analgesics. Proceedings of the 9th World Congress on Pain. Seattle (WA): 1999. p. 817–32.
76. Grant IS, Nimmo WS, Clements JA. Pharmacokinetics and analgesic effects of IM and oral ketamine. Br J Anaesth 1981;53:805–10.
77. Gehring R, Coetzee JF, Tarus-Sang J, et al. Pharmacokinetics of ketamine and its metabolite norketamine administered at a sub-anesthetic dose together with xylazine to calves prior to castration. J Vet Pharmacol Ther 2009;32(2):124–8.
78. Cheng JK, Chiou LC. Mechanisms of the antinociceptive action of gabapentin. J Pharmacol Sci 2006;100:471–86.
79. Hurley RW, Chatterjea D, Rose Feng M, et al. Gabapentin and pregabalin can interact synergistically with naproxen to produce antihyperalgesia. Anesthesiology 2002;97:1263–73.
80. Taylor CP. Mechanisms of analgesia by gabapentin and pregabalin–calcium channel alpha2-delta [Cavalpha2-delta] ligands. Pain 2009;142:13–6.
81. Sivenius J, Kälviäinen R, Ylinen A, et al. Double-blind study of gabapentin in the treatment of partial seizures. Epilepsia 1991;32(4):539–42.
82. Picazo A, Castañeda-Hernández G, Ortiz MI. Examination of the interaction between peripheral diclofenac and gabapentin on the 5% formalin test in rats. Life Sci 2006;79:2283–7.
83. Coetzee JF, Mosher RA, Kohake LE, et al. Pharmacokinetics of oral gabapentin alone or co-administered with meloxicam in ruminant beef calves. Vet J 2010. http://dx.doi.org/10.1016/j.tvjl.2010.08.008.
84. Bartoszyk GD, Wild A. B-vitamins potentiate the antinociceptive effect of diclofenac in carrageenin-induced hyperalgesia in the rat tail pressure test. Neurosci Lett 1989;101:95–100.
85. Fu QG, Carstens E, Stelzer B, et al. B vitamins suppress spinal dorsal horn nociceptive neurons in the cat. Neurosci Lett 1988;95:192–7.

86. Mauro GL, Martorana U, Cataldo P, et al. Vitamin B12 in low back pain: a randomised, double-blind, placebo-controlled study. Eur Rev Med Pharmacol Sci 2000;4:53–8.

87. Jolivalt CG, Mizisin LM, Nelson A, et al. B vitamins alleviate indices of neuropathic pain in diabetic rats. Eur J Pharmacol 2009;612(1–3):41.

Extralabel Use of Anesthetic and Analgesic Compounds in Cattle

Geof Smith, DVM, MS, PhD

KEYWORDS

- Anesthesia • Analgesia • Pain management • Residues • Pharmacology
- Withdrawal

KEY POINTS

- Lidocaine is the only anesthetic drug actually approved for cattle in the United States. Therefore, virtually all use of drugs for sedation is extralabel.
- There are no approved drugs for control of pain (analgesia) in the United States, so extralabel use of drugs is again very common.
- To legally use drugs in an extralabel manner, the practitioner must be able to establish a proper meat and/or milk withdrawal interval before administering the drug. If a withdrawal interval cannot be established, extralabel use of a drug is not permitted.
- Pharmacokinetic data are available for many of the common anesthesia and analgesia drugs used in cattle and, therefore, recommendations on meat and milk withdrawal intervals are provided.

The need for sedation or general anesthesia of cattle is relatively common in bovine practice. Inhalation anesthesia is occasionally used in calves, but in larger animals this can be difficult and requires expensive equipment. Therefore, injectable drugs are more frequently used for sedation and anesthesia. In the United States, the only anesthetic drug actually approved for use in cattle is 2% lidocaine hydrochloride. Therefore the administration of almost all anesthetic drugs represents extralabel drug use. Some of these compounds are also used by veterinarians as analgesic drugs in some cases. As the cattle industry is increasingly being tasked with improving animal welfare, pain management is gaining momentum and is becoming an important part of practice. There are no drugs currently approved for pain management in food animal species, and to date the Food and Drug Administration (FDA) has not been willing to consider the approval of drugs for use in food animal species strictly as analgesics. However, several products are available that can be used in an extralabel manner to manage pain. These agents can be used either preemptively (before a painful procedure) or in animals that have existing problems such as lameness or

Conflict of interest disclosure: The author has no conflicts of interest to report.
Department of Population Health & Pathobiology, North Carolina State University, 1060 William Moore Drive, Raleigh, NC 27607, USA
E-mail address: Geoffrey_Smith@ncsu.edu

Vet Clin Food Anim 29 (2013) 29–45
http://dx.doi.org/10.1016/j.cvfa.2012.11.003
0749-0720/13/$ – see front matter © 2013 Elsevier Inc. All rights reserved.

vetfood.theclinics.com

abdominal pain. The primary purpose of this article is to discuss the pharmacokinetics of the main drugs used for sedation, anesthesia, or analgesia in cattle, and include information on meat and milk withdrawal where possible. Efficacy of drugs to manage pain is discussed in an article by Stock ML and colleagues elsewhere in this issue.

ACEPROMAZINE

Acepromazine maleate is a phenothiazine derivative that is occasionally used as a sedative in cattle. Although not labeled for use in cattle in the United States, it is approved in both Canada and Australia. There are no published pharmacokinetic data on acepromazine administration in cattle, so recommended withdrawal intervals are primarily based on foreign approval information. In Canada, the drug (sold as Acevet) is approved for either intravenous or intramuscular administration as an aid in tranquilizing before loading for transportation; to help facilitate restraint; and as an aid in tranquilizing both bulls and cows during artificial insemination procedures. In Canada, acepromazine has a 7-day slaughter withdrawal time and a 48-hour milk withdrawal time. The Food Animal Residue Avoidance Databank (FARAD) has previously recommended the same withdrawal intervals following acepromazine use in the United States (**Table 1**).[1]

ASPIRIN

Aspirin (acetylsalicylic acid) remains a commonly used nonsteroidal anti-inflammatory drug (NSAID) in cattle for the control of pyrexia. It is available over the counter in 60-, 240-, or 480-grain tablets (1 grain = 65 mg). None of the products currently on the market in the United States are approved by the FDA for use in animals, and aspirin products do not have a new animal drug application number.[2] A study published in mid-1970s examined the pharmacokinetics of orally administered aspirin in cattle.[3] Animals received either 50 or 100 mg/kg orally every 12 hours for 5 days. Aspirin was slowly absorbed (absorption half-life was 3 hours) but rapidly eliminated (terminal half-life was 32 minutes). Steady-state concentrations were reached after 36 to 48 hours of dosing, and concentrations remained fairly consistent for the remainder of the 5-day study period. A more recent study examined the pharmacokinetics of aspirin

Table 1
Food Animal Residue Avoidance Databank recommended withdrawal intervals (WDI) for anesthesia and sedative drugs following extralabel use in cattle

Drug	Route of Administration	Meat WDI (d)	Milk WDI (d)
Acepromazine	IV or IM	7	2
Butorphanol	IV or IM	5	3
Detomidine	IV or IM	3	3
Guaifenesin	IV	3	2
Ketamine	IV or IM	3	3
Lidocaine	SC (volume >20 mL)	4	3
Propofol	IV	3	NA
Tolazoline	IV or IM	8	2
Xylazine	IV or IM	4	1
Yohimbine	IV	7	3

Abbreviations: IM, intramuscular; IV, intravenous; NA, not available; SC, subcutaneous.

in 4- to 6-month-old bull calves.[4] Calves were given aspirin orally at a dose of 50 mg/kg immediately before castration. Plasma concentrations of salicylate were only detectable in 3 of the 5 calves (approximately 2–3 hours after administration) and at no point did plasma concentrations exceed 10 μg/mL. Another recent study examined the pharmacokinetics of sodium salicylate when administered to Holstein calves through drinking water. Calves were given free-choice access to water containing between 2.5 and 5 mg of salicylate per milliliter (of drinking water) for several days before and after castration and dehorning.[5] The time to maximum plasma concentration (T_{max}) was 41.7 hours, and mean plasma concentrations achieved were 32.2 ± 1.6 μg/mL of salicylate. Plasma concentrations declined rapidly after sodium salicylate was removed from the drinking water, and plasma concentrations were undetectable within 24 hours. FARAD has previously recommended a 24-hour meat and milk withdrawal interval following administration of aspirin in beef and dairy cattle (**Table 2**).[2]

Two additional studies have been published in the last few years on the pharmacokinetics of compounded formulations of sodium salicylate administered intravenously in cattle. In one study, Angus bull calves received an intravenous bolus of sodium salicylate at a dose of 50 mg/kg immediately before castration.[4] The drug was rapidly cleared and plasma concentrations were below the limit of detection within 4 hours of administration. The volume of distribution was 0.18 ± 0.02 L/kg (mean ± SD), the clearance was 3.36 ± 0.55 mL/min/kg, and the terminal elimination half-life ($t_{1/2\lambda z}$) was 0.63 ± 0.10 hours. Another study used an amphotericin B model to induce arthritis in 4- to 6-month-old Holstein bull calves.[6] Sodium salicylate was given to calves at a dose of 50 mg/kg intravenously, and plasma concentrations were determined. As in the beef calf study, the drug was not widely distributed and was only detected for the first 4 hours after administration. The volume of distribution was 0.2 ± 0.005 L/kg (mean ± SD), the clearance was 4.3 ± 0.2 mL/min/kg, and the $t_{1/2\lambda z}$ was 36.9 ± 1.2 minutes.

BUTORPHANOL

Although there are limited published data on the clinical efficacy of butorphanol as an analgesic drug in cattle, it is commonly used either alone or in combination with other sedatives to relieve pain. It is the only opiate used in cattle with any regularity, and is also used by some veterinarians as an appetite stimulant. Whether butorphanol truly increases appetite in cattle is unknown, but its anecdotal use as a symptomatic treatment for anorexia is not uncommon. There are limited pharmacokinetic data available

Table 2
Recommended withdrawal intervals (WDI) for analgesic and nonsteroidal anti-inflammatory drugs following extralabel use in cattle

Drug	Route of Administration	Meat WDI (d)	Milk WDI (d)
Aspirin	Oral	1	1
Carprofen	IV or SC	21	0
Flunixin	IM	30	3
Gabapentin	Oral	21	3
Ketoprofen	IV or IM	7	1
Meloxicam	Oral	21	5
Phenylbutazone	Oral	55 (beef cattle only)	NA
Tolfenamic acid	IV (single dose)	7	1

for butorphanol in cattle. In one study 6 Jersey cows were given a single intravenous dose (0.25 mg/kg) of butorphanol and plasma concentrations were measured.[7] Overall the drug had rapid and extensive distribution followed by a slower elimination phase. The mean $t_{1/2\lambda z}$ for the 6 cows was 82 minutes. Apparent volume of distribution was 4.2 ± 1.2 L/kg (mean ± SD) and clearance was 34.6 ± 7.7 mL/min/kg. Another recently published study reported the pharmacokinetics of a lower dose of butorphanol given in combination with xylazine and ketamine.[5] A group of Holstein bull calves were given an intramuscular injection of butorphanol (0.025 mg/kg), xylazine (0.05 mg/kg), and ketamine (0.1 mg/kg) before castration. In this study, butorphanol was rapidly absorbed (T_{max} 9.5 ± 0.5 minutes) and rapidly cleared. The $t_{1/2\lambda z}$ of butorphanol was 71.3 ± 7.6 minutes and the total body clearance per fraction of drug absorbed was 64 ± 5 mL/min/kg. Based on these data, a conservative slaughter withdrawal interval for butorphanol would be 5 days; however, in the absence of tissue elimination data, longer withdrawal intervals might be warranted. A group of 3 Holstein cows were given an intravenous dose of butorphanol (0.045 mg/kg), and milk was collected twice a day for 4 days.[7] Trace amounts of butorphanol could be detected in milk for up to 36 hours after administration. Because these data are based on only 3 cows that received a fairly low dose of butorphanol, milk withdrawal intervals of at least 72 hours are generally recommended.

CARPROFEN

Carprofen is a newer NSAID commonly used in small animal veterinary medicine in the United States. This drug has a small volume of distribution (0.09 L/kg) and a much longer plasma elimination half-life (30–40 hours) in cattle in comparison with flunixin, and is poorly excreted in milk.[8,9] Carprofen is currently approved in several European and Asian countries for the control of inflammation associated with respiratory disease. The established maximum residue levels (MRL) for carprofen in the European Union (EU) are 500 µg/kg in muscle and 1000 µg/kg in liver and kidney.[10] Based on these concentrations, the drug has been given a meat withdrawal time of 21 days following single intravenous or subcutaneous doses of 1.4 mg/kg. In the EU, use of carprofen has recently been approved for the control of fever associated with toxic mastitis in dairy cattle. Minimal concentrations of the drug appear in milk following administration at approved doses (1.4 mg/kg). In a study of milk-residue depletion following either intravenous or subcutaneous administration in dairy cows, high-performance liquid chromatography revealed no drug concentrations of greater than 25 µg/kg in samples from any time point.[10] Therefore, this drug has been approved in the EU with no milk discard. However, it should be emphasized that because flunixin is approved in the United States for virtually the same indications in cattle, the use of carprofen would not be legal unless the veterinarian could provide justification as to why flunixin was not effective.

DETOMIDINE

Detomidine hydrochloride is approved for use in horses in the United States. Through its agonist action on α_2-receptors, it produces both analgesia and sedation in very low doses. Although xylazine is much more commonly used in ruminants, detomidine administration has been described as both an epidural and intramuscular sedative in cattle.[11,12] In a study done in dairy cattle, detomidine was rapidly absorbed following intramuscular administration, with peak concentrations occurring about 15 minutes after injection.[13] The $t_{1/2\lambda z}$ following either intravenous or intramuscular injections of detomidine at 80 µg/kg were 1.3 hours (intravenous) and 2.6 hours (intramuscular). It seemed that detomidine was cleared primarily by metabolism, as there were negligible concentrations of the drug in urine. Based on tissue concentrations determined 48 hours after detomidine administration in cattle, a meat withdrawal interval of 72 hours has been recommended.[1,13] Excretion of detomidine into milk was extremely low, but it could be detected in milk for 24 to 36 hours after administration. A milk withdrawal interval for detomidine of 72 hours has been recommended by FARAD.[1]

FLUNIXIN

In the United States, flunixin is the only NSAID labeled for use in beef and dairy cattle. It is indicated for the control of pyrexia associated with bovine respiratory tract disease and mastitis as well as for the control of inflammation associated with endotoxemia. Endotoxemia could potentially be associated with several diseases in cattle including toxic metritis, peritonitis, endocarditis, or acute salmonellosis. Following administration of the drug at the approved dose (2.2 mg/kg) and by the approved route (intravenous) in cattle, the meat withdrawal time is 4 days and the milk withdrawal time 36 hours. Despite being an approved drug, flunixin-residue violations in beef and dairy cattle as well as veal calves are common. For example, in the last 5 years flunixin has become the second most common residue violation behind penicillin in cull dairy cattle.[14]

It must be emphasized that flunixin is approved in beef and dairy cattle for intravenous use only. Multiple studies have demonstrated a longer plasma elimination half-life following intramuscular or subcutaneous administration of flunixin that could prolong the elimination of drug from tissue, possibly resulting in residue violations. A study in dairy cattle revealed that the $t_{1/2\lambda z}$ after administration of a single dose of flunixin (1.1 mg/kg) was longer when given intramuscularly (5.2 hours), than when given with intravenously (3.1 hours).[15] The bioavailability was reported to be 76% (range 44%–119%). Another study following repeated administration of flunixin at a dose of 2.2 mg/kg revealed that the $t_{1/2\lambda z}$ increased from a mean of 4.1 hours following intravenous administration to a mean of 26 hours after intramuscular administration.[16] In that study, flunixin could be detected for up to 8 days in plasma following multiple intramuscular doses. A more recent study compared the administration of flunixin (1.1 mg/kg given twice at a 12-hour interval) via the intravenous, intramuscular, and subcutaneous routes in lactating Holstein cattle.[17] The mean bioavailability following intramuscular and subcutaneous dosing was 84.5% and 104.2%, respectively and the mean $t_{1/2\lambda z}$ for flunixin were 3.42, 4.48, and 5.39 hours for intravenous, intramuscular, and subcutaneous routes, respectively.

When determining an extralabel withdrawal interval for a drug, tissue concentrations are more important than plasma concentrations. The elimination half-lives of flunixin in the tissues have been reported to be between 9 and 51 hours for liver and 22 and 37 hours in kidneys after 3 intravenous doses of 2.2 mg/kg every 24 hours.[18,19] These values represent up to a 10-fold increase in the elimination half-life in tissue compared with plasma. Given the significant increase in the plasma $t_{1/2\lambda z}$ after intramuscular injections, it is logical to assume that an increase in tissue half-life would also be seen, although the magnitude of the increase cannot currently be determined from available data. Because of the problems associated with intramuscular administration already outlined, FARAD has previously recommended a conservative 30-day slaughter withdrawal interval for flunixin products given intramuscularly.[2] If multiple doses are administered intramuscularly, the withdrawal interval may need to be extended to as long as 60 days. Few pharmacokinetic data are available on the subcutaneous administration of flunixin in cattle, so a withdrawal interval cannot be established.

Oral administration of flunixin has also been investigated in cattle. After receiving a single oral dose of 2.2 mg of granular flunixin per kilogram, the plasma $t_{1/2\lambda z}$ was similar after oral administration (6.2 hours) and after intravenous administration (5.2 hours).[20] Reported bioavailability was 60%. Other pharmacokinetic parameters were similar between these 2 routes of administration, but the effects on prostaglandin synthesis were significantly prolonged after oral versus intravenous dosing. FARAD recommends a slaughter withdrawal interval of 8 days and a milk withdrawal interval of 48 hours following a single oral dose of flunixin.[2]

Some veterinarians consider that flunixin does not distribute into the milk, therefore obviating the necessity to discard the milk. This opinion is based on older literature wherein concentrations of the drug were not detected in milk following intravenous or intramuscular administraton.[15] However, the current tolerance for flunixin concentrations in milk is set at 2 ppb (2 ng/mL), which is well below the limit of detection of the analytical technique used in that study. Newer research conducted during the drug-approval process revealed mean milk concentrations of 66, 20, and 14 ppb, respectively (0.066, 0.02, and 0.014 µg/mL) for the first, second, and third milkings in lactating dairy cows following intravenous administration of flunixin at a dosage of 2.2 mg/kg/d for 3 days.[21] Following administration by extralabel routes (intramuscular or subcutaneous), milk elimination of flunixin can be prolonged. When flunixin was given intravenously to 12 Holstein cattle (1.1 mg/kg given twice at a 12-hour interval), concentrations of the marker residue (5-hydroxy flunixin) were undetectable in all cows 36 hours after the second dose (which corresponds to the approved withdrawal time). However, 1 cow that had received intramuscular flunixin and 2 cows that had received subcutaneous flunixin still had milk concentrations above the tolerance limit (2 ppb) beyond the 36-hour withdrawal time.[17] Therefore, a milk withdrawal time of 72 hours is recommended following intramuscular injections of flunixin in dairy cattle. Because many drugs may be administered to cattle by farm personnel, veterinarians need to emphasize the importance of following label instructions for this product. Extended withdrawal intervals for meat and milk should be recommended when intramuscular (or subcutaneous) administration has already occurred.

GABAPENTIN

Gabapentin is a γ-aminobutyric acid (GABA) analogue that is used in humans and animals for the management of chronic pain of inflammatory or neuropathic origin. It has been reported that gabapentin can interact synergistically with NSAIDs to produce significant analgesia.[22] The pharmacokinetics of oral gabapentin (both by itself and coadministered with meloxicam) were recently described in 6- to 8-month-old beef calves.[23] Gabapentin capsules were given by stomach tube at a dose of 10 mg/kg. A maximum plasma concentration (C_{max}) of 2.97 ± 0.40 µg/mL (mean ± SD) was reached 9.33 ± 2.73 hours (T_{max}) after dosing. The plasma $t_{1/2\lambda z}$ was 11.02 ± 3.68 hours. After a 3-week washout period, a gabapentin dose of 15 mg/kg was given orally along with oral meloxicam tablets at a dose of 0.5 mg/kg. The C_{max} was 3.57 ± 1.04, and the $t_{1/2\lambda z}$ of gabapentin was 8.12 ± 2.11 hours.

In a study using lactating Holstein cows, gabapentin was given to 6 cows at a dose of 10 mg/kg orally (coadministered with oral meloxicam at a dose of 1 mg/kg) and another 6 cows at a dose of 20 mg/kg orally (coadministered with oral meloxicam at a dose of 1 mg/kg).[24] Gabapentin and meloxicam tablets were combined in a gelatin capsule and given at the same time. Milk samples were collected every 8 hours for

7 days after gabapentin administration. Plasma pharmacokinetics of gabapentin were comparable with those reported in beef calves. Following the 10 mg/kg dose, the plasma C_{max} was 2.87 ± 0.20 µg/mL, the T_{max} was 8 hours, and the half-life ($t_{1/2}$) was 5.50 ± 0.63 hours. After the 20 mg/kg dose the plasma C_{max} was 5.42 ± 0.69 µg/mL, the T_{max} was 9.33 ± 3.27 hours, and the $t_{1/2}$ was 5.26 ± 0.57 hours. Milk concentrations of gabapentin were depleted to below detectable concentrations by 48 hours following the 10 mg/kg dose (limit of quantitation was 10 ng/mL) and by 64 hours following the 20 mg/kg dose. Although an MRL has not been established for gabapentin in milk, it had depleted to below detectable levels in all cows by 64 hours. Therefore a milk withdrawal interval of 72 hours would be recommended in dairy cattle. More research is needed to determine an accurate meat withdrawal period. Gabapentin is a drug that would likely be used for several days in a row (perhaps weeks) in cattle, because it is primarily indicated for cattle with chronic pain (ie, lameness). Tissue concentrations following gabapentin administration are not available, and pharmacokinetic data following repeated administration of the drug at therapeutic concentrations are needed. Until then a conservative meat withdrawal interval of 21 days is recommended. It is also unlikely that gabapentin would be given to cattle without coadministration of an NSAID (ie, meloxicam), so the withdrawal interval of that drug must also be taken into consideration.

GUAIFENESIN

Guaifenesin is a centrally acting muscle relaxant that is occasionally used in some anesthetic protocols. Combined with xylazine and ketamine ("triple drip"), it has historically been used for field anesthesia. Pharmacokinetic data on guaifenesin are limited to horses, and elimination is fairly rapid. FARAD has previously recommended a meat withdrawal interval of 3 days and a milk withdrawal interval of 48 hours following guaifenesin administration in cattle.[1]

KETAMINE

Ketamine hydrochloride is a short-acting dissociative anesthetic drug that is commonly used either alone or in combination with other drugs for anesthesia or short-term sedation in cattle and other ruminants. Although no tissue-residue data have been published, several studies have examined the plasma pharmacokinetics of ketamine in cattle. In one study, the pharmacokinetics of ketamine were studied in 12 calves receiving ketamine before umbilical hernia repair. Four calves received an intravenous bolus of ketamine at a dose of 5 mg/kg.[25] The apparent volume of distribution was 4.04 ± 0.66 L/kg (mean $\pm$ SD), clearance was 40.4 ± 6.6 mL/min/kg, and the elimination half-life was 60.5 ± 5.4 minutes. Eight calves were given the same dose of ketamine 10 minutes after xylazine premedication (0.2 mg/kg). The volume of distribution was significantly reduced (2.15 ± 0.71 L/kg), clearance was reduced (28.8 ± 6.1 mL/min/kg), and the duration of anesthesia was prolonged. However, the $t_{1/2\lambda z}$ did not significantly change (56.4 ± 14.0 minutes). Similar results on the plasma pharmacokinetics of ketamine were also reported in 4- to 6-month-old Angus bull calves that received a lower dose of ketamine (0.1 mg/kg) combined in the same syringe with a low dose of xylazine (0.05 mg/kg) given intravenously immediately before castration.[26]

Another recent study examined the plasma pharmacokinetics and milk elimination of ketamine in lactating Holstein cows following a dose of 5 mg/kg given intravenously.[27] Plasma pharmacokinetics were similar to those described in calves, with an apparent volume of distribution of 3.23 ± 1.51 L/kg (mean $\pm$ SD), a clearance of

1.29 ± 0.70 L/h/kg, and a $t_{1/2\lambda z}$ of 1.8 ± 0.5 hours. Plasma concentrations of ketamine were not detected 8 hours after administration. Ketamine could be detected in milk from cows for up to 48 hours after administration. Of the 6 cows used for this study, 5 still had measurable ketamine concentrations in milk 48 hours after administration; however, concentrations were not detected in any cows at 60 hours after dosing. Despite the absence of tissue elimination data for ketamine, the recommended withdrawal interval for both meat and milk is 72 hours (3 days).

KETOPROFEN

Ketoprofen is another NSAID that has been used in ruminants for alleviating some of the clinical signs associated with endotoxemia. However, the use of this drug appears to have declined substantially in recent years because it does not offer an advantage over labeled drugs (ie, flunixin) and is much more expensive. Pharmacokinetic data in cattle following intravenous administration of ketoprofen indicates that the drug has a short plasma half-life (about 30 minutes) and a small volume of distribution (0.1 L/kg).[28] In 6 healthy lactating dairy cattle, very low concentrations (<90 ng/mL) of ketoprofen were detected in milk from 10 to 120 minutes following a single intravenous bolus of 3.3 mg/kg.[28] Ketoprofen is rapidly eliminated by the kidneys following intravenous or intramuscular administration,[29] and when injected intramuscularly is substantially less irritating to tissues than either flunixin or phenylbutazone.[30] After repeated intramuscular administrations of ^{14}C-ketoprofen at a dosage of 3 mg/kg for 3 days, radioactivity could only be measured in the kidneys 24 hours after the third injection.[29] In other tissues, concentrations were not detectable. Based on these data, FARAD has recommended a meat withdrawal interval of 7 days and a milk withdrawal interval of 24 hours following dosages of up to 3.3 mg/kg every 24 hours for 3 days.[2] However, with the approval of flunixin in the United States, the use of ketoprofen would not be allowed under the current guidelines for extralabel drug use, and it should not be considered appropriate for use in the supportive treatment of a cow with toxemia.

LIDOCAINE

Lidocaine hydrochloride (2%) is approved in the United States for use in cattle as a local anesthetic. It is labeled without any meat or milk withdrawal time, being approved only as an epidural (maximum of 15 mL) or for nerve blocks (up to 20 mL). However, practitioners often use much greater volumes of lidocaine to for paravertebral, inverted L, or other local infiltration blocks in cattle. In general, lidocaine is rapidly metabolized and eliminated after absorption. Following intravenous administration to adult beef cows at a dose of 1.5 mg/kg (over 1 minute), lidocaine had a plasma $t_{1/2}$ of 1.06 ± 0.70 hours, a volume of distribution of 4.6 ± 2.1 L/kg, a total body clearance of 2.5 ± 1.2 L/h/kg, and a $t_{1/2\lambda z}$ of 1.52 ± 0.94 hours.[31]

In another study with 9 lactating Holstein cows, lidocaine was given as either a caudal epidural (0.22 mg/kg of lidocaine or approximately 6 mL total volume) or an inverted-L local infiltration block (total volume 100 mL of 2% lidocaine).[32] There were no detectable lidocaine concentrations at any time point following the caudal epidural administration. Following the inverted-L nerve block, maximum lidocaine concentrations of 572 ± 207 ng/mL (mean ± SD) were achieved about 30 minutes following administration (T_{max} 0.52 ± 0.23 hours). The half-life of lidocaine (4.2 ± 1.7 hours) following the subcutaneous administration of 100 mL of 2% lidocaine was significantly longer than reported for intravenous use, and concentrations could be measured in plasma for 8.5 ± 1.4 hours. Concentrations of lidocaine in milk could be measured for up to 48 hours after administration by the inverted-L block. Out of the 9 cows in this study, 3 had measurable lidocaine concentrations in milk for up to 36 hours and 3 had measurable concentrations for as long as 48 hours. None of the cows had detectable concentrations at 60 hours. Based on these data, meat withdrawal intervals in cattle should be 4 days and milk should be dumped 3 days following the administration of lidocaine (particularly with large volumes). When lidocaine volumes less than 10 mL are given (ie, epidural), meat and milk withdrawal intervals of 24 hours are likely sufficient.[1]

MELOXICAM

Meloxicam is a newer NSAID in the oxicam group that has preferential (but not specific) binding to cyclooxygenase-2 receptors. It has been approved for use in cattle in several European countries and the United Kingdom as a single intravenous or subcutaneous dose of 0.5 mg/kg, with a withdrawal time of 15 days for meat and 5 days for milk. A small-animal formulation has been approved and is marketed in the United States. Several pharmacodynamic studies have shown that when given according to label directions there is no difference in the efficacy of meloxicam compared with flunixin for the treatment of respiratory tract disease in cattle; therefore, in the United States justifying the use of meloxicam in cattle as an anti-inflammatory would be difficult.[33,34]

However, the use of meloxicam as an analgesic drug is not uncommon in the United States. Research has shown that meloxicam can be effective in relieving pain associated with castration[35] and disbudding or dehorning.[36,37] Meloxicam has also been shown to help mitigate the pain associated with calf diarrhea.[38] Injectable formulations of meloxicam are marketed only for companion animals in the United States, and administration at therapeutic doses would be cost prohibitive. However, oral meloxicam tablets are readily available and represent a significant cost saving. The pharmacokinetics of oral meloxicam given at a dose of 1 mg/kg were investigated in a group of 3-month-old Holstein calves.[39] The drug had good bioavailability given orally and achieved a peak plasma C_{max} of 3.10 µg/mL (mean), which occurred 10 to 12 hours after administration. The $t_{1/2\lambda z}$ was 27.5 hours. In a similar study in 6- to 8-month-old beef calves, meloxicam tablets were given orally at 0.5 mg/kg (coadministered with gabapentin at a dose of 15 mg/kg).[23] The C_{max} was 2.12 ± 0.19 µg/mL, the T_{max} was 11.67 ± 3.44 hours, and the $t_{1/2\lambda z}$ was 20.47 ± 9.22 hours.

In a study comparing ruminant and preruminant dairy calves, 6 Holstein calves (4–7 months of age) received oral meloxicam at a dose of 0.5 mg/kg (delivered mixed in water via stomach tube), whereas another 6 calves (6–8 weeks old) received 0.5 mg/kg either by gavage or suspended in one feeding of milk replacer.[40] The C_{max} was significantly lower in preruminant calves that received meloxicam suspended in milk (1.27 ± 0.43 µg/mL) when compared with gavaged preruminant calves (2.20 ± 0.46 µg/mL) or ruminant calves (1.95 ± 0.96 µg/mL). The apparent volume of distribution per fraction of the dose absorbed was also considerably higher in preruminant calves that received meloxicam suspended in milk (365 ± 57 mL/kg) than in gavaged preruminant calves (177 ± 63 mL/kg) or ruminant calves (232 ± 83 mL/kg), likely indicating significant differences in drug bioavailability when meloxicam is fed directly with milk. Based on these data, when using oral meloxicam in preruminant calves (ie, before disbudding), it would be preferable to administer directly into the rumen (ie, stomach tube) or by waiting at least 1 to 2 hours after milk feeding.

In a study using lactating Holstein cows, meloxicam was given to 12 cows at a dose of 1 mg/kg (coadministered with oral gabapentin at doses of either 10 mg/kg or 20 mg/kg orally).[24] Meloxicam and gabapentin tablets were combined in a gelatin capsule and given orally at the same time. Milk samples were collected every 8 hours for 7 days after meloxicam administration. Plasma pharmacokinetics of meloxicam were comparable with those previously reported in calves. Following the 1 mg/kg dose, the plasma C_{max} was 2.89 ± 0.48 μg/mL (mean $\pm$ SD), the T_{max} was 11.33 ± 4.12 hours, and the $t_{1/2}$ was 14.58 ± 11.32 hours. Concentrations of meloxicam in milk were detectable for up to 80 hours after administration (assay limit of quantitation was 10 ng/mL), and the milk half-life was 10.38 ± 1.20 hours. Although milk concentrations that are safe for human consumption have not been established for meloxicam in the United States, there is an established MRL for meloxicam of 15 ng/mL (ppb) in the EU. Therefore, a milk withdrawal interval of 120 hours (5 days) would be recommended in dairy cattle, equivalent to the approved withdrawal time for meloxicam in Europe.

More research is needed to determine an accurate meat withdrawal period. Tissue concentrations following meloxicam administration are not available, and pharmacokinetic data following repeated administration of the drug at therapeutic concentrations is needed. Without tissue elimination data, one alternative for calculation of withdrawal intervals in food animal species is to multiply the terminal plasma half-life by 10.[41] Based on the plasma $t_{1/2\lambda z}$ of 40 hours reported in dairy calves,[40] a conservative meat withdrawal interval of 21 days is recommended.

PHENYLBUTAZONE

Phenylbutazone is another NSAID that has classically been used as an anti-inflammatory drug in ruminants. It has a much longer half-life than flunixin, and was preferred by some veterinarians because dosing once daily or every other day could achieve and maintain plasma drug concentrations within the therapeutic range.[42] However, in the past 10 years the FDA Center for Veterinary Medicine (FDA-CVM) has had substantial concerns about phenylbutazone residues in meat and milk. In 2000, the US Department of Agriculture and the FDA collaborated on a study looking at phenylbutazone residues in cull dairy cows. Over a 6-month period of sampling more than 2000 cows, residues were found in almost 0.1% of the animals. Because phenylbutazone is known to induce blood dyscrasias in humans, including aplastic anemia, leukopenia, agranulocytosis, and thrombocytopenia, there is a zero-tolerance policy for residues. Therefore, in 2003 the FDA-CVM instituted a ban on the use of phenylbutazone in dairy cattle.[43] The policy stated: "We are issuing this order based on evidence that extralabel use of phenylbutazone in female dairy cattle 20 months of age or older will likely cause an adverse event in humans. We find that such extralabel use presents a risk to the public health for the purposes of the Animal Medicinal Drug Use Clarification Act of 1994." The use of phenylbutazone in dairy cattle is now considered illegal, and a milk withdrawal interval therefore cannot be provided. The discussion on meat withdrawal that follows pertains to beef cattle only, because phenylbutazone cannot be used in dairy cattle.

The use of phenylbutazone in beef cattle is generally discouraged because of the long withdrawal time and high regulatory concern associated with this drug. The half-life of phenylbutazone in the plasma of cattle has been reported to be greatly prolonged compared with that in horses (5 hours) and dogs (4–6 hours).[44] Numerous studies have reported the elimination half-life of phenylbutazone in cattle via various routes of administration.[42,44–51] These times have ranged from a mean of 36 to 65 hours. Unlike flunixin, concentrations of phenylbutazone in tissues tend to parallel those in the plasma.[52]

Williams and colleagues[50] reported an upper limit of the 95% confidence interval of 95 hours for the elimination half-life of phenylbutazone following multiple oral doses in bulls. Assuming that it takes 10 elimination half-lives for 99.9% of a drug to be eliminated from the body, and taking into account the zero-tolerance policy for phenylbutazone residues in the United States, a 40- to 50-day withdrawal interval would be the minimum following oral or intravenous administration of phenylbutazone in beef cattle.[2] Following chronic oral administration (more than 10 days), a 55- to 60-day withdrawal interval is recommended.

Intramuscular administration is expected to cause tissue damage and possible prolonged absorption from the injection site, similar to that induced by flunixin.[30] Such damage may vary with the volume per injection site, as higher doses have been shown to cause an incremental increase in the amount of tissue damage.[53] Therefore, a minimum withdrawal interval of 55 days is recommended for phenylbutazone following intramuscular administration in beef cattle.[2]

Another factor to consider is the age of the animal being treated. Plasma half-lives of phenylbutazone in neonatal (24–36 hours) calves were typically 207 hours and 168 hours in healthy and endotoxemic animals, respectively.[48] Elimination half-lives have also been reported to be twice as long, with plasma clearances 40% to 50% lower in 1-month-old calves compared with 3- to 6-month old calves.[49] Phenylbutazone has also been shown to cross the blood-placenta barrier, and concentrations were detectable in calves born to cows treated with the drug. Continued exposure through the milk can lead to detectable plasma concentrations in newborn calves with elimination half-lives as long as 4 days.[54] Therefore, use of phenylbutazone in young animals is highly discouraged because the withdrawal interval would need to be considerably prolonged.

PROPOFOL

Propofol is a short-acting anesthetic drug that is administered intravenously to induce and/or maintain general anesthesia. Although it is rarely used in cattle, there are some pharmacokinetic data available. At the University of Milan in Italy, 5 Holstein calves (ranging from 60 to 120 kg) were given propofol at a dose of 3 mg/kg intravenously to induce anesthesia before umbilical hernia surgery.[55] Anesthesia was maintained with isoflurane, but blood was collected to determine the plasma pharmacokinetics of propofol. Although propofol concentrations declined rapidly, there was considerable variability between calves. Three of the calves had plasma levels that could be detected for up to 8 hours after administration, whereas in the other 2 calves propofol disappeared much more rapidly. The volume of distribution was 330 ± 171 mL/kg (mean ± SD), clearance was 1183 ± 443 mL/h/kg, and the elimination half-life was 3.3 ± 2.3 hours. Although tissue elimination data are not available to determine an accurate withdrawal interval, cattle should not be slaughtered for at least 72 hours after propofol administration. There are no data available on the elimination of propofol from lactating dairy cattle, and a milk withdrawal interval cannot be determined.

TOLAZOLINE

Tolazoline is an α-adrenergic receptor antagonist that is commonly used to reverse the pharmacologic effects of xylazine (or detomidine) and to decrease the recovery time associated with xylazine-induced sedation. A study has been done in both beef and dairy cattle that provides some data on the tissue elimination of tolazoline after intravenous administration at a dose of 4 mg/kg.[56] Samples of liver, kidney, muscle, and fat were collected from animals euthanized at 72, 96, and 120 hours after tolazoline administration. Either 3 or 4 of the cattle euthanized at all 3 time points still had detectable tolazoline residues (above 5 μg/kg) in liver and/or kidney samples. Based on these data, FARAD recommends a meat withdrawal interval of 8 days when tolazoline is given intravenously at doses between 2 and 4 mg/kg in cattle.[57] Following tolazoline administration to 10 lactating Holstein cows (4 mg/kg intravenously), residues were detected in milk samples from all cattle at the first milking (12 hours) after administration. Tolazoline residues greater than 10 μg/kg were still detectable in milk from 4 animals at the third milking (36 hours), with a mean concentration of 21 ± 14 μg/kg (ppb) of milk. No tolazoline residues were found in milk samples collected at 48, 60, or 84 hours after administration. Based on these data, the recommended milk withdrawal time following tolazoline administration in dairy cattle is 48 hours.[57]

TOLFENAMIC ACID

Tolfenamic acid is an NSAID in the anthracilic acid (fenamate) class that is approved in the EU and Canada for use in cattle with acute mastitis or respiratory tract disease. Although there are no data to indicate that tolfenamic acid is more effective than flunixin (which is approved in the United States), it has occasionally been used in an extralabel manner by veterinarians. Compared with other NSAIDs, tolfenamic acid has a large volume of distribution (about 1 L/kg) and a long elimination half-life (8–10 hours) in cattle.[58,59] The longer elimination half-life is likely a result of extensive enterohepatic recirculation in cattle, and a single injection can maintain therapeutic blood concentrations for at least 48 hours. The EU has set the MRL for tolfenamic acid as 50 μg/kg in muscle and milk, 100 μg/kg in the kidneys, and 400 μg/kg in the liver.[60] Based on these concentrations, the approved meat withdrawal time following subcutaneous injection of 2 mg tolfenamic acid per kg in beef cattle is 7 days. Extravascular administration is not permitted in dairy cattle, and the drug may only be given by the intravenous route. In Canada and the EU, a dose of 4 mg/kg is approved as a single intravenous injection, which is associated with a milk withdrawal time of 24 hours. However, this drug is not approved in the United States and its administration would not be legal unless a veterinarian could provide justification for its use.

XYLAZINE

Although not approved in the United States, xylazine hydrochloride is the most commonly used sedative in cattle. This α_2-agonist is approved in several countries, with withdrawal times ranging from 2 days (France) to 14 days (United Kingdom). It is approved in Canada at a dose of 0.11 to 0.33 mg/kg intramuscularly, with a meat withdrawal time of 3 days and a milk withdrawal time of 48 hours. Plasma pharmacokinetics of xylazine have previously been reported, and appear to be fairly similar across species (dog, horse, sheep and cattle). Following intravenous injection of xylazine at a dose of 0.2 mg/kg in cattle the $t_{1/2\lambda z}$ was 36 minutes, the volume of distribution was 1.9 L/kg, and the clearance was 42 mL/kg/min.[61] The pharmacokinetics of xylazine following intramuscular administration have been determined in sheep. Absorption is rapid (T_{max} = 14.7 minutes) with mean bioavailability of 41% ± 23% (mean ± SD). The elimination of the drug appeared to be very similar to that of intravenous administration in this study, with a $t_{1/2\lambda z}$ of 23 minutes following intravenous injection and 22 minutes following intramuscular administration. Another recently published study reported the pharmacokinetics of a lower dose of xylazine given in combination with butorphanol and ketamine.[5] A group of Holstein bull calves were given an intramuscular injection of butorphanol (0.025 mg/kg), xylazine (0.05 mg/kg), and ketamine (0.1 mg/kg) before castration. Xylazine was rapidly absorbed (T_{max} 9.5 ± 0.5 minutes), but the clearance rates were longer than previously reported. The $t_{1/2\lambda z}$ in this study was 96.4 ± 20.3 minutes, and the total body clearance per fraction of drug absorbed was 54 ± 5 mL/min/kg).

A study done in New Zealand reported the tissue pharmacokinetics of xylazine in both dairy and beef cattle.[56] Xylazine was given at a dose of 0.35 mg/kg intramuscularly to 13 steers and 10 lactating dairy cows. Samples of liver, kidney, muscle, and fat were collected from animals euthanized at 72, 96, and 120 hours after xylazine administration. Xylazine was not detected in any of the tissue samples (assay limit of detection 5 µg/kg) at these time points, and the approved meat withdrawal interval in New Zealand based on this work was set at 3 days. Xylazine residues were found in 3 of the 10 dairy cows 12 hours after administration but not at any time point after that. In the United States, FARAD recommends a meat withdrawal interval of 4 days and a milk withdrawal interval of 24 hours following xylazine administration in cattle.[57] However, when xylazine sedation is reversed using tolazoline, both the meat and milk withdrawal intervals need to be increased (see section on tolazoline).

YOHIMBINE

Yohimbine is an indole alkaloid that is occasionally used to reverse xylazine anesthesia in cattle. Minimal data are available on yohimbine in cattle, but in one study a dose of 0.25 mg/kg was given intravenously to a group of 5 steers.[62] The mean apparent volume of distribution at steady state was 4.9 ± 1.4 L/kg (mean ± SD), total body clearance was 69.6 ± 35.1 mL/min/kg, and $t_{1/2}$ was 46.7 ± 24.4 minutes. Based on these data, FARAD has recommended a meat withdrawal interval of 7 days.[1] Despite the lack of any milk elimination data in dairy cattle, the recommended milk withdrawal interval is 72 hours.

A drug that is occasionally used in cattle but for which there are no published pharmacokinetic data is Telazol (a combination of tiletamine hydrochloride and zolazepam). Neither meat nor milk withdrawal intervals can be provided for this drug because of the lack of any data on which to base them. Practitioners have many choices in the United States for both sedation and analgesia in bovine practice. However, most of these drugs do appear in edible tissues and milk for a period of time after administration. The rules and regulations regarding extralabel drug use should be emphasized to both veterinarians and livestock producers, one of the most important being that an accurate withdrawal time must be determined before the drug is administered to food-producing animals. Therefore certain drugs may not be appropriate for use in cattle, particularly in the United States, where regulations regarding extralabel drug use should be followed.

REFERENCES

1. Craigmill AL, Rangel-Lugo M, Damian P, et al. Extralabel use of tranquilizers and general anesthetics. J Am Vet Med Assoc 1997;211:302–4.
2. Smith GW, Davis JL, Tell LA, et al. Extralabel use of nonsteroidal anti-inflammatory drugs in cattle. J Am Vet Med Assoc 2008;232:697–701.
3. Gingerich DA, Baggot JD, Yeary RA. Pharmacokinetics and dosage of aspirin in cattle. J Am Vet Med Assoc 1975;167:945–8.
4. Coetzee JF, Gehring R, Bettenhausen AC, et al. Attenuation of acute plasma cortisol response in calves following intravenous sodium salicylate administration prior to castration. J Vet Pharmacol Ther 2007;30:305–13.
5. Baldridge SL, Coetzee JF, Dritz SS, et al. Pharmacokinetics and physiologic effects of intramuscularly administered xylazine hydrochloride-ketamine hydrochloride-butorphanol tartrate alone or in combination with orally administered

sodium salicylate on biomarkers of pain in Holstein calves following castration and dehorning. Am J Vet Res 2011;72:1305–17.

6. Kotschwar JL, Coetzee JF, Anderson DE, et al. Analgesic efficacy of sodium salicylate in an amphotericin B-induced bovine synovitis-arthritis model. J Dairy Sci 2009;92:3731–43.

7. Court MH, Dodman NH, Levine HD, et al. Pharmacokinetics and milk residues of butorphanol in dairy cows after single intravenous administration. J Vet Pharmacol Ther 1992;15:28–35.

8. Lohuis JA, van Werven T, Brand A, et al. Pharmacodynamics and pharmacokinetics of carprofen, a non-steroidal anti-inflammatory drug, in healthy cows and cows with Escherichia coli endotoxin-induced mastitis. J Vet Pharmacol Ther 1991;14:219–29.

9. Ludwig B, Jordan JC, Rehm WF, et al. Carprofen in veterinary medicine 1. Plasma disposition, milk excretion and tolerance in milk-producing cows. Schweiz Arch Tierheilkd 1989;131:99–106.

10. European Agency for the Evaluation of Medicinal Products—Committee for Veterinary Medicinal Products: Carprofen. Available at: www.emea.europa.eu/pdfs/vet/mrls/091404en.pdf. Accessed August 1, 2012.

11. Lin HC, Riddell M. Preliminary study of the effects of xylazine or detomidine with or without butorphanol for standing sedation in dairy cattle. Vet Ther 2003;4: 285–91.

12. Prado ME, Streeter RN, Mandsager RE, et al. Pharmacologic effects of epidural versus intramuscular administration of detomidine in cattle. Am J Vet Res 1999; 60:1242–7.

13. Salonen JS, Vähä-Vahe T, Vainio O, et al. Single-dose pharmacokinetics of detomidine in the horse and cow. J Vet Pharmacol Ther 1989;12:65–72.

14. United States Department of Agriculture—Food Safety Inspection Service. Red book. 2005-2010. Available at: http://www.fsis.usda.gov/Science/2005_Red_Book/index.asp. Accessed August 1, 2012.

15. Anderson KL, Neff-Davis CA, Davis LE, et al. Pharmacokinetics of flunixin meglumine in lactating cattle after single and multiple intramuscular and intravenous administrations. Am J Vet Res 1990;51:1464–7.

16. Odensvik K, Johansson IM. High-performance liquid chromatography method for determination of flunixin meglumine in bovine plasma and pharmacokinetics after single and repeated doses of the drug. Am J Vet Res 1995;56: 489–95.

17. Kissell LW, Smith GW, Leavens TL, et al. Plasma pharmacokinetics and milk residues of flunixin and 5-hydroxy flunixin following different routes of administration in dairy cattle. J Dairy Sci 2012;95:7151–7.

18. Lichtenwalner DM, Cameron BD, Young C. The metabolism and pharmacokinetics of flunixin meglumine in cows and steers. In: Hartigan PJ, Monaghan ML, editors. Proceedings of the 14th World Congress on Diseases of Cattle. Dublin (Ireland): Irish Cattle Veterinary Association; 1986. p. 1179–83.

19. Clement RP, Simmons RD, Christopher RJ, et al. Design and conduct of studies to meet residue chemistry requirements; residue depletion and metabolism of flunixin meglumine in cattle. In: Hutson DH, Hawkins DR, Paulson GD, editors. Xenobiotics and food-producing animals. New York: Oxford University Press; 1992. p. 37–48.

20. Odensvik K. Pharmacokinetics of flunixin meglumine and its effect on prostaglandin F2 alpha metabolite concentrations after oral and intravenous administration in heifers. J Vet Pharmacol Ther 1995;18:254–9.

21. Feely WF, Chester-Yansen C, Thompson K, et al. Flunixin meglumine residues in milk after intravenous treatment of dairy cattle with ^{14}C-flunixin meglumine. J Agric Food Chem 2002;50:7308–13.
22. Hurley RW, Chatterjea D, Rose Feng M, et al. Gabapentin and pregabalin can interact synergistically with naproxen to produce antiphyeralgesia. Anesthesiology 2002;97:1263–73.
23. Coetzee JF, Mosher RA, Kohake LE, et al. Pharmacokinetics of oral gabapentin alone or co-administered with meloxicam in ruminant beef calves. Vet J 2011; 190:98–102.
24. Malreddy PR, Coetzee JF, KuKanich B, et al. Pharmacokinetics and milk secretion of gabapentin and meloxicam co-administered orally with Holstein-Friesian cows. J Vet Pharmacol Ther, in press.
25. Waterman AE. The pharmacokinetics of ketamine administered intravenously in calves and the modifying effect of premedication with xylazine hydrochloride. J Vet Pharmacol Ther 1984;7:125–30.
26. Gehring R, Coetzee JF, Tarus-Sang J, et al. Pharmacokinetics of ketamine and its major metabolite norketamine administered at a sub-anesthetic dose together with xylazine to calves prior to castration. J Vet Pharmacol Ther 2008;32:124–8.
27. Sellers G, Lin HC, Riddell MG, et al. Pharmacokinetics of ketamine in plasma and milk of mature Holstein cows. J Vet Pharmacol Ther 2010;33:480–4.
28. DeGraves FJ, Riddell MG, Schumacher J. Ketoprofen concentrations in plasma and milk after intravenous administration in dairy cattle. Am J Vet Res 1996;57: 1031–3.
29. European Agency for the Evaluation of Medicinal Products—Committee for Veterinary Medicinal Products. Ketoprofen. Available at: www.emea.europa.eu/pdfs/vet/mrls/002095en.pdf. Accessed August 1, 2012.
30. Pyörälä S, Laurila T, Lehtonen S, et al. Local tissue damage in cows after intramuscular administration of preparations containing phenylbutazone, flunixin meglumine, ketoprofen and metamizole. Acta Vet Scand 1999;40:145–50.
31. Cox S, Wilson J, Doherty T. Pharmacokinetics of lidocaine after intravenous administration to cows. J Vet Pharmacol Ther 2011;35:305–8.
32. Sellers G, Lin HC, Riddell MG, et al. Pharmacokinetics of lidocaine in serum and milk of mature Holstein cows. J Vet Pharmacol Ther 2009;32:446–50.
33. Bednarek D, Zdzisinska B, Kondracki M, et al. A comparative study of the effects of meloxicam and flunixin meglumine (NSAIDs) as adjunctive therapy on interferon and tumor necrosis factor production in calves suffering from enzootic bronchopneumonia. Pol J Vet Sci 2003;6:109–15.
34. Friton GM, Cajal C, Ramirez Romero R, et al. Clinical efficacy of meloxicam (Metacam) and flunixin meglumine (Finadyne) as adjuncts to antibacterial treatment of respiratory disease in fattening cattle. Berl Munch Tierarztl Wochenschr 2004; 117:304–9.
35. Coetzee JF, Edwards LN, Mosher RA, et al. Effect of oral meloxicam on health and performance of beef steers relative to bulls castrated on arrival at the feedlot. J Anim Sci 2012;90:1026–39.
36. Theurer ME, White BJ, Coetzee JF, et al. Assessment of behavioral changes associated with oral meloxicam administration at time of dehorning in calves using a remote triangulation device and accelerometers. BMC Vet Res 2012; 8:48.
37. Heinrich A, Duffield TF, Lissemore KD, et al. The effect of meloxicam on behavior and pain sensitivity to dairy calves following cautery dehorning with a local anesthetic. J Dairy Sci 2010;93:2450–7.

38. Todd CG, Millman ST, McKnight DR, et al. Nonsteroidal anti-inflammatory drug therapy for neonatal calf diarrhea complex: effects on calf performance. J Anim Sci 2010;88:2019–28.

39. Coetzee JF, KuKanich B, Mosher R, et al. Pharmacokinetics of intravenous and oral meloxicam in ruminant calves. Vet Ther 2009;10:E1–8.

40. Mosher RA, Coetzee JF, Cull CA, et al. Pharmacokinetics of oral meloxicam in ruminant and preruminant calves. J Vet Pharmacol Ther 2011;35:373–81.

41. Riviere JE, Sundlof SF. Chemical residues in tissues of food animals. In: Riviere JE, Papich MG, editors. Veterinary pharmacology and therapeutics. 9th edition. Ames (IA): Wiley-Blackwell; 2009. p. 1453–62.

42. Martin K, Andersson L, Stridsberg M, et al. Plasma concentration, mammary excretion and side effects of phenylbutazone after repeated oral administration in healthy cows. J Vet Pharmacol Ther 1984;7:131–8.

43. Davis JL, Smith GW, Baynes RE, et al. Update on drugs prohibited from extralabel use in food animals. J Am Vet Med Assoc 2009;235:528–34.

44. Lees P, Ayliffe T, Maitho TE, et al. Pharmacokinetics, metabolism and excretion of phenylbutazone in cattle following intravenous, intramuscular and oral administration. Res Vet Sci 1988;44:57–67.

45. Arafat AK, Lees P. Pharmacodynamics and pharmacokinetics of phenylbutazone in calves. J Vet Pharmacol Ther 2002;25:299–309.

46. de Veau IF, Pedersoli W, Cullison R, et al. Pharmacokinetics of phenylbutazone in beef steers. J Vet Pharmacol Ther 2002;25:195–200.

47. de Veau EJ, Pedersoli W, Cullison R, et al. Pharmacokinetics of phenylbutazone in plasma and milk of lactating dairy cows. J Vet Pharmacol Ther 1998;21:437–43.

48. Semrad SD, McClure JT, Sams RA, et al. Pharmacokinetics and effects of repeated administration of phenylbutazone in neonatal calves. Am J Vet Res 1993;54:1906–12.

49. Volner Z, Nouws JF, Kozjek F, et al. Age-dependent pharmacokinetics of phenylbutazone in calves. Vet Q 1990;12:98–102.

50. Williams RJ, Boudinot FD, Smith JA, et al. Pharmacokinetics of phenylbutazone in mature Holstein bulls: steady-state kinetics after multiple oral dosing. Am J Vet Res 1990;51:371–5.

51. Williams RJ, Smith JA, Boudinot FD, et al. Pharmacokinetics of phenylbutazone given intravenously or orally in mature Holstein bulls. Am J Vet Res 1990;51:367–70.

52. Toutain PL, Alvinerie M, Ruckebusch Y. Pharmacokinetics and residue levels of phenylbutazone in the cow. Ann Rech Vet 1980;11:391–7.

53. Ferre PJ, Laroute V, Braun JP, et al. Simultaneous and minimally invasive assessment of muscle tolerance and bioavailability of different volumes of an intramuscular formulation in the same animals. J Anim Sci 2006;84:1295–301.

54. Chamberlain PL, Fowler BA, Sexton MJ, et al. Preliminary studies of offspring exposure to phenylbutazone and ivermectin during the perinatal period in a Holstein cow-calf model. Toxicol Appl Pharmacol 2003;187:198–208.

55. Cagnardi P, Zonca A, Gallo M, et al. Pharmacokinetics of propofol in calves undergoing abdominal surgery. Vet Res Commun 2009;33(Suppl 1):S177–9.

56. Delehant TM, Denhart JW, Lloyd WE, et al. Pharmacokinetics of xylazine, 2,6-dimethylaniline, and tolazoline in tissues from yearling cattle and milk from mature dairy cows after sedation with xylazine hydrochloride and reversal with tolazoline hydrochloride. Vet Ther 2003;4:128–34.

57. Haskell SR, Gehring R, Payne MA, et al. Update on FARAD food animal drug withholding recommendations. J Am Vet Med Assoc 2003;223:1277–8.

58. Landoni MR, Cunningham FM, Lees P. Pharmacokinetics and pharmacodynamics of tolfenamic acid in calves. Res Vet Sci 1996;61:26–32.
59. Sidhu PK, Landoni MF, Lees P. Influence of marbofloxacin on the pharmacokinetics and pharmacodynamics of tolfenamic acid in calves. J Vet Pharmacol Ther 2005;28:109–19.
60. European Agency for the Evaluation of Medicinal Products—Committee for Veterinary Medicinal Products: Tolfenamic acid. Available at: www.emea.europa.eu/pdfs/vet/mrls/018397en.pdf. Accessed August 1, 2012.
61. Garcia-Villar R, Toutain P, Alvinerie M, et al. The pharmacokinetics of xylazine hydrochloride: an interspecific study. J Vet Pharmacol Ther 1981;4:87–92.
62. Jernigan AD, Wilson RC, Booth NH, et al. Comparative pharmacokinetics of yohimbine in steers, horses and dogs. Can J Vet Res 1988;52:172–6.

Behavioral Responses of Cattle to Pain and Implications for Diagnosis, Management, and Animal Welfare

Suzanne T. Millman, BSc(Agr), PhD[a,b],*

KEYWORDS

- Animal welfare - Pain - Sickness behavior - Pressure algometry - Cognitive tests

KEY POINTS

- Pain and illness are key concepts for animal welfare in the eyes of the public. Practitioners and their clients must be current on this topic and able to defend husbandry practices. Practitioners have an important role in educating clients to recognize and respond to livestock pain.

- Pain is a subjective experience. Hence, one cannot truly know what another being (human or animal) experiences. Subjective experiences are challenging in medicine, but not unique to veterinary practice. Some techniques used in human medicine, particularly for nonverbal and preverbal patients, can be applied to animals.

- Veterinarians traditionally include behavior as components of subjective assessments performed during clinical examination, but objective measures of behavior are less common. Several techniques can be used to quantify behavior in the laboratory and in the field, including frequency and duration of behavioral elements (motor patterns). Objective assessment of pain-related behavior is important for developing and validating evidence-based interventions.

- Sensory discrimination tests, such as pressure algometry and thermal sensitivity devices, can be used to "ask" animals about the level of pain experienced and provide empirical data regarding efficacy of analgesic interventions.

- Affective or emotional responses to painful procedures can be assessed in preference and avoidance tests, but may be confounded with other negative states such as fear. Location avoidance responses from classical conditioning and self-selection of analgesia are 2 examples discussed.

[a] Department of Veterinary Diagnostic & Production Animal Medicine, Lloyd Veterinary Medical Center, Iowa State University, 2440, 1600 South 16th Street, Ames, IA 50011, USA; [b] Department of Biomedical Sciences, Lloyd Veterinary Medical Center, Iowa State University, 2440, 1600 South 16th Street, Ames, IA 50011, USA
* Lloyd Veterinary Medical Center, Iowa State University, 2440, 1600 South 16th Street, Ames, IA, 50011.
E-mail address: smillman@iastate.edu

Vet Clin Food Anim 29 (2013) 47–58
http://dx.doi.org/10.1016/j.cvfa.2012.11.007
0749-0720/13/$ – see front matter © 2013 Elsevier Inc. All rights reserved.

ATTITUDES ABOUT BOVINE PAIN

Inflicting and alleviating of pain are consistently cited as key societal concerns for farm animal welfare. Often concerns about farm animal welfare are assumed to be greater in Europe, but surveys of public attitudes in the United States report similar findings (**Table 1**).[1-3] In an Australian study, livestock producers, transporters, veterinarians, animal welfare scientists, and animal welfare advocates generally agreed that provision of pain relief for invasive procedures, such as castration, dehorning, and tail docking, was of greater importance than the techniques used to perform these procedures. However, animal welfare advocates placed more importance on pain as a factor of animal welfare assessment than did other groups, which prioritized general husbandry aspects such as stockmanship.[4] Similarly, a Belgian study revealed the potential for discord between farmers and citizens in their opinions about pain and stress.[5] Although both groups attached importance to these aspects of animal welfare, farmers perceived little opportunity for alleviating these problems without serious economic drawbacks, creating a conflict between interests and values at the level of the farmer. In the United States, dairy producers concede that routine surgeries such as dehorning are painful, but analgesia is rarely provided.[6,7] The discord between societal concerns about pain associated with customary livestock production practices is evident with the emergence of legislation, such as prohibitions on tail docking of cattle, in individual states in the United States, such as California and Rhode Island. Although concern about animal pain is a key component of public concern, opposition to routine surgeries, such as tail docking, has roots in further value-based concerns, such as disfiguring the animal's natural structure.[8] An expert committee in France proposed a "3S" approach to pain in food animals, "Suppress, Substitute, and Soothe," in which the first solution is to avoid painful procedures where possible, followed by the selection of the least painful technique, and last, intervention with analgesia.[9]

Veterinarians have important influence on the attitudes and behavior of livestock producers in regard to pain recognition and pain management. A survey of Danish dairy producers and veterinarians revealed general agreement about which diseases were painful and which diseases were not.[10] However, there was large variability in the level of pain believed to be associated with disease conditions. Interestingly, farmers ranked level of pain higher than veterinarians did, but were also less likely to provide analgesia. This finding is in contrast to other research in which veterinary respondents that rated levels of pain higher were also more likely to provide analgesia.[11,12] This discrepancy may reflect farmers' lack of awareness of or access to interventions that address pain.[5] In a Canadian survey, 13% of dairy producers reported being unaware of the opportunity for pain management, whereas producers that involved veterinarians in their management decision for disbudding and dehorning protocols

Table 1	
Examples of published surveys of public attitudes regarding the importance of pain in farm animals	
Statement	**Response**
"it is wrong to cause farm animals any pain, injury or stress"	83% agree[1]
"farm animals should be protected from feeling physical pain"	75% agreed[2]
"(i)t is of no concern to me whether farm animals feel emotional pain"	69% disagreed[2]
"(f)arm animals have roughly the same ability to feel pain and discomfort as humans"	81% agreed[3]

were 6.5 times more likely to provide analgesia.[7] Both bovine veterinarians and dairy producers cited pain relief as the primary reason for using analgesia. Similarly, 12% of dairy producers in northeast and north central United States used anesthetics when dehorning calves, indicating a potential interest in pain mitigation interventions should bovine practitioners offer it.[13]

Consensus among veterinary practitioners about appropriate pain management is unlikely, because attitudes vary considerably among individuals. The decision to use analgesics for particular conditions seems to have a dichotomous distribution, with practitioners choosing to use analgesics for all cases or for none.[7,12] Several surveys indicate that cesarean section and claw amputation are believed to be the most painful conditions in cattle, but differ for severity of castration pain.[12,14,15] In a national Canadian survey, dairy calves were more likely to be provided with analgesia for dehorning than beef calves, even when dehorned at the same ages,[16] and dairy cattle were also more likely to be treated with analgesia in a US survey.[15] Female practitioners rate pain higher when assessing bovine clinical conditions than male practitioners in some surveys[17] but not others,[7] or was observed only in association with particular clinical conditions.[14,15] Several surveys indicate that younger practitioners or more recent graduates report higher pain scores than their older colleagues.[12,14,15] For example, practitioners who graduated in the 1970s or earlier were more likely to agree that analgesics mask deteriorations in the condition of an animal, whereas those graduating in the 2000s were more likely to agree that cattle recover more quickly after the use of analgesics.[17] These differences may relate to training provided in the veterinary curriculum. A canine acute pain teaching tool, providing guidance on behavioral indicators of acute pain, was found to increase student knowledge and skill in terms of confidence in their own performance and for mentoring technicians for canine pain assessment.[18] Interesting, these researchers found students tracking in large animal practice reported less confidence in their ability to mentor technicians in pain management, supporting the need for development of tools for assessing behavioral indicators of pain in livestock species.

RECOGNIZING PAIN-SPECIFIC BEHAVIORAL RESPONSES

In psychology, pain processing includes sensation and perception. Sensation refers to the lower level of neurologic and biochemical components (nociception), whereas higher cognitive processing, such as interpretation, is associated with perception. A modification to the International Association for the Study of Pain definition of pain was suggested for application to animals: "an aversive sensory experience caused by actual or potential injury that elicits progressive motor and vegetative reactions, results in learned avoidance behavior, and may modify species specific behavior, including social behavior."[19] Physical signs of pain are the most reliable,[20,21] because these often include specificity that is lacking in biochemical measures (catecholamines, glucocorticoids, opioids, etc) and electrophysical measures (electroencephalograms, evoked potentials, etc). However, pain signs vary between species, type of insult, and stage of development. Basic motor responses, such as withdrawal, occur in response to acute pain stimuli and are associated with protection from further tissue damage. However, simple withdrawal responses can occur consciously or unconsciously, in awake and in anesthetized animals. More organized behavioral responses involving higher cognitive processing include aggression or escape attempts. There are 3 functions of nociception: (1) to warn the animal of actual damage to its tissues, (2) to predict when tissue damage is likely to occur, and (3) to warn conspecifics of the presence of danger.[22]

Pain is an affective state and hence can only truly be known by the individual experiencing it. Hence, pain can only be measured indirectly, in both humans and animals, presenting challenges for decision-making about pain management. The Gold Standard in human medicine is verbal self-reporting, and tools have been developed to describe the severity of pain, such as global pain scales in which patients are asked to numerically rate their pain experience on a scale of 1 to 10. Similarly, for the visual analogue scale, patients place a mark on a line, for which 1 extreme is "no pain" and the other extreme is "worst pain imaginable." These scales have the value of simplicity, but are problematic when assessing pain by proxy for preverbal and nonverbal human patients because of the lack of transparency for criteria used in this assessment. Refinements include defined checklists, such as descriptions of behavioral and facial expressions commonly associated with postsurgical pain in infants and children.[23] Several of these pain indices have been shown to correlate with procedure pain intensity and invasiveness. For example, the COMFORT scale, which includes physiologic and behavioral components, was found to have strong performance in terms of variance of scores that were associated with surgery invasiveness and levels of analgesia. Furthermore, the behavioral components explained the greatest proportion of this variance.[24] Hence behavior parameters can provide robust assessment tools for pain whereby they are clearly explained and validated.

Cattle behavior can be measured objectively or subjectively. Subjective assessments traditionally have been the most practical for clinical application, but advances in technology provide opportunities for objective assessments outside the laboratory. Pain assessment in veterinary practice has typically relied on subjective global pain scales, with clinicians or animal caretakers providing proxy assessments for the animals in their care. Intangible measures, such as demeanor, attitude, or lethargy, are often cited for clinical scoring of pain, but are poorly defined. Hence, challenges are likely to occur with interobserver and intraobserver reliability and interpretation. Subjective scoring systems may be improved when descriptions, photographic images, or videoclips of behaviors are provided for training clinicians and animal caretakers (**Fig. 1**). A Web site developed by Dr Joyce Kent and Dr Vince Molony, Royal (Dick) School of Veterinary Studies, provides an excellent resource with photographic images and videoclips of pain responses in several livestock species to common clinical situations ("Guidelines for the Recognition and Assessment of Animal Pain," http://www.link.vet.ed.ac.uk/animalpain/Default.htm). Validation of subjective scoring systems for animal subjects is emerging and is a positive step in the evolution of pain research. For example, a standardized facial grimace scale has been validated for assessing pain in mice, including 5 distinct components, of which 3 components are also observed in the human facial pain grimace.[25] Facial expressions in cattle have received little attention, but where there are similarities in anatomy, bovine equivalents to some of the mouse grimace components are worth exploring— such as orbital tightening and ear position. Subjective pain scoring is most refined in terms of bovine lameness and locomotion scoring, with excellent training resources available for practitioners, producers, and researchers. A locomotion scoring system that provides detailed descriptions of the observable changes in gait and allows observers to score components of the gait separately was received, validated, and found to be sufficiently sensitive to identify cows with severe hoof lesions,[26] as well as lame cows that were provided with a local anesthetic.[27]

Pain behavior responses are also measured objectively, particularly in experimental applications where detailed observations are collected during live observations or more frequently from videorecordings. Videorecordings provide advantages of eliminating the influence of observers on the animal's behavior as well as opportunities to

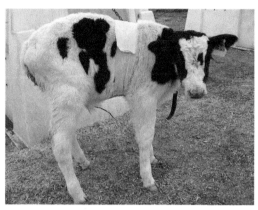

Fig. 1. Subjective scoring of pain associated with calf diarrhea, including back arch and abnormal tail position postures. Calf postures were scored from digital photographs presenting lateral standing profiles of each calf on days 0 to 5, relative to the onset of naturally occurring diarrhea. Observers were blinded to the treatment and the experimental day. Calves that received meloxicam were significantly less likely to display an abnormal tail hang posture versus saline-treated calves.[28] This (intact) calf also displays the easing quarters and an abnormal hind leg standing posture described as indicators of visceral pain. (*Data from* Molony V, Kent JE, Robertson IS. Assessment of acute and chronic pain after different methods of castration of calves. Appl Anim Behav Sci 1995;46:33–48.)

play back and to alter image size and speed for more accurate observations. In ethology, the science of animal behavior, a key component of research methodology is the development of an appropriate ethogram, which consists of a list of definitions for mutually exclusive behaviors.[29] For transparency and to avoid inherent bias associated with interpretation, definitions that focus on motor patterns or movements that an animal performs are preferred over those described in terms of an underlying motivation. Behaviors can then be quantified, such as frequency and duration of occurrence. Experiments can also be designed to provoke behavior and to be quantified in terms of latency to respond and thresholds of stimulus required for response. Manual collection of empirical behavioral data is labor intensive. New technologies are emerging for automated data collection, such as accelerometers for frequency and duration of activity and resting behavior, and show promise for detecting behavioral changes associated with lameness.[30] However, these technologies are currently not sufficiently sensitive to detect subtle and specific pain-related behaviors, such as head shaking.

Pain behaviors can be described as those that occur when pain is present versus absent and are absent or decreased when animals are provided with appropriate analgesia treatments versus placebo treatments, such as saline. Postsurgical somatic pain following cautery disbudding or dehorning of calves was associated with increased head-related motor patterns, such as head shaking and ear flicking, and calves receiving the nonsteroidal anti-inflammatory drug (NSAID) meloxicam performed fewer of these responses.[31] Conversely, somatic and visceral postsurgical castration pain is associated with increased foot stomping or kicking, and easing of quarters.[32] The animal may also direct its attention to the site of injury through licking. Pain associated with inflammation that occurs days after rubber ring castration is associated with lesion licking and is performed twice as frequently when calves are castrated surgically or using a Burdizzo.[32]

Specific postural changes are also associated with painful conditions, such as limb guarding. Visceral pain associated with castration has been characterized by statue standing, in which calves remain immobile, and abnormal standing with the hind legs stretched back or apart, and lying with hind legs extended.[32] Abnormal standing posture seems to be a more robust measure of castration pain, because it is observed more frequently than abnormal lying and is less frequently performed by castrated calves that received an NSAID.[33] Although pain-specific behaviors and postures are relatively straightforward to observe and quantify when detailed definitions are provided, these behaviors are more difficult to record when observing the hospital pen directly because they occur at low frequencies and when the animal is undisturbed by activity in the barn.

NONSPECIFIC BEHAVIORAL RESPONSES TO PAIN

In addition to specific pain responses, general and nonspecific pain responses are associated with painful conditions. During painful procedures, cattle typically struggle or attempt to escape. Because neonatal dairy calves typically do not display fear responses to handlers, their passive standing posture and absence of escape attempts when disbudded with a local anesthetic provides sufficiently compelling evidence in support of analgesia for veterinary practitioners and producers. Escape attempts can be quantified using exit velocity, determined by the latency for the animal to break an infrared beam, by strain gauges measuring the force the animal exerts on the restraint chute, or by software analysis of head movements captured with video-images.[34] Hot-iron branding was associated with greater maximum exertion force, greater head movement distances, and greater head movement velocities than freeze branding or sham branding. In this experiment, image analysis was a more sensitive technique for detecting treatment differences than frequency counts or exertion forces; it was quick and inexpensive, but its application depends on animal restraint methods. Other researchers also found hot-iron branding to be associated with greater escape responses than cattle that were subjected to restraint or freeze branding.[35]

Similarly, in some livestock species distress calls are performed during painful procedures and can be discriminated from other vocalizations, such as contact calls, by the increase in rate, pitch, and volume.[36] However, vocalizations may not be a very robust measure of pain because cattle rarely vocalize because of their stoic nature. Approximately 50% of cattle vocalized during branding,[35] 14% during castration,[37] and 13% during disbudding[38] versus 100% of goats that vocalized during disbudding.[39] Furthermore, differences have been observed between beef breeds for propensity to vocalize when experiencing the same intervention, perhaps because of variations in temperament.[40] Nonetheless, calls given during painful procedures are distinct from other calls. Hot-iron branding resulted in 60% of the cattle emitting vocalizations and these calls were of greater intensity than calves that were only restrained.[41] In contrast, the acoustic properties of contact calls, that cattle emit when isolated, are short calls at lower fundamental frequencies.

TECHNIQUES TO "ASK" ANIMALS TO RATE THEIR PAIN

Several standard tests have been developed for assessing nociception in animal models for biomedical research, including von Frey filaments for mechanoreceptors and the Hargreaves' or plantar test for thermoreceptors. Nociception tests are being modified increasingly or applied increasingly to livestock to ask about the sensory discriminatory perception of pain. To tease apart pain from other aversive experiences, such as fear or distress, attenuation of the response should occur when relevant analgesia is applied. Whereever possible, local anesthesia is preferable to opioids or sedatives because of the confounding that results from direct impacts of the latter on animal behavior.

Pressure algometry is an example of a mechanical nociception test that has proven useful for assessing pain in livestock. This tool measures the amount of force applied to a surface, and painful thresholds are determined using a withdrawal response. When applied around the horn buds, calves displayed significantly lower nociception thresholds following disbudding when compared with pressure tolerated on the day before surgery.[30] Furthermore, calves that received meloxicam displayed less pressure sensitivity than calves that received a placebo solution. Pressure algometry also suggests that the duration of postsurgical pain is greater than estimates using neuroendocrine markers, with significantly lower nociception thresholds observed for 3 days following surgery relative to baseline values.[42] Refinements to the technique, such as the use of a calf head-restraint device and blindfolding the calf to avoid responses associated with anticipation or fear, facilitate interobserver and intraobserver reliability (**Fig. 2**). Pressure algometry seems to be a robust tool, with the potential for clinical application because it is inexpensive and easy to use and the differences in response are often large. When pressure algometry was applied to the coronary band on sows with chemically induced lameness, nociception thresholds were reduced by 50% on the lame leg compared with the day prior to lameness induction or compared with the sound leg.[42]

Thermal sensitivity tests are typically performed in a research laboratory by immersing the animal's foot in a heated water bath or by directing a radiant light source or a CO_2 laser thermal stimulator at the skin. Nociception threshold is quantified by the amount of time (latency) for a vocalization or avoidance (limb withdrawal) response. In cattle, a radiant thermal source directed at the coronary band was used as a thermal nociception test and revealed that ingestion of placenta or amniotic fluid attenuated the pain response postpartum.[43] A laser thermal nociception device was found to stimulate withdrawal and kicking responses that corresponded with increasing power outputs when applied to the caudal aspect of the metatarsus of dairy cows restrained in a tie-stall.[44] This technique was sufficiently robust to detect hypoalgesia associated with environmental stressors.[45] Similarly, a CO_2 laser thermal

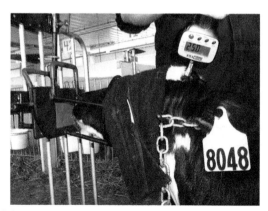

Fig. 2. A head withdrawal response is used with pressure algometry to determine mechanical threshold stimulus that a calf will tolerate near the horn bud. Calves tolerate significantly less pressure.

stimulator was found to provoke a foot lift or kicking withdrawal response when skin temperature reached 45°C to 55°C.[46] These researchers found that at least 3 replications of the test were required to control for individual variation. Unlike radiant thermal sources, CO_2 laser stimulators have the advantage of using a monochromatic, long wavelength infrared source of radiation, and hence, absorption is not affected by pigmentation of the skin. However, standard operating procedures for all thermal nociception tests require the skin surface to be free of hair, manure, and moisture.[44] Furthermore, validation is needed for safety precautions, such as maximum duration of stimulus application, to avoid tissue damage on different skin surfaces. A ceiling value of 20 seconds was used successfully as a safety precaution when a radiant thermal nociception stimulus (constant 80% beam intensity, 200°C) was used during a lameness study in sows.[42] However, these same criteria were insufficient when the thermal test was used in a disbudding study, resulting in blisters on 2 calves.[42]

TECHNIQUES TO "ASK" ANIMALS TO RATE THEIR PAIN EXPERIENCE

Classical pain tests, quantifying reflexive nociceptive withdrawal responses to mechanical or thermal stimuli, provide information about the sensory-discriminatory aspects of pain, but not the affective (emotional) components. In humans, anxiety, depression, and anhedonia may occur in association with chronic pain, such as inflammation, due to the affective component of pain rather than actual pain sensation.[47,48] Although animals cannot self-report pain verbally, cognitive tests can be used to "ask" animals about their affective states, such as pain.

Conditioned avoidance tests are based on an animal's ability to recall an association of a stimulus, such as a location or a person, with a previous aversive experience. Conditioned place avoidance is commonly observed whereby livestock have previously experienced painful interventions, such as branding, dehorning, or castration. Similarly, cattle may associate the appearance or odor of a veterinary practitioner with a previous aversive experience, resulting in difficulties with handling. However, it is often difficult to tease apart an aversion arising because of experiences associated with pain versus fear. This aversion is especially problematic with extensively managed livestock that are unfamiliar with handlers and equipment. Hence, inclusion of sham-handled controls is important for experimental design. In several species, electrical stimulation results in startle and withdrawal reflexive behaviors, as well as higher pain processes associated with aggression and avoidance behaviors. However, it is used in livestock to facilitate movement (electric prods), for restraint (electroimmobilization), and for semen collection (electroejaculation). Aversiveness of electroimmobilization was determined using condition place preference[49] and sheep took twice as long to move through a handling race that was associated with electroimmobilization when compared with their flock mates that received only physical restraint in a chute. Similarly, sheep that received an electrical shock during feeding performed escape responses and displayed longer latencies to return to the feeder in a dose-dependent manner, avoidance responses that were associated with a transient increase in electroencephalogram power spectrum.[50] These results have been used to advise against the practice of electroimmobilization, such as animal welfare policies of the American Veterinary Medical Association and Canadian Veterinary Medical Association.

One of the most elegant experiments designed to "ask" animals about their pain experience was a preference test conducted by researchers at the University of Bristol.[51] Lame and sound broiler chickens were trained to discriminate between 2 feeds, one containing the NSAID carprofen, by presenting the feed in different colored hoppers on alternate days. After the training period, birds were provided free access to both diets. Consumption of the diet resulted in improved gait scores in the lame birds in a dose-dependent manner. Lame birds consumed significantly more drugged feed than sound birds, and higher proportions of drugs were consumed as the severity of lameness increased. Although this experimental design provides compelling evidence of pain and analgesia, its utility may be influenced by phylogeny. Chickens are scavengers and have evolved to investigate and make decisions about novel foods, whereas cattle are grazers. However, sheep were found to self-medicate, preferentially consuming sodium bentonite, polyethylene glycol, and dicalcium phosphate when treated with grains, tannins, and oxalic acid, respectively.[52] Hence, experiments using self-selection of analgesia are warranted for evaluating pain responses by cattle.

SUMMARY

In conclusion, understanding the behavioral changes associated with pain is important for veterinary practitioners to respond to the increased scrutiny of painful husbandry procedures and care provided for painful clinical conditions. Subjective and objective techniques can be used to measure cattle behavior, with opportunities to improve diagnosis and provide empirical evidence for the assessment of interventions. Nociception tools, such as pressure algometry, have the potential for application to the field based on ease and speed of data collection, as well as low cost. Management of cattle during painful procedures and convalescence can have long-lasting impacts on associations with particular locations and caretakers, posing challenges for handling.

REFERENCES

1. Bennett RM, Anderson J, Blaney RJ. Moral intensity and willingness to pay concerning farm animal welfare issues and implications for agricultural policy. J Agric Environ Ethics 2002;15:187–202.
2. Rauch A, Sharp JS. Ohioans' attitudes about animal welfare. A topical report from the 2004 Ohio Survey of Food, Agricultural and Environmental Issues. Columbus (OH): Department of Human and Community Resource Development, The Ohio State University; 2005.
3. Lusk JL, Norwood FB. A survey to determine public opinion about the ethics and governance of farm animal welfare. J Am Vet Med Assoc 2008;233:1121–6.
4. Phillips CJ, Wojciechowska J, Meng J, et al. Perceptions of the importance of different welfare issues in livestock production. Animal 2009;3:1152–66.
5. Vanhonacker F, Verbeke W, Van Poucke E, et al. Do citizens and farmers interpret the concept of farm animal welfare differently? Livest Sci 2008;116:126–36.
6. Hoe FG, Ruegg PL. Opinions and practices of Wisconsin dairy producers about biosecurity and animal well-being. J Anim Sci 2006;82:1553–63.
7. Misch LJ, Duffield TF, Millman ST, et al. An investigation into the practices of dairy producers and veterinarians in dehorning dairy calves in Ontario. Can Vet J 2007; 48:1249–54.
8. Weary DM, Schuppli CA, von Keyserlingk MA. Tail docking dairy cattle: responses from an online engagement. J Dairy Sci 2011;89:3831–7.
9. Guatteo R, Levionnois O, Fournier D, et al. Minimizing pain in darm animals: the 3S approach – "suppress, substitute, soothe". Animal 2012;6:1261–74.
10. Thomsen PT, Anneberg I, Herskin MS. Differences in attitudes of farmers and veterinarians towards pain in dairy cows. Vet J 2012;194:94–7. http://dx.doi.org/10.1016/j.tvjl.2012.02.025.

11. Huxley JN, Whay HR. Current attitudes of cattle practitioners to pain and the use of analgesics in cattle. Vet Rec 2006;159:662–8.

12. Hewson CJ, Dohoo IR, Lemke KA, et al. Canadian veterinarians' use of analgesics in cattle, pigs, and horses in 2004 and 2005. Can Vet J 2007;48:155–64.

13. Fulwider WK, Grandin T, Rollin BE, et al. Survey of dairy management practices on 113 north Central and northeastern United States dairies. J Dairy Sci 2008;91:1686–92.

14. Laven RA, Huxley JN, Whay HR, et al. Results of a survey of attitudes of dairy veterinarians in New Zealand regarding painful procuedres and conditions in cattle. N Z Vet J 2009;57:215–20.

15. Fajt VR, Wagner SA, Norby B. Analgesic drug administration and attitudes about analgesia in cattle among bovine practitioners in the United States. J Am Vet Med Assoc 2011;238:755–67.

16. Hewson CJ, Dohoo IR, Lemke KA, et al. Factors affecting Canadian veterinarians' use of analgesics when dehorning beef and dairy calves. Can Vet J 2007;48:1129–36.

17. Thomsen PT, Gidekull M, Kerskin MS. Scandinavian bovine practitioners' attitudes to the use of analgesics in cattle. Vet Rec 2010;167:2256–8.

18. Mich PM, Hellyer PW, Kogan L, et al. Effects of a pilot training program on veterinary students' pain knowledge, attitude, and assessment skills. J Vet Med Educ 2010;37:358–68.

19. Zimmermann M. Behavioural investigations of pain in animals. In: Duncan IJ, Molony V, editors. Assessing pain in farm animals. Bruxelles (Belgium): Office for Official Publications of the European Communities; 1986. p. 16–29.

20. Molony V. Assessment of pain by direct measurement of cerebro cortical activity. In: Duncan IJ, Molony V, editors. Assessing pain in farm animals. Bruxelles (Belgium): Office for Official Publications of the European Communities; 1986. p. 79–88.

21. Le Bars D, Gozariu M, Cadden SW. Animal models of nociception. Pharmacol Rev 2001;53:597–652.

22. Bateson P. Assessment of pain in animals. Anim Behav 1991;42:827–39.

23. Chambers CT, Finley GA, McGrath PJ, et al. The parents' postoperative pain measure: replication and extension to 2-6-year-old children. Pain 2003;105:437–43.

24. Franck LS, Ridout D, Howard R, et al. A comparison of pain measures in newborn infants after cardiac surgery. Pain 2011;152:1758–65.

25. Langford DJ, Bailey AL, Chanda ML. Coding of facial expressions of pain in the laboratory mouse. Nat Methods 2010;7:447–9.

26. Flowers FC, Weary DM. Effects of hoof pathologies on subjective assessments of dairy cow gait. J Dairy Sci 2006;89:139–46.

27. Rushen J, Pombourcq E, de Passille AM. Validation of two measures of lameness in dairy cows. Appl Anim Behav Sci 2007;106:173–7.

28. Todd CG, McKnight DR, Millman ST, et al. Meloxicam therapy for calves with neonatal calf diarrhea complex. Proceedings of the International Congress of the International Society of Applied Ethology. Merida, July 31–August 3, 2007. p. 175.

29. Martin P, Bateson P. Measuring behaviour: an introductory guide. 3rd edition. Cambridge, UK: Cambridge University Press; 2007. p. 187.

30. Higginson JH, Millman ST, Leslie KE, et al. Validation of the new pedometry system for use in behaviour research and lameness detection in dairy cattle. In: Proceedings of the 1st North American Conference on Precision Dairy

Management. Toronto: 2010. p. 132–3. Available at: http://www.precisiondairy 2010.com/conferenceproceedings.htm. Accessed December 4, 2012.

31. Heinrich A, Duffield TF, Lissemore KD. The effect of meloxicam on behavior and pain sensitivity of dairy calves following cautery dehorning with a local anesthetic. J Dairy Sci 2010;93:2450–7.

32. Molony V, Kent JE, Robertson IS. Assessment of acute and chronic pain after different methods of castration of calves. Appl Anim Behav Sci 1995;46:33–48.

33. Ting ST, Earley B, Crowe MA. Effect of repeated ketoprofen administration during urgical castration of bulls on cortisol, immunological function, feed intake, growth and behavior. J Anim Sci 2003;81:1253–64.

34. Schwartzkopf-Genswein KS, Stookey JM, Crowe TG, et al. Comparison of image analysis, exertion force, and behavior measurements for use in the assessment of beef cattle responses to hot-iron and freeze branding. J Anim Sci 1998;76:972–9.

35. Lay DC, Friend TH, Grissom KK, et al. Effects of freeze or hot-iron branding of angus calves on some physiological and behavioral indicators of stress. Appl Anim Behav Sci 1992;33:137–47.

36. Weary DM, Braithwaite LA, Fraser D. Vocal response to pain in piglets. Appl Anim Behav Sci 1998;56:161–72.

37. Currah JM, Hendrick SH, Stookey JM. The behavioral assessment and alleviation of pain associated with castration in beef calves treated with flunixin meglumine and causal lidocaine epidural anesthesia with epinephrine. Can Vet J 2009;50: 375–82.

38. Stewart M, Stafford KJ, Dowling SK, et al. Eye temperature and heart rate variability of calves disbudded with or without local anesthetic. Physiol Behav 2008;93:789–97.

39. Alvarez L, Gutierrez J. A first description of the physiological and behavioural responses to disbudding in goat kids. Anim Welfare 2010;19:55–9.

40. Watts JM, Stookey JM. The propensity of cattle to vocalize during handling and isolation is affected by phenotype. Appl Anim Behav Sci 2001;74:81–95.

41. Watts JM, Stookey JM. Effects of restraint and branding on rates and acoustic parameters of vocalization in beef cattle. Appl Anim Behav Sci 1999;62:125–35.

42. Tapper TR. An investigation of pressure algometry and thermal sensitivity for assessing pain associated with a sow lameness model and calf disbudding [masters of science thesis]. Ames (IA): Department of Biomedical Science, Iowa State University; 2011.

43. Pinheiro Machado LC, Hurnik JF, Burton JH. The effect of amniotic fluid ingestion on the nociception of cows. Physiol Behav 1997;62:1339.

44. Herskin MS, Muller R, Schrader L, et al. A laser-based method to measure thermal nociception in dairy cows: short-term repeatability and effects of power output and skin condition. J Anim Sci 2003;81:945–54.

45. Herskin MS, Munksgaard L, Ladewig J. Effects of acute stressors on nociception, adrenocortical responses and behavior of dairy cows. Physiol Behav 2004;83: 411–20.

46. Veissier I, Rushen J, Colwell D, et al. A laser-based method for measuring thermal nociception of cattle. Appl Anim Behav Sci 2000;66:289–304.

47. Rhudy JL, Meagher MW. Fear and anxiety: divergent effects on human pain thresholds. Pain 2000;84:65–75.

48. Vlaeyen JW, Linton SJ. Fear-avoidance and its consequences in chronic musculo-skeletal pain: a state of the art. Pain 2000;85:317–32.

49. Rushen J. Aversion of sheep to electro-immobilization and physical restraint. Appl Anim Behav Sci 1986;15:315–24.

50. Ong RM, Morris JP, O'Dwyer JK, et al. Behavioural and EEG changes in sheep in response to painful acute electrical stimuli. Aust Vet J 1997;75:189–93.
51. Danbury TC, Weeks CA, Chambers JP, et al. Self-selection of the analgesic drug carprofen by lame broiler chickens. Vet Rec 2000;46:307–11.
52. Villalba JJ, Provenza FD, Shaw R. Sheep self-medicate when challenges with illness-inducing foods. Anim Behav 2006;71:1131–9.

Remote Noninvasive Assessment of Pain and Health Status in Cattle

Miles E. Theurer, BS[a], David E. Amrine, DVM[b],
Brad J. White, DVM, MS[c],*

KEYWORDS

- Behavior monitoring • Remote sampling • Animal welfare

KEY POINTS

- Cattle behavior is frequently monitored to determine health and wellness state.
- Available remote monitoring systems include
  - Clinical illness scores
  - Visual monitoring
  - Accelerometers
  - Pedometers
  - Feed intake and behavioral monitoring
  - Global position systems
  - Real time location systems
  - Thermography images
  - Rumen telemetry temperature bolus.
- Selection of remote behavioral monitoring system is influenced by
  - The behavior of interest (frequency and type)
  - Labor required to monitor the animals
  - Monitoring expenses.
- Interpretation of multiple behavioral responses as an aggregate indicator of animal wellness status instead of as individual outcomes may be a more accurate measure of true state of animal pain or wellness status.

The authors have nothing to disclose.
[a] Department of Diagnostic Medicine and Pathobiology, Kansas State University, Mosier Hall J 118, 1800 Denison Avenue, Manhattan, KS 66506, USA; [b] Department of Diagnostic Medicine and Pathobiology, Kansas State University, Mosier Hall I 111, 1800 Denison Avenue, Manhattan, KS 66506, USA; [c] Department of Clinical Sciences, Kansas State University, Mosier Hall Q 211, 1800 Denison Avenue, Manhattan, KS 66506, USA
* Corresponding author.
E-mail address: bwhite@vet.k-state.edu

INTRODUCTION

The ability to remotely identify cattle that require an intervention due to pain or disease is important for animal health providers and researchers. Behavior is frequently monitored to measure potential changes in animal well-being.[1] Stress, pain, or disease may alter animal behavior relative to optimal wellness status, but monitoring these changes is challenging without a clear definition of the expected behavioral response to an adverse event.[2] Some behavioral definitions are vague and are not specifically tied to one pain or disease response. Improvement in behavioral monitoring techniques is needed for remote monitoring of activity to be useful as diagnostic or research tools.

Multiple methods are available to monitor cattle behavior, including subjective visual observation, objective measures of cattle activity, or determination of cattle location within the housing area. Subjective measurements of pain and cattle well-being include behavioral, depression, or illness scores based on observer impression of the animal's current wellness state. The challenges with using subjective measures to determine cattle wellness state are related to potential differences between observers and among observers over time.

An opportunity exists to more discretely identify potential behavioral changes via collection of data using remote sensing technologies. Objective, continuous behavioral monitoring using accelerometers and pedometers has been used to assess cattle behavior in a variety of scenarios.[3–9] Monitoring cattle location within a defined environment has also been used in an effort to identify and monitor potential behavioral changes.[8,10]

The objective of this article is to describe potential benefits and challenges of remotely monitoring cattle behavior with available methodologies, including clinical illness scores (CISs), visual monitoring, accelerometers, pedometers, feed intake and behavioral monitoring, global position systems (GPSs), and real-time location systems (RTLSs). Although all of these remote monitoring systems are not directly applicable in a clinical setting, the results from research based on these technologies provides valuable insights to practitioners on the associations between behavioral changes and pain and wellness states.

OBSERVER MONITORING CLINICAL ILLNESS

One of the most common methods to determine wellness or painful state of an animal is having a trained observer monitor cattle for clinical signs of pain or disease. Multiple clinical signs and subjective assessments can be used to determine the animal's overall wellness status. Often a combination of findings can be categorized into a single value, or CIS, which represents the current state of the animal. The potential benefit of determining a CIS is presumably that it correlates with the need for an intervention or the probability of a specific outcome.[11] Scoring systems that assign a value based on degrees of illness are relatively common[12] and are frequently used in disease research.[3,10,13] Even when quantitative measurements, such as rectal temperature, are combined with subjective assessment, the final disease classification remains subjective.[14,15] This subjectivity may affect how the results are interpreted if the CIS is used as one of the criteria in a treatment or preventative health program.

Research has shown limited agreement among observers using the same CIS to identify calves with respiratory disease.[16] Potential sources of variation include differences among the experience and training of observers, cattle type, and environmental conditions. When a subjective scoring system is applied and interpreted by more than one individual, it should be repeatable among those individuals. Other research has evaluated agreement among veterinarians assigning body condition scores to cows and determined that even small amounts of training among the observers can increase the overall agreement.[17] A clear case definition and educational programs can decrease the variation between observers and make the results more clinically applicable.

Although CISs are frequently used, true accuracy relative to disease state is difficult to determine. There is no gold standard to diagnose respiratory disease in cattle, but the presence or absence of pulmonary lesions at harvest has been compared with ante mortem diagnoses of clinical respiratory disease.[18–20] Results from these studies illustrate low correlations between lung scores and diagnosis of clinical illness. White and Renter[21] estimated the sensitivity and specificity of using clinical signs of illness combined with rectal temperature to diagnose respiratory disease to be 61.8% and 62.8%, respectively. A test with imperfect sensitivity and specificity can underestimate or overestimate morbidity, leading to errors in the interpretation of preventative or therapeutic treatment efficacy.[16]

One way to improve CIS agreement among observers is the implementation of a refined scoring system with limited categories. The objective of assigning CIS to cattle is to accurately identify those animals that need an intervention (sensitivity) and those that do not (specificity); therefore, the system could be condensed to those two categories. If calves are deemed to require an intervention, the selection of the intervention would be based on clinician's judgment of the case. For example, a calf that was deemed to have clinical respiratory disease may require an intervention with an antimicrobial; whereas euthanasia may be a more appropriate intervention for an animal severely ill enough to become moribund and nonresponsive to human approach. Dichotomizing the results would increase agreement among observers and could potentially increase accuracy of comparison of CIS among individual observers. As previous research has illustrated, distinguishing illness severity based on CIS is challenging.[10,16] Much of the analysis of CIS data is based on the dichotomization of an animal into healthy or sick; therefore, systems that have more than two main levels serve a limited purpose.

Monitoring clinical illness by visual appraisal is a common procedure and the specific implementation of the scoring system influences final data interpretation. Although CIS are quantitative, they may not be repeatable between or among observers and do not provide an objective measure of the degree of clinical illness. Care should be taken to limit potential sources of variability among observers through training and selection of the appropriate scoring system for the situation.

OBSERVER MONITORING FREQUENCY OF SPECIFIC BEHAVIOR

Comparing calf wellness status among treatment groups in a research environment or over time in a clinical application can also be performed by monitoring the frequency of specific behaviors associated with pain or disease. Researchers have noted increases in specific behaviors, such as the number of head shakes, ear twitches, and foot stomps, after a painful procedure, such as castration.[22–24] Other researchers have documented a difference in head shakes and ear twitches following dehorning.[25–29]

The frequency of all these behaviors has been associated with increased cortisol concentrations, and increased cortisol concentrations are often associated with stress and fearful events.[30,31] However, neither cortisol nor counts of these behavior measurements have been determined to be specific indicators of pain. Calves may increase counts of ear flicks, tail switches, and foot stomps following painful procedures but these behaviors may also increase with high insect burden.[32,33] These behavioral counts are not specific for pain or wellness status but they are cost-effective and relatively easy to obtain through live observations or video analysis.

The most cost-effective method to determine the frequency of these behaviors is having an observer document the activities as they occur in the field. A limitation of this method is that behavioral activities occurring at rapid rates (eg, ear flicks) can be challenging to accurately record as they occur.[34] In a population environment, recording these behaviors on more than one animal simultaneously can also be challenging. Cattle activity may also be difficult to interpret when the observer is in close enough proximity to document specific behaviors because, as studies have shown, the presence of a human observer may alter cattle behavior.[35,36] Cattle behavioral patterns change throughout the day following a circadian rhythm,[37] but it is difficult for an observer to continuously document cattle behavior for 24 hours a day. Due to these limitations, monitoring of these behaviors is commonly performed through video analysis.

The use of the video collection technology allows observers to analyze cattle behavior at their leisure and enables observation of tail flicks, ear twitches, stomping, postural behavior, and positional location just as collected during live observation. Video recording systems are relatively easy to set up and can be used in most scenarios. The output files can be viewed on a variety of common electronic devices, including laptop computers and DVD players, allowing for minimal additional input costs to view the videos. The required quality of the video recording system is based on the specific behavior desired to document, the number of animals to observe, and environmental conditions.

Limitations of video analysis include the need to clearly identify and visualize individual animal activity, as well as the labor required to document the frequency of specific behaviors. Identification of individual animals is important to document while observing multiple animals in a pen-level setting when the experimental unit is the individual, but identification on the video may be difficult using only a visual identification ear tag or coat coloration patterns. Animals may be uniquely marked with all-weather paint sticks, spray paint, and hair dye to ease the ability to identify animals on video; however, all of these markings will wear away making it necessary to apply multiple times. Determining frequency of behavioral counts is difficult in low ambient light; however, adding artificial lights has shown to increase the amount of time dairy cows spend lying down and to reduce distance traveled.[38] Depth perception is decreased while watching video footage compared with live observation, making it challenging to determine if animals are actually eating or drinking or just spending time near the feeder or water. Another issue with video observation is the labor involved to view and document all the behavior activity desired.

Video viewing is a time-consuming and tedious task. Software exists to make data recording of animal behavior easier for the viewer while watching the video.[39,40] Video sampling methods have been evaluated to reduce the amount of labor required to analyze the video. Continuous, scan, time, and focal animal sampling have all been used to minimize the labor required to classify segments of video, yet still accurately determine animal behavior.

Continuous sampling is observing animal activity for the entire period that data were captured at the same speed that video was recorded. Scan sampling is observing animal behavior for a brief period, and then repeating the observation after a period of time.[41] The portion of time passed between recording samples is the scan interval and is set at a predetermined length. The frequency of behavioral activity monitored during the observation period is used to represent the percentage of behavior activity over the entire period of time.[42] Scan sampling has been shown to accurately evaluate frequency of cattle behaviors compared with continuous sampling; however, when the scan interval was greater than or equal to 30 minutes (a 30 minute gap between sampling periods), correlation to continuous sampling decreased.[41]

Time sampling is identifying behavior for a period of 10 minutes at the beginning of each hour and then multiplying the frequency of behavioral activity by 6 to represent activity for the entire hour.[43] Time sampling has low correlation coefficients compared with continuous monitoring for describing standing, lying, feeding, drinking, and walking activity.[41] This low correlation makes time sampling a less accurate method for classifying cattle behaviors based on recorded video.

Focal sampling is the monitoring of a portion of animals within the group for the entire period to determine behavioral activity for the group. Focal sampling of 1 animal out of 10 animals per pen was accurate for describing all 10 animals' standing, lying, feeding, and walking behaviors; however, watering behavior required observing 4 out of 10 animals per pen to accurately describe drinking behavior.[41] Individual animal variation in the behaviors of interest may influence accuracy of focal sampling; however, this technique may be appropriate for some pen-level studies. Observing video clips at the rate of four times faster than recorded speed has accurately depicted swine feeding and watering behavior in confined settings compared with real-time recording speed.[43]

Video recording and documenting counts of specific behaviors can be used to monitor potential changes related to pain or wellness status; however, the process is time and labor intensive. The use of scan and focal sampling will reduce the amount of labor required to accurately determine animal behavior. Despite potential limitations, continuous video monitoring is considered the gold standard by which other behavior monitoring devices are evaluated.

MONITORING ACTIVITY WITH ACCELEROMETERS

Accelerometers are devices that continuously measure gravitational force in multiple axes; these values can be processed to determine activity and postural behaviors. **Fig. 1**A, B show a three-dimensional accelerometer attached with the horizontal, vertical, and diagonal axes the accelerometer monitors gravitational force. Before remote continuous monitoring technology can be used to assess the physiologic and behavioral patterns that cattle display, the technology requires validation.[44,45] Accelerometers have been shown to accurately monitor calf behaviors of standing, lying, or walking with 97.7% agreement to video analysis.[6] This high accuracy allows the user to effectively rely on the accelerometers to determine posture behavior compared with using a labor intensive process of analyzing video.

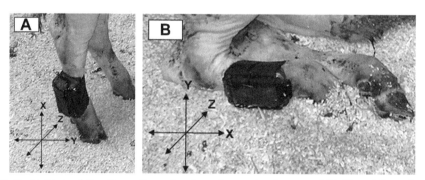

Fig. 1. Position of the three-dimensional accelerometer (measured X, Y, and Z axes) on the lateral aspect of the right rear limb in a standing (A) and lying (B) calf. (*From* Robert B, White BJ, Renter DG, et al. Evaluation of three-dimensional accelerometers to monitor and classify behavior patterns in cattle. Comput Electron Agr 2009;67(1–2):80–4; with permission.)

Assessing postural changes may be important in evaluating calf wellness or pain status and several studies have illustrated differences in postural behavior following painful stimuli. Calves have been shown to increase the percentage of time standing in the hours immediately following castration based on accelerometer analysis.[46] However, Pauly and colleagues[5] determined that calves spent more time lying down and less time walking in the 5-day period following castration. The difference between these two studies may be due to the length of the monitoring period and a potential time-dependent change in behaviors. Theurer and colleagues[8] determined that calves administered the nonsteroidal, antiinflammatory drug, meloxicam, before cautery dehorning spent more time lying down for 5 days after dehorning compared with control calves that did not receive analgesia as commonly performed in production practice.[47] Lying behavior decreased in calves after being induced with experimental lameness using an amphotericin B synovitis-arthritis induction model.[48] Accelerometers are an effective tool for continuous monitoring of behavior changes in response to pain.

Accelerometers (GP1 SENSR, Reference LLC, Elkader, IA, USA) have also been used to monitor disease and wellness state of cattle. Calves challenged with *Mannheimia haemolytica* spent more time lying down compared with unchallenged control calves.[7] This agrees with a common assumption that a primary clinical sign of respiratory disease is depression. In another respiratory disease trial, there was no difference in the amount of time morbid calves spent lying down or walking compared with baseline data collected before challenge.[3] These findings suggest that the postural activity of cattle may be influenced by disease or pain state, but changes in standing and lying behavior may not be a specific response to changes in wellness status.

Daily environmental conditions, differences among individual calves, and circadian rhythms also affect the amount of time calves spend lying[37]; therefore, it is important to make comparisons of behavioral activities of calves housed in the same environmental conditions. Monitoring control animals allows the observer to distinguish between the behavioral changes associated with administering a procedure from daily variation due to environmental conditions.[37,49,50] The placement of the accelerometer on the animal and accelerometer size and weight may transiently alter normal gait and behavior. A brief acclimation period may be needed for the cattle to adjust to having the accelerometer attached to their legs.

Limitations of using accelerometers to monitor behavior include cost, data processing, and technological constraints. Accelerometers are relatively expensive compared with other behavior monitoring techniques, such as video analysis. Transforming the accelerometer into useable behavioral measurements can be achieved with validated algorithms; however, generating the data processing technique is time consuming. The accelerometers must have sufficient battery life, on-board memory storage (or the ability to wirelessly transmit data), and be small enough to be easily affixed to the animal in some method. The objective quantification of cattle postural behavior as determined by accelerometers provides valid data to compare potential changes in behavioral patterns associated with pain or wellness status.

MONITORING STEP-COUNT FREQUENCY WITH PEDOMETERS

Pedometers have been used to objectively quantify the number of steps traveled and total distance traveled. An on-board algorithm calculating the number of steps from the raw data is contained within the pedometer. Pedometers are relatively easy to attach and use, but the number of steps each calf travels varies considerably among days and environmental conditions.

The distance calves travel may be associated with painful and stressful procedures. The amount calves travel following a painful procedure such as castration may vary because some research demonstrated calves traveled fewer steps for 4 days after castration[51] whereas other work was unable to detect a difference in the number of steps traveled in calves after castration.[52] Stress may also influence the distance traveled because calves have been shown to take more steps for 3 days after weaning.[53] Bulls travel more steps than steers per day indicating the need for accounting for gender in the analysis.[51] In properly designed experiments, pedometers may be useful in determining changes in behavior following a painful procedure.

Pedometers have been used to detect early lameness in dairy cattle, but a 15% decrease in activity was needed before the pedometer could accurately identify 92% of lame cattle.[54] The biologic significance of a 15% decrease in activity has not been established, but there may be clinical implications in detecting cattle before a change this large is detected. O'Callaghan and colleagues[55] demonstrated that lame dairy cows traveled 22.5 fewer steps per hour compared with cows that were not lame based on visual locomotion score throughout most of the lactating period. Because pedometers are directly measuring locomotion, they are a valuable tool in identifying and monitoring musculoskeletal pain. However, changes in step counts as measured by pedometers are not only specific for identifying pain; due to increased activity levels, pedometer technology has also been able to accurately detect the onset of estrus in cows.[56,57]

Pedometers can be effective monitoring devices for evaluating pain response and health status of cattle. The relative lower cost of investment and labor intensity compared with other technologies makes pedometers an attractive tool to objectively monitor potential behavioral changes.

FEED INTAKE AND BEHAVIORAL MONITORING

Systems are available to measure individual cattle feeding behavior and intake in group-housed situations. These systems have been used to identifying morbid cattle from healthy cattle based on differences in feeding behaviors.[58] Feed and water intake, duration, and frequency are specific behaviors that can be monitored with these systems. Systems that monitor feeding and watering behaviors that are commercially available include GrowSafe (GrowSafe Systems Ltd, Airdrie, AB, Canada) and Insentec (Repelweg, Marknesse, Netherlands). GrowSafe uses radio frequency identification (RFID) ear tags to identify individual animals. Insentec, on the other hand, uses transponder collars to identify when animals are at feeding or watering stations. Both systems have integrated software that allows for real-time monitoring and analysis of animal feeding or watering behavior.

RFID technology has been used to document a reduction in the frequency of visits to feeders.[24] Researchers evaluating residual feed intake found distinct differences in feeding behaviors among high and low residual feed intake calves using both the GrowSafe and Insentec monitoring systems.[59,60] Because feed inputs represent one of the largest costs in producing beef, monitoring behaviors that may identify calves with less than ideal feed efficiencies may be beneficial.[61] Monitoring the feeding behavior of an animal over a period of time allows establishment of a baseline against which deviations in subsequent behavioral patterns can be evaluated. Investigators have used algorithms with 7-day rolling average feeding times as baselines to identify behavioral changes correlated with painful locomotive conditions in dairy cows days before farm staff were able to diagnose lameness.[62]

Monitoring animal feeding behavior and intake can provide insight into potential changes in wellness or pain status. Setup, maintenance, training, and expense are all potential disadvantages that must be considered when evaluating remote feed intake and behavior systems. However, the feed intake and frequency data collection capabilities make these systems an attractive monitoring tool to use because feed costs are important to the producer.

LOCATION DETERMINATION: GPSS

GPSs have been used to remotely monitor movement of wildlife and domestic animals.[63,64] Advances in GPS technology have created lighter and more accurate receivers, but monitoring multiple animals in varied geographic regions is often cost-prohibitive.[64] Three of the largest challenges when monitoring cattle with GPS technology are the ability to have real-time updates, decreased battery life, and spatial accuracy.

Current technology allows for the location of a GPS receiver to be updated every second, but this update rate exceeds the power sources available in most animal monitoring units.[65] Custom units with real-time updates once every minute have been developed. However, battery life was only 3.7 days.[66] Others using non–real-time receivers have successfully monitored cattle for longer durations (11 days) by only waking the system up from a deep sleep mode every 600 seconds; however, depending on the environment, these infrequent readings may not provide the level of data necessary to define specific behaviors.[67]

Positional accuracy of the systems are also an issue and some research shows a discrepancy between visual and tag positions of an average plus or minus standard deviation of 9 m plus or minus 7 m.[66] Other work illustrates that 99.9% of positional fixes fell within 20 m and 97.3% within 10 m of a known point.[67] Based on these accuracies, the GPS can give approximate location of individuals, but readings are not discrete enough to delineate specific activities such as eating or drinking.

The tradeoffs of battery life and positional update frequency limit the potential uses of GPS systems in situations in which the behavior needs to be continually monitored for longer periods of time. Accuracy of 10 m may be sufficient for questions of pasture usage and grazing activities, but is not sufficient for monitoring feeding and watering behaviors. These limitations make GPS difficult to use to monitor changes in pain or wellness status in cattle.

MONITORING MOVEMENT IN A DEFINED SYSTEM WITH RTLSS

RTLS are designed to locate the position of an item anywhere within a defined area. The architecture of an RTLS consists of receivers spaced around the desired monitoring space, active or passive tags that are placed on the objects to be monitored, computer hardware, and software to receive and translate positional data. Tags used with most RTLSs are smaller and have considerably longer battery life than current GPS technology. Like GPS, most RTLSs require line-of-sight from tags to sensors for accurate readings. **Fig. 2** demonstrates a calf within the sensor area and shows how three receivers locate the animal and triangulate its position. Amount of time is calculated by subtracting the time of arrival at that location from the previous time of arrival documented. Although similar to RFID behavior and intake systems, RTLS has the distinct advantage of being able to monitor an animal's location anywhere within the pen, thus not restricting evaluation to only feeding and drinking behaviors.

The system monitors location within the pen at preset intervals and not the specific behavior the calf is engaged in while at that position. Therefore, for data to be useful, the positions must be matched with a known diagram of the facility structure with

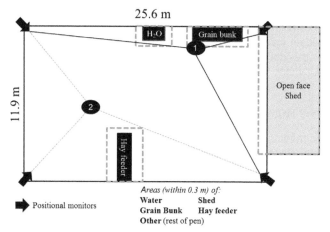

Fig. 2. A remote triangulation system with positional monitors (*arrows*) able to triangulate animal position and compare with marked areas of interest including grain bunk, hay feeder, shed, and water. Calf position is determined by the relative distance between the calf tag and at least three readers (lines from the readers to the points within the pen). Amount of time at a location is determined by calculating the difference between time of arrival at specific coordinates and previous triangulation time point. (*Circle 1*) Calf at the grain bunk. (*Circle 2*) Calf in the pen, but not next to a location of interest. (*Adapted from* Theurer ME, White BJ, Coetzee JF, et al. Assessment of behavioral changes associated with oral meloxicam administration at time of dehorning in calves using a remote triangulation device and accelerometers. BMC Vet Res 2012;8(1):48; with permission.)

specific areas of interest (proximity to feed, water, shelter) identified on the same scale of axes as measured by the RTLS. Depending on the frequency of measurements, the RTLS can be used to document the percent of time animals spend in specific locations within the housing environment.

An advantage of RTLS is the ability to measure levels of activity such as distance traveled and time spent within a given proximity to other calves. By measuring location over discrete time intervals, the data can be compared to determine the distance an animal traveled over a given period with results similar to measurements taken using pedometers. Social interactions with other calves (or the lack thereof) can be monitored by comparisons of the proximity of individual calves to other animals within the pen. Real-time location systems have been used to monitor potential changes in cattle behavior that may be associated with pain or alterations in wellness status.

Investigators have used RTLS technology (Ubisense, Denver, CO, USA) to determine that certain behaviors, such as time spent at the feed bunk and distance traveled, were associated with CISs.[10] The distance traveled by calves as monitored with RTLS was also associated with the level of lung consolidation, indicating that monitoring movement may be a reasonable tool for wellness status evaluation.[10] Theurer and colleagues[8] identified calves that were dehorned and given pain medication had different feeding behaviors when measured by RTLS technology compared with calves dehorned without pain medications. These associations with behavior changes indicate that RTLS technology is a valid tool to generate quantitative measurements of cattle activities that can be used to monitor potential changes in wellness or pain status in response to an intervention.

Limitations of RTLS technology include expense and technological constraints. The RTLSs are able to monitor animal behavior within a specific area, but those areas need to be equipped with multiple sensors to accurately monitor behavioral activity; this may be cost prohibitive in many situations. Installation and calibration of an RTLS requires significant investment in time and resources and, although the use of this technology for monitoring animals is relatively new, these systems have been used successfully for many years for monitoring assets in large complex manufacturing environments.

THERMOGRAPHY IMAGES

Thermography imaging can be used to monitor and record surface temperatures in multiple species. This technology has been used to noninvasively monitor welfare in cattle[68] and monitor nasal mucosal temperatures.[69] Using thermography in cattle housed in high ambient temperatures has been shown to result in low sensitivity (70.7%) and adequate specificity (89.5%) of identifying animals above or below a rectal temperature cutoff value.[70]

Corneal surface temperatures have been monitored using thermography based on the hypothesis that changes in corneal temperature may be reflective of changes in core temperature resulting from pain or disease. In one study, there was no difference in surface temperature 2 to 3 hours after dehorning procedure.[71] Maximum surface corneal temperature has been shown to decrease $0.27^{\circ}C$ from baseline 2 to 5 minutes in calves after disbudding without local anesthesia.[72] However, disbudded cattle had higher surface temperatures 5 to 15 minutes after disbudding compared with controls that were not disbudded.[72] Temporal relationships need to be taken into account when analyzing thermography images.

Cattle infected with foot-and-mouth disease virus have been monitored using infrared thermography imaging; however, this system resulted in a low sensitivity (61.1%) and adequate specificity (87.7%) of correctly identifying infected animals with foot-and-mouth disease.[73] There was not a strong correlation between face surface temperature and rectal temperature, but there was a positive correlation between foot surface temperature and rectal temperature, indicating peripheral extremities may be more illustrative of core body temperature. The use of infrared thermography imaging has also resulted in low sensitivity (67.6%) and adequate specificity (86.8%) of identifying calves with bovine respiratory disease.[74]

Thermography images can be relatively easy to capture; however, to capture the images correctly the distance from the camera and the animal needs to be relatively consistent. Environmental conditions affect the relative temperatures recorded on images and need to be standardized to collect images for comparison when designing a research trial. Interpretation of the thermography images needs to include the temporal relationship related to the procedure performed (establishment of a baseline reading in similar environmental conditions) to detect changes. Thermography imaging needs to have refinement of the cutoff values used to detect morbid or painful animals before becoming implemented into industry practice.

RUMEN TELEMETRY TEMPERATURE BOLUS

Rumen telemetry temperature boluses have been used to noninvasively monitor the health parameters of cattle.[75] Rumen temperatures have been shown to increase in calves challenged with *Mannheimia haemolytica*, and rumen temperatures have also been shown to have a strong correlation ($R^2 = 0.80$) to rectal temperatures.[76] The use of reticulorumen boluses has a positive predictive value of 73% for identifying animals infected with bovine respiratory disease when compared with a physical examination.[77] The pyrogenic effect of lipopolysaccharide was shown to only transiently increase rectal temperatures when administered to dairy calves[50]; however, rumen temperature increased 2°C when administered lipopolysaccharide to beef heifers.[75]

Limitations of rumen bolus telemetry system include the expense and administration of the bolus into the animal. The continued automatic thermal documentation has potential advantages related to remote monitoring of temperature changes. Overall effectiveness of the rumen telemetry temperature bolus is affected by specific facets of the system, including ability to use telemetry in the specific environment (interference, geographic distribution), data collection, and management plan.

TYMPANIC BULLA AND INTRAVAGINAL TEMPERATURE MONITORS

Tympanic bulla temperature can be monitored using a portable data logger attached to a thermistor. Temperature readings obtained with tympanic bulla thermometers have been correlated to rectal temperature,[78,79] and tympanic temperature has been shown to increase 0.78°C and 0.65°C by moving cattle around in the summer and winter, respectively.[80] The increase in body temperature due to processing needs to also be taken into consideration when evaluating the health status of an individual animal.

Intravaginal temperature can be monitored using a thermistor modified with finger-like projections to prevent expulsion from the vagina.[56] The onset of estrus has been able to be determined using intravaginal temperature moinitors.[56,81] However, there is little published literature describing the use of tympanic bulla and intravaginal temperature monitors to determine health or wellness states.

SUMMARY

Determining animal wellness status is frequently based on visual appraisal or performance parameters. The use of multimodal, remote, quantitative monitoring techniques will become more critical in determining the physiologic, behavioral, and performance responses cattle experience in different scenarios. Interpretation of multiple behavioral responses as an aggregate indicator of animal wellness status instead of as individual outcomes may be a more accurate measure of true state of well-being. Individual animals differ greatly in behavior and accurate interpretation of behavioral changes depends on the ability to establish normal baseline activity in calves in a specific housing environment.

Behavioral data should be interpreted carefully because none of the commonly monitored behaviors are truly specific for one type of illness or pain response. Statistical analyses should account for the hierarchy of repeated measures on individual calves, the effect of having multiple observers, housing effects, time of day, and seasonality. If these potential sources of variability are not included in statistical analysis, differences between treatment groups may be falsely detected or there may be differences that are undetected.

There are numerous remote monitoring methods available to assess the pain or well-being status of an animal; however, determination of the specific behavior needed to monitor, labor, and expense all need to be taken into consideration before deciding which behavioral monitoring device to use. The selection of the appropriate system for the situation depends on the expected benefits compared with costs of operating the system. Use of a remote monitoring system provides basic information on cattle behavioral changes that can be translated to other aspects of clinical practice and animal wellness evaluation.

REFERENCES

1. Gonyou HW. Why the study of animal behavior is associated with the animal welfare issue. J Anim Sci 1994;72(8):2171–7.
2. Levitis D, Lidlicker WZ, Freund G. Behavioural biologists do not agree on what constitutes behaviour. Anim Behav 2009;78(1):103–10.
3. Hanzlicek GA, White BJ, Mosier DA, et al. Serial evaluation of physiologic, pathological, and behavioral changes related to disease progression of experimentally induced *Mannheimia haemolytica* pneumonia in postweaned calves. Am J Vet Res 2010;71(3):359–69.
4. Theurer ME, White BJ, Anderson DE, et al. Effect of transportation during periods of high ambient temperature on physiology and behavior of beef heifers. Am J Vet Res, in press.
5. Pauly C, White BJ, Coetzee JF, et al. Evaluation of analgesic protocol effect on calf behavior after concurrent castration and dehorning. Inter J App Res Vet Med 2012;10(1):54–61.
6. Robert B, White BJ, Renter DG, et al. Evaluation of three-dimensional accelerometers to monitor and classify behavior patterns in cattle. Comput Electron Agr 2009;67(1–2):80–4.
7. Theurer ME, Anderson DE, White BJ, et al. Effect of *Mannheimia haemolytica* pneumonia on behavior and physiologic responses of calves experiencing hyperthermal environmental conditions Paper presented at: XXVII World Buiatrics Conference 2012. Lisbon (Portugal), June 3–8, 2012.
8. Theurer ME, White BJ, Coetzee JF, et al. Assessment of behavioral changes associated with oral meloxicam administration at time of dehorning in calves using a remote triangulation device and accelerometers. BMC Vet Res 2012; 8(1):48.
9. Dockweiler J, Bergamasco L, Coetzee J, et al. Effect of age and castration method on physiological stress indicators in calves. Paper presented at Phi Zeta Sigma Chapter. Manhattan, March 6, 2012.
10. White BJ, Anderson DE, Renter DG, et al. Clinical, behavioral, and pulmonary changes following *Mycoplasma bovis* challenge in calves. Am J Vet Res 2012; 73(4):490.
11. Hayes G, Mathews K, Kruth S, et al. Illness severity scores in veterinary medicine: what can we learn? J Vet Intern Med 2010;24(3):457.
12. Perino LJ, Apley M. Clinical trial design in feedlots. Vet Clin North Am Food Anim Pract 1998;14(3):243–66.
13. Coetzee JF, Edwards LN, Mosher RA, et al. Effect of oral meloxicam on health and performance of beef steers relative to bulls castrated on arrival at the feedlot. J Anim Sci 2012;90(3):1026.
14. Sanderson MW. Designing and running clinical trials on farms. Vet Clin North Am Food Anim Pract 2006;22(1):103–23.
15. Wenz JR, Garry FB, Barrington GM. Comparison of disease severity scoring systems for dairy cattle with acute coliform mastitis. J Am Vet Med Assoc 2006;229(2):259.
16. Amrine DE, White BJ, Larson RL, et al. Determining precision and accuracy of clinical illness scores compared to pulmonary consolidation scores in Holstein calves with induced Mycoplasma bovis pneumonia. Am J Vet Res, in press.
17. Kristensen E, Dueholm L, Vink D, et al. Within- and across-person uniformity of body condition scoring in Danish Holstein cattle. J Dairy Sci 2006;89(9): 3721–8.

18. Wittum TE, Woollen NE, Perino LJ, et al. Relationships among treatment for respiratory tract disease, pulmonary lesions evident at slaughter, and rate of weight gain in feedlot cattle. J Am Vet Med Assoc 1996;209(4):814–8.
19. Schneider MJ, Tait RG, Busby WD. An evaluation of bovine respiratory disease complex in feedlot cattle: impact on performance and carcass traits using treatment records and lung lesion scores. J Anim Sci 2009;87(5):1821–7.
20. Thompson PN, Stone A, Schultheiss WA. Use of treatment records and lung lesion scoring to estimate the effect of respiratory disease on growth during early and late finishing periods in South African feedlot cattle. J Anim Sci 2006;84(2): 488–98.
21. White BJ, Renter DG. Bayesian estimation of the performance of using clinical observations and harvest lung lesions for diagnosing bovine respiratory disease in post-weaned beef calves. J Vet Diagn Invest 2009;21(4):446–53.
22. Robertson IS, Kent JE, Molony V. Effect of different methods of castration on behaviour and plasma cortisol in calves of three ages. Res Vet Sci 1994;56(1): 8–17.
23. Mellor DJ. Effects of castration on behaviour and plasma cortisol concentrations in young lambs, kids and calves. Res Vet Sci 1991;51(2):149.
24. Gonzalez LA, Schwartzkopf-Genswein KS, Caulkett NA, et al. Pain mitigation following band castration of beef calves and its effects on performance, behavior, E. coli, and salivary cortisol. J Anim Sci 2009;88:802–10.
25. Morisse JP, Cotte JP, Huonnic D. Effect of dehorning on behaviour and plasma cortisol responses in young calves. Appl Anim Behav Sci 1995;43(4):239–47.
26. McMeekan C, Stafford K, Mellor D, et al. Effects of a local anaesthetic and a non-steroidal anti-inflammatory analgesic on the behavioural responses of calves to dehorning. N Z Vet J 1999;47(3):92–6.
27. Graf B. Behavioural and physiological responses of calves to dehorning by heat cauterization with or without local anaesthesia. Appl Anim Behav Sci 1999; 62(2–3):153.
28. Stilwell G, Carvalho RC, Carolino N, et al. Effect of hot-iron disbudding on behaviour and plasma cortisol of calves sedated with xylazine. Res Vet Sci 2010;88(1): 188–93.
29. Vickers KJ, Niel L, Kiehlbauch LM, et al. Calf response to caustic paste and hot-iron dehorning using sedation with and without local anesthetic. J Dairy Sci 2005;88(4):1454–9.
30. Grandin T. Assessment of stress during handling and transport. J Anim Sci 1997; 75(1):249–57.
31. Mormede P, Soissons J, Bluthe RM, et al. Effect of transportation on blood serum composition, disease incidence, and production traits in young calves. Influence of the journey duration. Ann Rech Vet 1982;13(4):369–84.
32. Hillerton JE, Bramley AJ. Variability between Muscidae populations of dairy heifers on two different types of pasture in southern England. Br Vet J 1986; 142(2):155–62.
33. Harris JA, Hillerton JE, Morant SV. Effect on milk production of controlling muscid flies, and reducing fly-avoidance behaviour, by the use of fenvalerate ear tags during the dry period. J Dairy Res 1987;54(2):165–71.
34. Altmann J. Observational study of behavior: sampling methods. Behaviour 1974; 49(3):227.
35. Ishiwata T, Kilgour RJ, Uetake K, et al. Choice of attractive conditions by beef cattle in a Y-maze just after release from restraint. J Anim Sci 2006;85(4): 1080.

36. Grignard L. The social environment influences the behavioural responses of beef cattle to handling. Appl Anim Behav Sci 2000;68(1):1.
37. Robért BD, White BJ, Renter DG, et al. Determination of normal beef cattle activity patterns utilizing wireless accelerometers: circadian rhythms, variation among days, and differences between individual calves. Am J Vet Res 2011; 72(4):467.
38. Phillips CJ, Schofield SA. The effect of supplementary light on the production and behaviour of dairy cows. Anim Prod 1989;48(2):293–303.
39. Hänninen L. CowLog: open-source software for coding behaviors from digital video. Behav Res Meth 2009;41(2):472.
40. Morrow-Tesch JL, Dailey JW, Jiang H. A video data base system for studying animal behavior. J Anim Sci 1998;76(10):2605.
41. Mitlohner FM, Morrow-Tesch JL, Wilson SC, et al. Behavioral sampling techniques for feedlot cattle. J Anim Sci 2001;79(5):1189–93.
42. Colgan PW. Quantitative ethology. Wiley; 1978.
43. Arnold-Meeks C, McGlone JJ. Validating techniques to sample behavior of confined, young pigs. Appl Anim Behav Sci 1986;16(2):149.
44. Duff GC, Galyean ML. Board-invited review: recent advances in management of highly stressed, newly received feedlot cattle. J Anim Sci 2007;85(3):823–40.
45. Weary DM, Huzzey JM, von Keyserlingk MA. Board-invited review: using behavior to predict and identify ill health in animals. J Anim Sci 2009;87:770–7.
46. White BJ, Coetzee JF, Renter DG, et al. Evaluation of two-dimensional accelerometers to monitor behavior of beef calves after castration. Am J Vet Res 2008;69(8): 1005–12.
47. Coetzee J, Nutsch A, Barbur L, et al. A survey of castration methods and associated livestock management practices performed by bovine veterinarians in the United States. BMC Vet Res 2010;6(1):12.
48. Schulz KL, Anderson DE, Coetzee JF, et al. Effect of flunixin meglumine on the amelioration of lameness in dairy steers with amphotericin B-induced transient synovitis-arthritis. Am J Vet Res 2011;72(11):1431.
49. Fuquay JW. Heat stress as it affects animal production. J Anim Sci 1981;52(1): 164.
50. Theurer ME, Anderson DE, White BJ, et al. Physiological and behavioral changes with variations in ambient temperature and exposure to lipopolysaccharides in cattle. Paper presented at: American Association of Bovine Practitioners. St. Louis, 2011.
51. Devant M, Marti S, Bach A. Effects of castration on eating pattern and physical activity of Holstein bulls fed high-concentrate rations under commercial conditions. J Anim Sci 2012. [Epub ahead of print].
52. Currah JM, Hendrick SH, Stookey JM. The behavioral assessment and alleviation of pain associated with castration in beef calves treated with flunixin meglumine and caudal lidocaine epidural anesthesia with epinephrine. Can Vet J 2009;50(4): 375–82.
53. Haley DB, Bailey DW, Stookey JM. The effects of weaning beef calves in two stages on their behavior and growth rate. J Anim Sci 2005;83(9):2205–14.
54. Mazrier H, Tal S, Aizinbud E, et al. A field investigation of the use of the pedometer for the early detection of lameness in cattle. Can Vet J 2006; 47(9):883–6.
55. O'Callaghan KA, Cripps PJ, Downham DY, et al. Subjective and objective assessment of pain and discomfort due to lameness in dairy cattle. Anim Welfare 2003; 12(4):605.

56. Redden KD, Kennedy AD, Ingalls JR, et al. Detection of estrus by radiotelemetric monitoring of vaginal and ear skin temperature and pedometer measurements of activity. J Dairy Sci 1992;76:713–21.
57. Roelofs JB, van Eerdenburg FJ, Soede NM, et al. Pedometer readings for estrous detection and as predictor for time of ovulation in dairy cattle. Theriogenology 2005;64(8):1690–703.
58. Sowell BF, Branine ME, Bowman JG, et al. Feeding and watering behavior of healthy and morbid steers in a commercial feedlot. J Anim Sci 1999;77(5):1105–12.
59. Nkrumah JD, Basarab JA, Price MA, et al. Different measures of energetic efficiency and their phenotypic relationships with growth, feed intake, and ultrasound and carcass merit in hybrid cattle. J Anim Sci 2004;82(8):2451.
60. Kelly AK, McGee M, Crews DH, et al. Effect of divergence in residual feed intake on feeding behavior, blood metabolic variables, and body composition traits in growing beef heifers. J Anim Sci 2010;88(1):109.
61. Bingham GM, Friend TH, Lancaster PA, et al. Relationship between feeding behavior and residual feed intake in growing Brangus heifers. J Anim Sci 2009;87(8):2685–9.
62. Gonzalez LA, Tolkamp BJ, Coffey MP, et al. Changes in feeding behavior as possible indicators for the automatic monitoring of health disorders in dairy cows. J Dairy Sci 2008;91(3):1017–28.
63. Moen R, Pastor J, Cohen Y. Effects of animal activity on GPS telemetry location attempts. Alces 2001;37(1):207–16.
64. Davis JD, Darr MJ, Xin H, et al. Development of a GPS herd activity and well-being kit (GPS HAWK) to monitor cattle behavior and the effect of sample interval on travel distance. Appl Eng Agr 2011;27(1):143–50.
65. Tomkiewicz SM, Fuller MR, Kie JG, et al. Global positioning system and associated technologies in animal behaviour and ecological research. Philos Trans R Soc Lond B Biol Sci 2010;365(1550):2163.
66. Schleppe JB, Lachapelle G, Booker CW, et al. Challenges in the design of a GNSS ear tag for feedlot cattle. Comput Electron Agr 2010;70(1):84–95.
67. Trotter MG, Lamb DW, Hinch GN, et al. Global navigation satellite system livestock tracking: system development and data interpretation. Anim Prod Sci 2010;50(6):616.
68. Stewart M, Webster JR, Schaefer AL, et al. Infrared thermography as a non-invasive tool to study animal welfare. Anim Welfare 2005;14:319–25.
69. Willatt DJ. Continuous infrared thermometry of the nasal mucosa. Rhinology 1993;31(2):63–7.
70. Gomez A, Vergara C, Cook NB, et al. Is thermography a possible new method to evaluate body temperature in fresh cows? Paper presented at: American Association of Bovine Practitioners. St. Louis, 2011.
71. Stewart M, Stookey JM, Stafford KJ, et al. Effects of local anesthetic and a nonsteroidal antiinflammatory drug on pain responses of dairy calves to hot-iron dehorning. J Dairy Sci 2009;92(4):1512–9.
72. Stewart M. Eye temperature and heart rate variability of calves disbudded with or without local anaesthetic. Physiol Behav 2008;93(4–5):789.
73. Rainwater Lovett K. Detection of foot-and-mouth disease virus infected cattle using infrared therm0ography. Vet J 2009;180(3):317.
74. Schaefer AL, Cook NJ, Church JS, et al. The use of infrared thermography as an early indicator of bovine respiratory disease complex in calves. Res Vet Sci 2007;83(3):376–84.

75. Small JA. Core body temperature monitoring with passive transponder boluses in beef heifers. Can Vet J 2008;88(2):225.
76. Rose Dye TK. Rumen temperature change monitored with remote rumen temperature boluses after challenges with bovine viral diarrhea virus and *Mannheimia haemolytica*. J Anim Sci 2010;89(4):1193.
77. Timsit E. Early detection of bovine respiratory disease in young bulls using reticulo-rumen temperature boluses. Vet J 2011;190(1):136.
78. Davis MS, Mader TL, Holt SM, et al. Strategies to reduce feedlot cattle heat stress: effects on tympanic temperature. J Anim Sci 2003;81(3):649–61.
79. Mader TL, Holt SM, Hahn GL, et al. Feeding strategies for managing heat load in feedlot cattle. J Anim Sci 2002;80(9):2373–82.
80. Mader T, Davis M, Kreikemeier W. Case study: tympanic temperature and behavior associated with moving feedlot cattle. Prof Anim Sci 2005;21:339–44.
81. Rorie RW, Bilby TR, Lester TD. Application of electronic estrus detection technologies to reproductive management of cattle. Theriogenology 2002;57(1):137–48.

Assessment and Management of Pain Associated with Castration in Cattle

Johann F. Coetzee, BVSc, Cert CHP, PhD

KEYWORDS

- Castration • Cattle • Pain assessment • Analgesia • Animal welfare

KEY POINTS

- Validated pain assessment tools are needed to support approval of analgesic compounds to alleviate pain associated with castration.
- Accelerometers, videography, heart rate variability determination, electroencephalography, thermography, and plasma neuropeptide measurement have been used to assess behavioral, physiologic, and neuroendocrine changes associated with castration.
- Preemptive administration of a nonsteroidal antiinflammatory drug (NSAID) and local anesthesia significantly decreases peak serum cortisol concentration after castration.
- Local anesthesia alone tends to decrease peak cortisol concentrations more than NSAIDs, whereas NSAIDs alone tend to decrease the area under the cortisol-time curve more than local anesthesia alone.

INTRODUCTION

Castration of male calves destined for beef production is one of the most common livestock management practices performed in the United States amounting to approximately 7 million procedures per year.[1] Methods of castration are typically associated with physical, chemical, or hormonal damage to the testicles.[2] In most production settings, physical castration methods are the most common. These can be subdivided into procedures involving surgical removal of the testes, or methods that irreparably

Dr Coetzee is supported by Agriculture and Food Research Initiative Competitive Grants #2008-35204-19238 and #2009-65120-05729 from the USDA National Institute of Food and Agriculture.

Conflict of Interest Statement: Dr Coetzee has been a consultant for Intervet-Schering Plough Animal Health, Norbrook Laboratories Ltd, and Boehringer Ingelheim Vetmedica.

Portions of this review previously appeared in Coetzee JF. A review of pain assessment techniques and pharmacological approaches to pain relief after bovine castration in the United States. (2011) Invited Review. Applied Animal Behavioral Science 135(4);192–213. Used with permission.

Department of Veterinary Diagnostic and Production Animal Medicine, College of Veterinary Medicine, Iowa State University, 1600 S. 16th Street, Ames, IA 50011, USA

E-mail address: hcoetzee@iastate.edu

damage the testicles by interruption of the blood supply using a castration clamp (bur-dizzo castration), a rubber ring, or a latex band.[3]

The benefits of castration include a reduction in aggression and mounting behavior of males resulting in fewer injuries in confinement operations and reduced dark-cutting beef.[4] Steers also have higher meat quality with increased tenderness and marbling. Carcasses from steers therefore command higher prices at market compared with bulls.[3] Castration also prevents physically or genetically inferior males from reproducing and prevents pregnancy in commingled pubescent groups.[2] Although the benefits of castration are widely accepted in most countries, all castration methods have been demonstrated to produce physiologic, neuroendocrine, and behavioral changes indicating pain and distress.[2,5–10]

Societal concern about the moral and ethical treatment of animals is becoming more prevalent.[11] In particular, negative public perception of pain associated with castration procedures is mounting, with increasing calls for the development of practices to relieve pain and suffering in livestock.[12] Preemptive analgesia can be applied in advance of the painful stimulus thereby reducing sensitization of the nervous system to subsequent stimuli that could amplify pain. Agents that could be used to provide preemptive analgesia include local anesthetics, nonsteroidal antiinflammatory drugs (NSAIDs), opioids, α2-agonists, and N-methyl-D-aspartate receptor antagonists.[13] The American Veterinary Medical Association "supports the use of procedures that reduce or eliminate the pain of dehorning and castrating of cattle" and proposes that "available methods of minimizing pain and stress include application of local anesthesia and the administration of analgesics." Despite this, a recent survey of bovine veterinarians conducted by our research group found that only 1 in 5 survey respondents use anesthesia or analgesics at the time of castration.[14] Furthermore, 90% of respondents indicated that they castrate and dehorn cattle at the same time although there are few studies examining the effect of this on the animal in the literature.

It is remarkable that although administration of local anesthesia before castration and dehorning is legislated in several European countries,[15] there are currently no analgesic drugs specifically approved for pain relief in livestock by the US Food and Drug Administration (FDA).[16] FDA Guidance Document 123 for the development of effectiveness data for NSAIDs states that "validated methods of pain assessment must be used in order for a drug to be indicated for pain relief in the target species."[17] The identification and validation of robust, repeatable pain measurements is therefore fundamental for the development and approval of effective analgesic drug regimens for use in livestock.

The development of robust biomarkers for the objective measurement of pain is necessary for evaluating the efficacy of analgesic treatment regimens during routine animal husbandry procedures such as castration and dehorning. This process is especially complex in a prey species, such as cattle, that inherently conceal pain.[18] Pain is defined as "an aversive feeling or sensation associated with actual or potential tissue damage resulting in physiologic, neuroendocrine, and behavioral changes that indicate a stress response."[19] In previous research, markers for the evaluation of pain and distress associated with noxious animal husbandry procedures have focused on assessing behavioral, physiologic, and neuroendocrine changes. A change in animal behavior has been assessed using visual pen scoring,[20] videography,[9] vocalization,[9,21] measurement of chute exit speed,[22–24] pedometers,[9] and accelerometers.[25] Physiologic changes have been assessed using serum cortisol measurement,[2] heart rate determination,[26] feed intake, and average daily gain (ADG).[27,28] Neuroendocrine changes have been assessed through measurement of the neuropeptide substance

P[21], infrared thermography,[29,30] heart rate variability (HRV),[29–31] skin electrical imped-ance (electrodermal activity),[24,32] and electroencephalography (EEG).[33,34] Several of these tools have also been used to assess the efficacy of analgesic compounds.

This review discusses the options for providing analgesia to calves before castration and the tools that have been used to assess analgesic drug efficacy. Published evidence to support the effect of analgesic compounds on physiologic, neuroendo-crine, and behavioral changes associated with castration is also reviewed. Publica-tions were identified on PubMed using the search terms "Castration" and "Bovine" and "Analgesia." Studies that compared pain biomarkers in castrated control calves with calves treated with an analgesic before castration were used to determine a percent change associated with drug treatment (**Tables 1** and **2**).

ASSESSMENT TOOLS USED TO DETERMINE THE EFFICACY OF ANALGESIC DRUGS IN CATTLE AFTER CASTRATION
Assessment of Behavioral Changes After Castration

Assessment tools that have been used to quantify changes in animal behavior following castration include visual scoring systems,[26] videography,[9,10] vocalization,[9] chute behavior,[9] pedometers,[9] and accelerometers.[25]

The literature on behavioral responses associated with castration has been summarized in a review by Stafford and Mellor.[2] The investigators concluded that assessments of individual animal behavioral changes in response to pain are highly subjective. Escape behaviors demonstrated at castration but not seen afterward may reflect a pain response[35] or a desire to escape confinement.[36] Fell and colleagues[36] reported that surgically castrated calves struggle and kick during the procedure but calves castrated with rubber rings are quieter. Macauley and colleagues[37] found that calves castrated surgically were less active than control calves or calves castrated using a burdizzo. Robertson and colleagues[38] found that rubber ring, burdizzo, and surgical castration caused significant behavioral responses indicating pain during the first 3 hours after castration. Fisher and colleagues[39] found that 14-month-old bulls castrated surgically stamped their hind feet, swished their tails, and grazed less after castration than control bulls and bulls castrated using bands. Behaviors indicating a painful sensation such as turning the head toward the hindquarters, alternate lifting of the hind legs, abnormal postures, and slow movement of the tail have been reported weeks after rubber ring castration.[40]

Currah and colleagues[9] and González and colleagues[10] used videography to deter-mine the stride length of calves before and after surgical and band castration, respec-tively. Both studies reported that stride length was significantly shortened after castration. Furthermore, Currah and colleagues[9] concluded that calves took signifi-cantly fewer steps after surgical castration in a study that used pedometers to compare step count before and after the procedure. In the same study, only 10 of 71 calves (14%) vocalized during castration and no difference in chute behavior assessed using load cells was reported. White and colleagues[25] used accelerometers to evaluate standing and laying behavior in calves before and after surgical castration. The study concluded that calves spent significantly more time standing after castration.

Assessment of Physiologic Changes After Castration

Physiologic changes after castration have been assessed using serum cortisol, heart rate, feed intake, and ADG measurements.

Table 1
Summary of the scientific literature examining the effect of analgesic drug administration on plasma cortisol response in castrated calves

References	Procedure	Study Population	Analgesic Regimen	Outcome Parameter	Percent Change in Cortisol (%)	Significance (P Value)
Faulkner et al,[63] 1992	Surgical Castration	6–9 mo beef	Xylazine 0.02 mg/kg and butorphanol 0.07 mg/kg IV 90 s before castration	Cortisol (day 3)	−10.03	NS
Fisher et al,[5] 1996	Burdizzo clamp castration	5.5 mo dairy	Lidocaine local anesthesia, 8 mL/testicle, 15 min before castration	Cortisol (Cmax)	−15.61	NS
				Cortisol AUEC	−13.15	NS
	Surgical castration		Lidocaine local anesthesia, 8 mL/testicle, 15 min before castration	Cortisol (Cmax)	−23.04	<0.05
				Cortisol AUEC	−21.97	<0.05
Earley and Crowe,[42] 2002	Surgical castration	5.5 mo dairy	Ketoprofen 3 mg/kg IV, 20 min before castration	Cortisol (Cmax)	−46.07	<0.05
				Cortisol AUEC	−55.65	<0.05
			Lidocaine local anesthesia, 6 mL/testicle, 20 min before castration	Cortisol (Cmax)	−51.75	<0.05
				Cortisol AUEC	−25.72	NS
			Ketoprofen 3 mg/kg IV and lidocaine local anesthesia, 6 mL/testicle administered 20 min before castration	Cortisol (Cmax)	−37.12	<0.05
				Cortisol AUEC	−33.22	<0.05
Stafford et al,[43] 2002	Rubber ring castration	2–4 mo dairy	Lidocaine local anesthesia, 3 mL/testicle, 20 min before castration	Cortisol (Cmax)	−68.42	<0.05
			Ketoprofen 3 mg/kg IV and lidocaine local anesthesia, 3 mL/testicle administered 20 min before castration	Cortisol (Cmax)	−55.26	<0.05
	Band castration		Lidocaine local anesthesia, 3 mL/testicle, 20 min before castration	Cortisol (Cmax)	−72.28	<0.05
			Ketoprofen 3 mg/kg IV and lidocaine local anesthesia, 3 mL/testicle administered 20 min before castration	Cortisol (Cmax)	−74.26	<0.05

Study	Age/Type	Treatment	Measure	Value	P
Stafford et al,[43] 2002					
Surgical castration (pull)	2–4 mo dairy	Lidocaine, 3 mL/testicle, 20 min before castration	Cortisol (Cmax)	−2.94	NS
		Ketoprofen 3 mg/kg IV and lidocaine local anesthesia, 3 mL/testicle administered 20 min before castration	Cortisol (Cmax)	−55.88	<0.05
Surgical castration (cut)		Lidocaine, 3 mL/testicle, 20 min before castration	Cortisol (Cmax)	52.73	<0.05
		Ketoprofen 3 mg/kg IV and lidocaine local anesthesia, 3 mL/testicle administered 20 min before castration	Cortisol (Cmax)	−43.64	<0.05
Burdizzo clamp castration		Lidocaine local anesthesia, 3 mL/testicle, 20 min before castration	Cortisol (Cmax)	−17.19	NS
		Ketoprofen 3 mg/kg IV and lidocaine local anesthesia, 3 mL/testicle administered 20 min before castration	Cortisol (Cmax)	−67.19	<0.05
Ting et al,[59] 2003 Burdizzo clamp castration	13 mo dairy	Ketoprofen 3 mg/kg IV, 20 min before castration	Cortisol (Cmax)	−33.76	<0.001
			Cortisol AUEC	−52.47	<0.001
		Lidocaine, 8 mL/testicle, 20 min before castration	Cortisol (Cmax)	−34.55	<0.001
			Cortisol AUEC	1.14	NS
		Xylazine 0.05 mg/kg and lidocaine 0.4 mg/kg Epidural, 10 min before castration	Cortisol (Cmax)	−24.65	<0.001
			Cortisol AUEC	14.07	NS
Ting et al,[60] 2003 Surgical castration	11 mo dairy	Ketoprofen 3 mg/kg IV, 20 min before castration	Cortisol (Cmax)	11.82	NS
			Cortisol AUEC	−41.67	<0.05
		Ketoprofen 1.5 mg/kg IV twice; 20 min before castration and repeated at castration	Cortisol (Cmax)	−2.95	NS
			Cortisol AUEC	−42.59	<0.05
		Ketoprofen 1.5 mg/kg IV, 20 min before castration, repeated at castration and 3 mg/kg at 24 h after castration	Cortisol (Cmax)	0.00	NS
			Cortisol AUEC	−26.54	<0.05

(continued on next page)

Table 1
(continued)

References	Procedure	Study Population	Analgesic Regimen	Outcome Parameter	Percent Change in Cortisol (%)	Significance (P Value)
Pang et al,[6] 2006	Band castration	5.5 mo dairy	Carprofen 1.4 mg/kg IV, 20 min before castration	Cortisol (Cmax)	−18.74	NS
				Cortisol AUEC	−22.99	NS
	Burdizzo clamp castration		Carprofen 1.4 mg/kg IV, 20 min before castration	Cortisol (Cmax)	−4.07	NS
				Cortisol AUEC	−25.85	NS
Coetzee et al,[45] 2007	Surgical castration, Henderson castration tool	4–6 mo beef	Sodium salicylate 50 mg/kg IV <30 s before castration	Cortisol (Cmax)	−11.44	NS
				Cortisol AUEC	−6.33	NS
			Acetylsalicylic acid 100 mg/kg by mouth <30 s before castration	Cortisol (Cmax)	23.29	NS
				Cortisol AUEC	17.72	NS
Thüer,[66] 2007	Burdizzo clamp castration	<1 mo dairy	Lidocaine, 10 mL local anesthesia 5 min before castration	Cortisol (Cmax) estimated	−35.38	P = .014
	Band castration		Lidocaine, 10 mL local anesthesia 5 min before castration	Cortisol (Cmax) estimated	−25.00	NS
Stilwell,[8] 2008	Burdizzo clamp castration	6 mo old dairy	Lidocaine, 4 mL	Cortisol (6 h)	−41.38	NS
			Epidural administered 5 min before castration	Cortisol (24 h)	−22.41	NS
				Cortisol (48 h)	45.76	NS
			Flunixin meglumine 2.2 mg/kg SC and lidocaine, 4 mL	Cortisol (6 h)	−51.90	<0.05
				Cortisol (24 h)	−30.69	NS
			Epidural administered 5 min before castration	Cortisol (48 h)	30.37	NS
			Carprofen 1.4 mg/kg SC and lidocaine, 4 mL	Cortisol (6 h)	−58.89	<0.05
			Epidural administered 5 min before castration	Cortisol (24 h)	−47.52	<0.05
				Cortisol (48 h)	−36.48	<0.05
Boesch et al,[56] 2008	Burdizzo clamp castration	1 wk dairy	Lidocaine, 10 mL local anesthesia 20 min before castration	Cortisol (Cmax) estimated	−35.00	P = .061
			Bupivacaine, 10 mL local anesthesia 20 min before castration	Cortisol (Cmax) estimated	−29.17	NS

Study	Castration type	Age/breed	Treatment	Measure	Value	P
Gonzalez et al,[10] 2010	Band castration	210 d beef	Xylazine 0.07 mg/kg epidural and IV flunixin meglumine at 1.1 mg/kg	Salivary cortisol (4 h)	−59.84	0.03
				Salivary cortisol (24 h)	−26.04	0.31
				Salivary cortisol (14 d)	0.00	0.77
Coetzee et al,[14,65] 2010	Surgical castration, Henderson castration tool	4–6 mo beef	Xylazine 0.05 mg/kg IV <30 s before castration	Cortisol (Cmax)	−8.21	NS
				Cortisol AUEC	28.70	NS
			0.05 mg/kg xylazine and 0.1 mg/kg ketamine IV <30 s before castration	Cortisol (Cmax)	−8.69	NS
				Cortisol AUEC	22.50	NS
Stewart et al,[30] 2010	Surgical castration	4 mo dairy	Lidocaine, 5 mL into the scrotum followed by 7 mL at the neck of the scrotum	Cortisol (Cmax)	−39.67	P<.05
Webster et al,[61] 2010	Surgical castration, Henderson castration tool	2–3 mo dairy	Flunixin meglumine, 1.1 mg/kg IV, 20 min before castration	Cortisol (Cmax)	−26.37	NS
				Cortisol AUEC	−33.55	NS
			2% Lidocaine ring block (20 mL) and intratesticular (5 mL/testes), 20 min before castration	Cortisol (Cmax)	−10.56	NS
				Cortisol AUEC	−21.94	NS
			2% Lidocaine ring block (20 mL) and intratesticular (5 mL/testes) and flunixin meglumine 1.1 mg/kg IV, 20 min before castration	Cortisol (Cmax)	−48.16	NS
				Cortisol AUEC	−48.26	NS
Baldridge et al,[24] 2010	Surgical castration followed by surgical dehorning (Barnes)	2–4 mo dairy	Sodium salicylate at 2.5–5 mg/mL in the drinking water (13.62–151.99 mg of salicylate/kg bodyweight)	Cortisol (Cmax)	1.60	NS
				Cortisol AUEC (0–1 h)	−9.27	NS
				Cortisol AUEC (1–6 h)	−36.90	P<.05
				Cortisol AUEC (6–24 h)	−22.83	NS

(continued on next page)

Table 1
(continued)

References	Procedure	Study Population	Analgesic Regimen	Outcome Parameter	Percent Change in Cortisol (%)	Significance (P Value)
			0.025 mg/kg butorphanol, 0.05 mg/kg xylazine, 0.1 mg/kg ketamine coadministered IM immediately before castration	Cortisol (Cmax)	−12.00	NS
				Cortisol AUEC (0–1 h)	−28.90	P<.05
				Cortisol AUEC (1–6 h)	−5.82	NS
				Cortisol AUEC (6–24 h)	−0.01	NS
			Sodium salicylate at 2.5–5 mg/mL in the drinking water (13.62–151.99 mg of salicylate/kg bodyweight) and 0.025 mg/kg butorphanol, 0.05 mg/kg xylazine, 0.1 mg/kg ketamine coadministered IM immediately before castration	Cortisol (Cmax)	−3.46	NS
				Cortisol AUEC (0–1 h)	−20.89	NS
				Cortisol AUEC (1–6 h)	−24.19	NS
				Cortisol AUEC (6–24 h)	−15.69	NS

Percent change in cortisol was calculated using the formula [(Mean of analgesic group/Mean of castrated control group) − 1] × 100.
Abbreviations: AUEC, area under the effect curve for cortisol; Cmax, maximum plasma concentration; IM, intramuscularly; IV, intravenously; SC, subcutaneously.

Table 2
Summary of scientific literature examining the effect of analgesic drug administration on other outcomes in castrated calves

References	Procedure	Study Population	Analgesic Regimen	Outcome Parameter	Percent Change (%)	Significance (P Value)
Faulkner et al,[63] 1992	Surgical castration	6–9 mo beef	Xylazine 0.02 mg/kg and butorphanol 0.07 mg/kg IV 90 s before castration	ADG (day 0–27)	−11.11	NS
				Feed intake (day 0–27)	−5.00	NS
				Gain/feed	−11.11	NS
				Morbidity (day 0–27)	−4.17	NS
				Mortality (day 0–27)	0.00	NS
Fisher et al,[5] 1996	Burdizzo clamp castration	5.5 mo dairy	Lidocaine local anesthesia, 8 mL/testicle, 15 min before castration	Feed intake (day 1–20)	0.49	NS
				ADG (day 0–35)	−1.15	NS
	Surgical castration		Lidocaine local anesthesia, 8 mL/testicle, 15 min before castration	Feed intake (kg) (day 1–20)	0.96	NS
				ADG (day 0–35)	32.79	$P<.05$
Earley and Crowe,[42] 2002	Surgical castration	5.5 mo dairy	Ketoprofen 3 mg/kg IV, 20 min before castration	Fibrinogen (day 35)	−8.43	$P<.05$
				Haptoglobin (day 35)	50.00	NS
				Feed intake (day 1–35)	−4.64	NS
				ADG (day 0–35)	71.43	NS
			Lidocaine local anesthesia, 6 mL/testicle, 20 min before castration	Fibrinogen (day 35)	−13.79	$P<.05$
				Haptoglobin (day 35)	50.00	NS
				Feed intake (day 1–35)	−2.79	NS
				ADG (day 0–35)	17.86	NS
			Ketoprofen 3 mg/kg IV and lidocaine local anesthesia, 6 mL/testicle administered 20 min before castration	Fibrinogen (day 35)	−28.93	$P<.05$
				Haptoglobin (day 35)	0.00	NS
				Feed intake (day 1–35)	−2.48	NS
				ADG (day 0–35)	96.43	$P<.05$
Ting et al,[59] 2003	Burdizzo clamp castration	13 mo dairy	Ketoprofen 3 mg/kg IV, 20 min before castration	Feed intake (day −1 to 33)	4.66	NS
				ADG (day −1 to 35)	46.51	NS
			Lidocaine, 8 mL/testicle, 20 min before castration	Feed intake (day −1 to 33)	−0.26	NS
				ADG (day −1 to 35)	0.00	NS
			Xylazine 0.05 mg/kg and lidocaine 0.4 mg/kg Epidural, 10 min before castration	Feed intake (day −1 to 33)	−0.26	NS
				ADG (day −1 to 35)	20.93	NS

(continued on next page)

Table 2
(continued)

References	Procedure	Study Population	Analgesic Regimen	Outcome Parameter	Percent Change (%)	Significance (P Value)
Ting et al,[60] 2003	Surgical castration	11 mo dairy	Ketoprofen 3 mg/kg IV, 20 min before castration	Feed intake (day −1 to 33)	−0.82	NS
				ADG (day −1 to 35)	7.69	NS
			Ketoprofen 1.5 mg/kg IV twice; 20 min before castration and repeated at castration	Feed intake (day −1 to 33)	6.28	NS
				ADG (day −1 to 35)	−9.23	NS
			Ketoprofen 1.5 mg/kg IV, 20 min before castration, repeated at castration and 3 mg/kg at 24 h after castration	Feed intake (day −1 to 33)	2.73	NS
				ADG (day −1 to 35)	−18.46	NS
Pang et al,[6] 2006	Band castration	5.5 mo dairy	Carprofen 1.4 mg/kg IV, 20 min before castration	Fibrinogen (day 35)	−19.25	NS
				Haptoglobin (day 35)	−76.19	P<.05
				Rectal temperature	0.00	NS
	Burdizzo clamp castration		Carprofen 1.4 mg/kg IV, 20 min before castration	Fibrinogen (day 35)	−2.13	NS
				Haptoglobin (day 35)	0.00	NS
				Rectal temperature	0.26	NS
Gonzalez et al,[10] 2010	Band castration	210 d beef	Xylazine 0.07 mg/kg epidural and IV flunixin meglumine at 1.1 mg/kg	ADG (day 0–42)	0.00	0.21
				Feed intake (day 0–42)	−1.54	0.02
				Fecal *Escherichia coli*, log (cfu)	−10.16	0.9
				Lying time, %	29.65	0.1
				Step length (back)	−3.83	0.04
				Step length (front)	−1.03	0.38
Stewart et al,[30] 2010	Surgical castration	4 mo dairy	Lidocaine, 5 mL into the scrotum followed by 7 mL at the neck of the scrotum	Heart rate (0–2 min)	−58.82	<0.05
				Eye temperature (5–20 min after castration)	−40.43	<0.05
				HRV: LF power	−7.34	NS
				HRV: HF power	−7.34	NS
				HRV: LF/HF ratio	−76.19	NS

Study	Procedure	Animal	Treatment	Outcome	Value	P value
Baldridge et al,[24] 2010	Surgical castration followed by surgical dehorning (Barnes)	2–4 mo dairy	Sodium salicylate at 2.5–5 mg/mL in the drinking water (13.62–151.99 mg of salicylate/kg bodyweight)	ADG (day 0–13)	1111.22	<0.05
				Chute exit speed	−0.97	NS
			0.025 mg/kg butorphanol, 0.05 mg/kg xylazine, 0.1 mg/kg ketamine coadministered IM immediately before castration	ADG (day 0–13)	729.98	NS
				Chute exit speed	77.81	<0.05
			Sodium salicylate at 2.5–5 mg/mL in the drinking water (13.62–151.99 mg of salicylate/kg bodyweight) and 0.025 mg/kg butorphanol, 0.05 mg/kg xylazine, 0.1 mg/kg ketamine coadministered IM immediately before castration	ADG (day 0–13)	1095.92	<0.05
				Chute exit speed	94.97	<0.05
Coetzee et al,[62] 2011	Surgical castration	8–10 mo (193–285 kg) beef	Meloxicam tablets at 1 mg/kg suspended in 50 mL of water in a dosing syringe and administered orally, 24 h before castration	ADG (day 1–14)	21.79	NS
				DMI (day 1–14)	2.13	NS
				G/F ratio (day 1–14)	18.75	NS
				ADG (day 15–28)	−2.6	NS
				DMI (day 15–28)	0.86	NS
				G/F ratio (15–28 d)	−4.55	NS
				Pull rate (%)	−42.92	<0.05
				Bovine respiratory disease treatment rate (%)	−49.11	<0.05

Percent change in cortisol was calculated using the formula [(Mean of analgesic group/Mean of castrated control group) − 1] × 100.

Abbreviations: ADG, average daily gain in body weight; cfu, colony forming units; DMI, Dry Matter Intake; G/F, Gain to Feed Ratio; HF, high frequency; HRV, heart rate variability; LF, low frequency.

Several studies have evaluated acute cortisol response as a method of determining the extent and duration of distress associated with castration in cattle.[19,40–43] Studies reviewed by Stafford and Mellor[2] indicate that surgical and latex band castrations, especially when performed in older cattle, seem to elicit higher plasma cortisol responses that remain higher than pretreatment levels for longer. The peak cortisol concentration after surgical castration occurs within the first 30 minutes after castration and ranges from 45 nmol/L after rubber ring castration to 129 nmol/L after surgical castration. The duration of plasma cortisol response higher than pretreatment levels typically ranges from 60 minutes after burdizzo castration to 180 minutes after surgical castration.

Cortisol has been widely used as a measurement of distress because its response magnitude, as indicated by peak height, response duration, and/or integrated response usually accords with the predicted noxiousness of different procedures.[35,44] At each end of the cortisol response range, however, interpretation is less straightforward. At the lower end, for example, studies have shown that tail docking with a ring and tail docking with a docking iron cause similar cortisol responses to control handling in older lambs.[19] At the upper end of the range, there are several examples in which cortisol responses do not increase proportionally to the severity of different treatments as might be expected. There may be a ceiling effect on plasma cortisol responses.[19,45] Other studies have shown that plasma cortisol concentration after surgical castrations varies greatly between animals.[43] Based on these data, it has been hypothesized that low responses may be due to individuals having a high pain threshold.[2] Variations may also come about because of differences in the way in which a particular castration method is performed by different operators. These data suggest that plasma cortisol levels may not always accurately reflect the extent of the pain response in animals.

Schwartzkopf-Genswein and colleagues[26] evaluated the heart rate in 15 calves before and after surgical castration. Heart rates were significantly lower at 15 and 30 minutes after castration compared with precastration rates. However, there was a significant increase in heart rate at 120 minutes after castration. The investigators concluded that castration had little effect on heart rate. However, these results may have been confounded because calves had been dehorned 21 days previously and the overall heart rates were higher before and after castration than they were in the period before the dehorning.

Production parameters are often too imprecise to reflect the pain experienced by animals after castration.[2] Furthermore, weight gain after castration may be negatively influenced by a decrease in testosterone after removal of the testes.[46] However, assessment of production parameters is critical if research on animal well-being is to have relevance to livestock producers. In studies reviewed by Stafford and Mellor,[2,46,47] burdizzo or surgical castration was found to have no effect on ADG over a 3-month period after castration. However, the ADG of 7-week-old calves during the 5 weeks after castration using rubber rings, a clamp, or surgery was found to be lower than noncastrated calves but similar between the different castration methods.[46] Rubber ring and surgical castration were reported to cause a decrease in ADG of 50% and 70%, respectively, in cattle aged 8 to 9 months.[48] When 8-, 9-, and 14-month-old cattle were castrated surgically or using latex bands, cattle castrated later had poorer growth rates than those castrated at weaning. Cattle castrated with latex bands also had lower growth rates than those castrated surgically during the following 4 to 8 weeks.[39,47]

In a study conducted by Oklahoma State University, 162 bull calves were used to determine the effects of latex banding of the scrotum or surgical castration on growth rate. Bulls that were banded at weaning gained less weight than bulls that were banded or surgically castrated at 2 to 3 months of age.[27] In a second study, 368 bull calves were used in 2 separate experiments to examine the effect of the method of castration on health and performance. In the first experiment, latex banding of intact males shortly after arrival was found to decrease daily gain by 19% compared with purchasing steers, and by 14.9% compared with surgically castrating intact males shortly after arrival. In the second experiment, purchased castrated males gained 0.26 kg (0.58 lb) more and consumed 0.57 kg (1.26 lb) more feed per day than intact males surgically castrated shortly after arrival.[28]

Assessment of Neuroendocrine Changes After Castration

Neuroendocrine changes have been assessed through measurement of the neuropeptide substance P,[21] infrared thermography,[29,30] HRV,[29–31] electrodermal activity,[24,32] and EEG.[33,34]

Substance P is an 11-amino acid prototypic neuropeptide that regulates the excitability of dorsal horn nociceptive neurons and is present in areas of the neuroaxis involved in the integration of pain, stress, and anxiety. One study found that plasma substance P concentrations are up to 27-fold greater in human patients with soft tissue injury than healthy controls.[49] In a recent study to evaluate plasma substance P and cortisol response after castration, no significant difference in plasma cortisol response between castrated and uncastrated calves was observed over time ($P =$ .644).[21] In contrast, mean plasma substance P concentrations were significantly higher in castrated calves compared with uncastrated controls over the course of the study ($P = .042$). Significant increases in plasma substance P concentration after castration suggest that this measurement may be associated with nociception although further investigation is necessary.

Infrared thermography evaluates changes in surface temperature.[29] Epinephrine release associated with castration causes changes in sympathetic tone. The adrenergic effects on cutaneous blood flow cause changes in skin temperature that can be quantified with a thermography camera (**Fig. 1**). A decrease in eye temperature observed after castration of calves without local anesthetic has been attributed to sympathetically mediated alterations in blood flow in capillary beds.[30]

HRV measurement assesses the variation in the intervals separating consecutive heart beats.[31] HRV is used to investigate the functioning of the autonomic nervous system, especially the balance between sympathetic and vagal activity.[31] It has been hypothesized that HRV measurement provides a more detailed measure of a stress response than heart rate alone.[29] This is because HRV makes it possible to measure the balance between sympathetic and parasympathetic tone, therefore

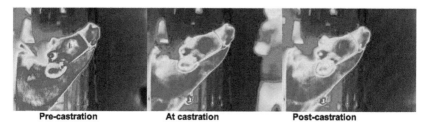

| Pre-castration | At castration | Post-castration |

Fig. 1. Time sequence thermography images taken before castration, at the time of castration, and immediately after castration in a Holstein calf. Color changes likely indicate changes in peripheral perfusion associated with catecholamine release following castration.

providing a more detailed interpretation of autonomic activity.[31] HRV data are analyzed using frequency domain measures including high-frequency (HF) power (0.30–0.80 Hz), low-frequency (LF) power (0.04–0.30 Hz), and the LF/HF ratio. These outcomes are calculated by fast Fourier transformation.[29,30]

Recently, Stewart and colleagues[30] observed a significant increase in HF power from baseline in calves castrated surgically without local anesthesia. In contrast, a significant decrease in LF power compared with baseline was observed in calves castrated surgically with local anesthesia. The investigators concluded that an increase in HF power indicates an increase in parasympathetic activity that may be associated with deep visceral pain, as might occur when the spermatic cords are torn.

Electrodermal activity (EDA) is the electrical resistance between 2 electrodes applied to the skin.[50] EDA can be influenced by changes in resistance as a result of changes in sympathetic outflow. The Pain Gauge (Public Health Information Systems, Inc, Dublin, OH) is purported to be capable of measuring EDA although there is a paucity of data to support this use in livestock species. A study that used the Pain Gauge in rats found it ineffective for accurately assessing postoperative pain because pain scores did not decrease with increasing dosages of analgesic regimens.[51] Similar results were reported by Kotschwar and colleagues[32] in calves subjected to an amphotericin B lameness model. Baldridge and colleagues[24] observed a significant decrease in EDA measurement coinciding with the presence of quantifiable plasma xylazine, ketamine, and butorphanol concentrations. After 90 minutes, EDA increased and was not significantly different from other treatment groups. A difference in EDA between a sham and actual castration and dehorning period both with analgesia was not observed. Therefore, it was concluded that EDA measurement was not a reliable indicator of pain associated with dehorning and castration in calves and that EDA effects were likely associated with other physiologic changes associated with drug exposure.

EEG responses of calves to noxious stimuli associated with scoop dehorning using a minimal anesthesia model have been studied.[33] However, the use of general anesthesia may have confounded these results. Further studies are needed to determine the relevance of this research to understanding pain in conscious calves. Our research group is currently investigating the effect of age and method of castration on EEG response in conscious calves.[34] **Fig. 2** represents the EEG taken from a fully conscious, 12-week-old Holstein calf before and after surgical castration. Before castration, a distinct, low-frequency wave pattern predominates. Immediately after castration, there is a significant shift toward high-frequency, low-amplitude brain activity (beta frequency). The relative power of the low-frequency and high-frequency waves decreased and increased between baseline and castration periods, respectively. This activity is known as desynchronization of waves and is associated with nociception.[33] Delta bands showed a tendency toward an increase during the first recovery period suggesting attempted synchronization within 5 to 10 minutes after castration. The results of this study suggest that EEG may be a sensitive and specific measure of changes in brain electrical activity associated with castration.

ANALGESIC STRATEGIES AND THEIR EFFECTS ON PAIN BIOMARKERS
Local Anesthesia

One technique for providing local anesthesia of the testicles before castration has been previously described by Skarda.[52] Proper restraint and scrotal disinfection are recommended before commencing this procedure. In this approach, the testicle is grasped individually within the scrotum so that the overlying skin is tensed, which

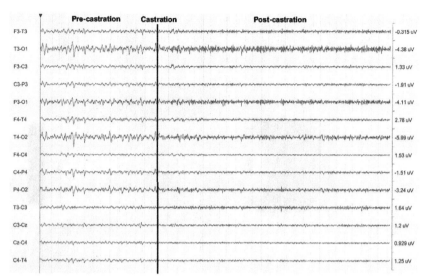

	Pre-castration	Castration	Post-castration	
F3-T3				-0.315 uV
T3-O1				-4.38 uV
F3-C3				1.33 uV
C3-P3				-1.91 uV
P3-O1				-4.11 uV
F4-T4				2.78 uV
T4-O2				-5.99 uV
F4-C4				1.53 uV
C4-P4				-1.51 uV
P4-O2				-3.24 uV
T3-C3				1.64 uV
C3-Cz				1.2 uV
Cz-C4				0.929 uV
C4-T4				1.25 uV

Fig. 2. Example of an EEG trace (30 s duration) illustrating brain electrical activity in a 6-week-old calf at castration. Note the transition in wave activity between the precastration period (calf restrained into the chute), castration (beginning of the procedure), and the postcastration period. There is a shift from a medium high-amplitude slow-frequency wave activity to low-amplitude fast-frequency EEG wave pattern (bipolar montage; time constant = 0.3 s; high-frequency filter = 70 Hz; notch filter inserted, amplitude-integrated EEG 2–30). (*Courtesy of* Dr Luciana Bergamasco, Kansas State University.)

facilitates the infiltration of 3 to 5 mL of 2% lidocaine subcutaneously along the line of incision. In bulls that weigh more than 200 kg, a 16 to 18 gauge needle measuring 3.75 to 7.5 cm is inserted below the tail of the epididymis toward the center of the testicle at an angle approximately 30° from perpendicular and 10 to 15 mL of 2% lidocaine are injected into each testicle (**Fig. 3**). In calves less than 200 kg, a 20 gauge needle measuring 2.5–3.75 cm is used to inject 2 to 10 mL of local anesthetic into the center of the testicle.

A second approach described by Rust and others involves the administration of 10 mL of 2% lidocaine subcutaneously along the circumference of the neck of the scrotum (**Fig. 4**A, B) followed by placement of 5 mL of a 2% lidocaine solution into each spermatic cord (see **Fig. 4**C, D).[53] After administration of lidocaine blocks, the bulls are released and run back through the chute for the treatment procedure after a 10-min waiting period to allow for the local anesthesia to take effect.

An overdose of local anesthesia can occur after accidental intravenous injection resulting in cardiac sodium channels becoming blocked so that conduction and automaticity become adversely depressed.[54] Generally, bupivacaine is considered more cardiotoxic than lidocaine. Aspiration before administration of local anesthetics is recommended to avoid accidental intravascular administration. The toxic dose of lidocaine and bupivacaine in cattle is considered to be 10 mg/kg and 3 to 4 mg/kg, respectively. Signs of overdose include sedation, twitching, convulsions, coma, and death.

Effect of Local Anesthesia on Biomarkers of Pain and Distress in Cattle at Castration

Lidocaine and bupivacaine have been examined as potential local anesthetics for use before bovine castration (see **Table 1**). Lidocaine has a fairly rapid onset of activity

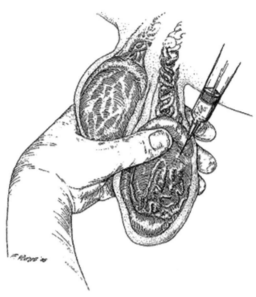

Fig. 3. Placement of an intratesticular local anesthetic injection for testicular block before castration. (*From* Skarda RT. Techniques of local analgesia in ruminants and swine. Vet Clin North Am Food Anim Pract 1986;2:621–63; with permission.)

(2–5 minutes), an intermediate duration of action (90 minutes), and a lower toxicity than bupivacaine.[55] Bupivacaine is the most potent long-acting amide local anesthetic with a slower onset of activity (20–30 minutes) but a longer duration of action (5–8 hours).[55] Boesch and colleagues[56] reported a similar reduction in plasma cortisol concentrations

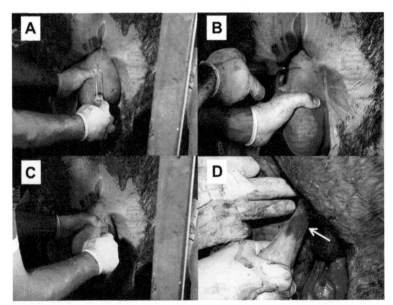

Fig. 4. Administration of 10 mL of 2% lidocaine subcutaneously along the circumference of the neck of the scrotum (*A*, *B*) followed by placement of 5 mL of a 2% lidocaine solution into each spermatic cord (*C*, *D*). (*Courtesy of* Dr Dan Thompson, Kansas State University.)

in 1-week-old dairy calves treated with lidocaine and bupivacaine before burdizzo clamp castration. This result suggests that bupivacaine may not offer significant clinical advantages over lidocaine possibly because of the slower onset of activity.

Surveys report that 10% of New Zealand producers,[57] 43% of British veterinarians,[58] and 22% of US veterinarians[14] administer local anesthetics before castration. A review of the literature identified 8 studies evaluating the effect of local anesthesia on plasma cortisol concentration after surgical and nonsurgical castration (see **Table 1**). The average percent reduction in peak plasma cortisol concentration (Cmax) in calves receiving local anesthesia alone before castration compared with castrated controls was 25.8% (95% confidence interval [CI] 2.46%–49.1%). However, the average area under the effect curve (AUEC) for cortisol was only reduced by 16.3% (95% CI 2.91%– 29.7%) (**Fig. 5**). This result suggests that local anesthetics alone are effective in reducing acute distress associated with castration. However, the overall AUEC is only modestly reduced in calves receiving local anesthesia before castration likely due to the absence of analgesic and antiinflammatory effects extending into the postoperative period.

Several studies have evaluated the effect of local anesthetic administration before castration on feed intake, average daily weight gain, and inflammatory mediators (see **Table 2**). In most cases, the results of these studies have not shown a significant difference in performance between treated and control calves.[5,59,60] Recently, Stewart and colleagues[30] observed significant differences in heart rate and eye temperature in calves castrated with local anesthesia compared with untreated castrated controls. Changes were also observed in HRV, however the extent of this change from baseline levels in the castrated groups was not statistically significant.

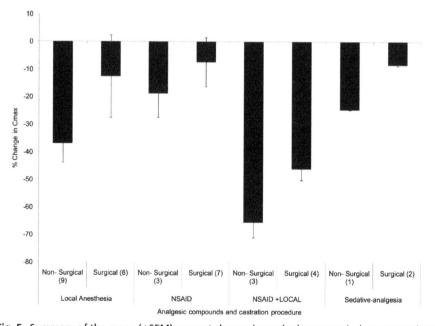

Fig. 5. Summary of the mean (±SEM) percent change in peak plasma cortisol concentrations (Cmax) in calves treated with analgesic compared with untreated castrated control calves in the published literature. The number of treatment groups evaluated is indicated in parentheses. Percent change in cortisol was calculated using the formula [(Mean of analgesic group/Mean of castrated control group) − 1] × 100.

NONSTEROIDAL ANTIINFLAMMATORY DRUGS (NSAIDs)

A review of the literature identified 8 studies evaluating the effect of NSAIDs alone on plasma cortisol concentration after surgical and nonsurgical castration (see **Fig. 5**). The average percent reduction in peak plasma cortisol concentration (Cmax) in calves receiving only an NSAID before castration compared with castrated control calves was 10.8% (95% CI 4.2% increase to 25.9% decrease in cortisol). However, the AUEC for cortisol was reduced by an average of 29% (95% CI 13.2%–44.8% reduction) (**Fig. 6**). This result suggests that NSAIDs alone are not effective in reducing acute distress associated with castration. However, the reduction in overall AUEC was greater in calves receiving an NSAID compared with calves administered only local anesthesia before castration. This result is likely due to the analgesic and antiinflammatory effects of NSAIDs extending into the postoperative period.

Most studies examining the effect of NSAIDs on pain biomarkers after bovine castration have involved administration of the analgesic 20 minutes before the start of the procedure. This procedure was presumably used to ensure adequate analgesic drug concentrations in the tissues at the time of castration. However, this significantly diminishes the external validity of these studies because such a delay is impractical in field situations. Future studies should examine the effect of drug administration at the time of the procedure so that the results are relevant to typical livestock production settings.

Earley and Crowe[42] and Stafford and colleagues[43] demonstrated a significant reduction in peak plasma cortisol concentrations in calves that were administered a combination of local anesthesia and an NSAID before castration compared with calves receiving either drug alone (see **Table 1**). The average percent reduction in peak plasma cortisol

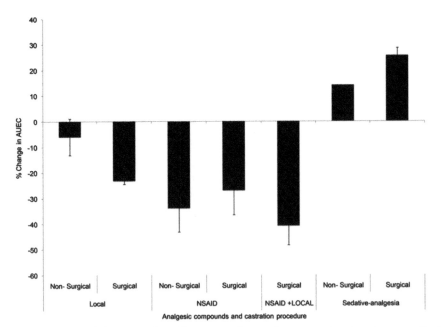

Fig. 6. Summary of the mean (±SEM) percent change in area under the plasma cortisol concentration over time curve (AUEC) in calves treated with analgesic compared with untreated castrated control calves in the published literature. The number of treatment groups evaluated is indicated in parentheses. Percent change in cortisol was calculated using the formula [(Mean of analgesic group/Mean of castrated control group) − 1] × 100.

concentration (Cmax) in calves receiving local anesthesia and an NSAID before castration compared with castrated control calves was 54.5% (95% CI 42.5%–66.53% decrease in cortisol) compared with 25.8% (95% CI 2.46%–49.1%) for local anesthesia alone and 10.8% (95% CI 4.2% increase to 25.9% decrease in cortisol) for NSAID alone (see **Fig. 5**). These results indicate that a multimodal analgesic approach using drugs that act on different receptors in the nociceptive pathway is more effective in mitigating pain associated with castration than a single analgesic agent.

Flunixin Meglumine

Stillwell and colleagues[8] reported that flunixin meglumine (2.2 mg/kg) combined with lidocaine epidural administration 5 minutes before burdizzo clamp castration decreased plasma cortisol concentration at 6 hours after castration by 50% compared with castrated control calves (see **Table 1**). However, at 48 hours after castration, the plasma cortisol concentration was 30% higher in flunixin-treated calves compared with control calves although this difference was not statistically significant. Currah and colleagues[9] observed that beef calves receiving 2.2 mg/kg flunixin meglumine combined with a lidocaine epidural took significantly more steps after surgical castration than castrated control calves. Furthermore, stride length was significantly greater in calves receiving flunixin than untreated calves at 4 and 8 hours after castration; however, at 12 hours there was no difference in the treatment groups.

González and colleagues[10] reported that salivary cortisol concentrations were 60% lower at 4 hours after band castration in calves receiving xylazine epidural and flunixin meglumine (1.1 mg/kg) compared with castrated controls. However, this difference was less evident at 24 hours and 14 days after castration. Stride length and feed intake were also significantly less in flunixin-treated calves compared with castrated controls. Webster and colleagues[61] found that peak plasma cortisol concentrations were 26% lower in calves receiving 2.2 mg/kg flunixin intravenously (IV) at 20 minutes before surgical castration compared with untreated calves. Calves that were administered a combination of lidocaine local anesthesia and flunixin meglumine IV had 48% lower peak plasma cortisol concentrations compared with castrated control calves. Neither of these differences was statistically significant.

Ketoprofen

Single or multiple doses of ketoprofen administered alone or in combination with local anesthesia before castration in cattle have been studied (see **Tables 1** and **2**).[42,59,60] Administration of ketoprofen without local anesthesia before castration reduced plasma cortisol concentrations by an average of 14% (95% CI 16.2% increase to 44.63% decrease in cortisol). However, the combination of local anesthesia and ketoprofen markedly reduced plasma cortisol concentrations by an average of 56% (95% CI 41% to 70% decrease) compared with castrated controls. These studies suggest that ketoprofen is more effective if combined with local anesthesia as part of a multimodal analgesic protocol.

Salicylic Acid Derivatives

A study was conducted to examine the effect of oral aspirin and intravenous sodium salicylate on plasma cortisol response after surgical castration in bulls.[45] Twenty bulls were randomly assigned to 1 of 4 groups (n = 5 bulls per treatment): (1) uncastrated, untreated control group; (2) castrated, untreated group; (3) castrated group receiving 50 mg/kg sodium salicylate IV immediately before castration; and (4) castrated group receiving 50 mg/kg aspirin (acetylsalicylic acid) orally immediately before castration. After castration or simulated castration, blood samples for salicylate and cortisol determination were collected at 3, 10, 20, 30, 40, 50 minutes and 1, 1.5, 2, 4, 6, 8, 10, and 12 hours after castration using a preplaced jugular catheter.

Oral aspirin administered at 50 mg/kg did not achieve quantifiable plasma salicylate concentrations in cattle. Mean plasma cortisol concentrations in this group were also the highest. In contrast, IV sodium salicylate significantly mitigated the mean plasma cortisol response at 30, 50, and 120 minutes after administration ($P<.05$). This effect was negated when plasma salicylate concentrations decreased to less than 20 µg/mL. Plasma sodium salicylate concentration decreased to less than the limit of quantitation by 240 minutes after IV injection. These results demonstrate that oral aspirin administered at 50 mg/kg does not achieve therapeutic concentrations in cattle. Furthermore, a sodium salicylate–mediated decrease in plasma cortisol response occurred in animals treated with IV sodium salicylate immediately before castration. This effect became less evident once plasma salicylate concentrations decreased to less than 20 µg/mL suggesting that this may be the minimum pain inhibitory concentration for salicylate in plasma.

Salicylate is more soluble than aspirin and may offer a convenient and cost-effective means of providing free-choice access to an NSAID in drinking water. Baldridge and colleagues[24] found that calves receiving 2.5 to 5 mg of sodium salicylate/mL of water beginning 72 hours before concurrent surgical castration and dehorning and continuing for 48 hours after surgery had a higher average daily weight gain for 13 days after castration/dehorning than untreated calves. However, water consumption decreased over the course of treatment suggesting that the inclusion of sodium salicylate had a negative effect on water palatability. Calves receiving sodium salicylate also has a significantly lower AUEC for cortisol in the period 1 to 6 hours after castration/dehorning.

Carprofen

Pang and colleagues[6] observed that carprofen administered at 1.4 mg/kg IV, 20 minutes before band castration reduced peak plasma cortisol concentrations by 19% compared with castrated control calves (see **Table 1**). However, this difference was not statistically significant. Carprofen-treated calves demonstrated a significant reduction in plasma haptoglobin concentrations (see **Table 2**). These effects were less in calves castrated with a burdizzo clamp. Stilwell and colleagues[8] reported a 59% reduction in plasma cortisol concentrations at 6 hours and a 36% reduction at 48 hours after burdizzo clamp castration in calves receiving 1.4 mg/kg carprofen combined with a lidocaine epidural compared with castrated controls.

Meloxicam

In a recent study, our group reported that meloxicam administration before castration in post weaning calves reduced the incidence of respiratory disease at the feedlot.[62] These findings have implications for developing NSAID protocols for use in calves at castration with respect to addressing animal health and welfare concerns.

SEDATIVE-ANALGESIC DRUGS
Opioid Analgesics

Faulkner and colleagues[63] investigated the health and performance effects of intravenous butorphanol (0.07 mg/kg) and xylazine (0.02 mg/kg) coadministration to weanling bulls at the time of castration. Coadministration of xylazine and butorphanol resulted in reduced chute activity and clinical sedation characterized by muscle relaxation and occasional (<15%–20%) difficulty in exiting the chute. Cortisol concentrations immediately after castration were not evaluated in this study. However, treated calves were found to have significantly higher cortisol concentrations at 3 days after castration compared with castrated controls. The investigators concluded that butorphanol and xylazine did not reduce stress or improve performance.

α-2 Adrenergic Agonists

Caulkett and others described the used of xylazine hydrochloride as an epidural injection to provide analgesia at the time of castration.[64] Xylazine (0.07 mg/kg) was diluted in 0.9% sodium chloride to a volume of 7.5 mL, which was administered by caudal epidural injection.[61] In this experiment, 30 ± 14 minutes elapsed from the time of injection to castration in the 77 animals on trial. The investigators observed that 97% of animals demonstrated some degree of sedation with 2.6% of animals showing profound depression. In 80.5% of cases, the animal showed no response to surgical stimulation after epidural anesthesia. Only 14.3% of animals showed moderate ataxia after anesthesia; severe ataxia was observed in 2.6% of animals.

The technique for caudal epidural anesthesia has been described elsewhere.[52] Briefly, the location for epidural anesthesia is identified by lowering the tail and palpating the depression and movement between the respective vertebrae (**Fig. 7**). The overlying skin is disinfected and an 18 gauge needle measuring 3.57 to 5 cm is inserted in the center of the C1-C2 joint space while the needle is directed ventrocranially at an angle of 10° to vertical; essentially perpendicular to the general contour of the tail. The needle is inserted until it contacts the floor of the vertebral canal at which time it is withdrawn approximately 0.5 cm to avoid injection into the intervertebral disc. The correct placement of the needle is confirmed by observing a droplet of anesthetic in the hub of the needle being aspirated once the needle punctures the epidural space (the hanging drop technique). In addition, minimal resistance is encountered on the plunger of the syringe during the injection procedure when the needle is located in the epidural space. A dose of 1 mL of 2% lidocaine hydrochloride per 100 kg bodyweight provides local anesthesia of the perineum after 5 to 20 minutes and the effect lasts for 30 to 150 minutes.[52] Complications from caudal epidural anesthesia are rare and are most often associated with infection or injury if the animal becomes recumbent on a slippery surface.[52]

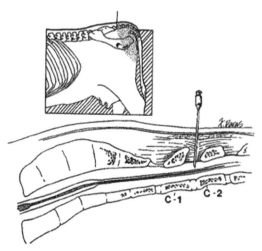

Fig. 7. Needle placement for caudal epidural analgesia in cattle. (*From* Skarda RT. Techniques of local analgesia in ruminants and swine. Vet Clin North Am Food Anim Pract 1986;2:621–63; with permission.)

Ting and colleagues[59] found that peak plasma cortisol concentrations were not significantly attenuated in calves administered a combination of 0.05 mg/kg xylazine and 0.4 mg/kg lidocaine epidural before burdizzo clamp castration. However, the integrated cortisol response (AUEC) was 26.5% less than in untreated calves (P<.05) (see **Table 1**). González and colleagues[10] observed that salivary cortisol concentrations were 60% lower at 4 hours after band castration in calves receiving xylazine epidural and flunixin meglumine (1.1 mg/kg) compared with castrated controls. Coetzee and colleagues[65] found that xylazine alone at 0.05 mg/kg IV or in combination with ketamine at 0.1 mg/kg reduced peak plasma cortisol concentrations by 8% compared with surgically castrated control calves. However, the integrated cortisol response was higher in treated calves compared with untreated controls. These data suggest a rebound in plasma cortisol concentrations once the effect of the drug wears off. Similar findings were reported in calves receiving a combination of xylazine, ketamine, and butorphanol before concurrent dehorning and castration in calves.[24]

N-Methyl-D-Aspartate Receptor Antagonists

Coetzee and colleagues[65] found that ketamine administered at 0.1 mg/kg in combination with xylazine at 0.05 mg/kg IV reduced peak plasma cortisol concentrations by 8% compared with surgically castrated control calves. However, the integrated cortisol response (AUEC) tended to be higher in treated calves compared with untreated controls. In this study, the half-life of xylazine and ketamine after IV administration was approximately 11 minutes. This result suggests that plasma cortisol concentrations likely rebounded in treated calves after the sedative-analgesic effect of the drug diminished. In this study, higher plasma norketamine concentrations were associated with lower plasma substance P concentrations compared with lower norketamine concentrations (**Fig. 8**).

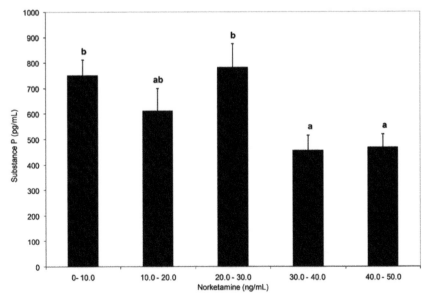

Fig. 8. Comparison between plasma substance P concentrations (pg/mL) and plasma norketamine concentrations (ng/mL) in calves receiving 0.1 mg/kg of ketamine before surgical castration. Columns with different letters are significantly different (P<.05).

SUMMARY

Castration of cattle is considered necessary to reduce aggression, prevent injuries in confinement operations, and to improve meat quality. However, all methods of castration have been shown to produce physiologic, neuroendocrine, and behavioral changes indicating pain and distress. Direct and indirect measurement of these changes using accelerometers, videography, HRV determination, electroencephalography, thermography, and plasma neuropeptide assessment may provide information that would lead to regulatory approval of analgesic drugs in livestock.

Administration of a local anesthetic alone effectively mitigates acute distress associated with castration but the integrated cortisol response is only modestly reduced. NSAID administration alone is not effective in reducing acute distress associated with castration, however the reduction in overall AUEC reported is greater in NSAID-treated calves compared with calves receiving only local anesthesia. The combination of local anesthesia and an NSAID achieved the greatest reduction in cortisol response in published reports, suggesting that a multimodal analgesic approach is more effective in mitigating the pain associated with castration than the use of a single analgesic agent. Lidocaine and flunixin meglumine are the only compounds with analgesic properties that are approved by the FDA for use in cattle. However, flunixin requires IV administration and at least once daily dosing to be effective. In the absence of compounds specifically licensed for pain relief in cattle, extra-label drug use regulations allow for unapproved analgesic drugs to be administered by or under the supervision of a veterinarian provided such use does not result in a violative tissue residue. Accordingly, a combination of local anesthesia with oral administration of a long-acting NSAID such as meloxicam may provide the optimum balance of convenience and analgesic efficacy at the time of castration.

Regulatory concerns combined with unease about the cost and convenience of drug administration at the time of castration is an impediment to the routine adoption of analgesic protocols in production systems. Although administration of multimodal analgesic protocols is associated with a significant decrease in plasma cortisol concentration after castration, most studies have not addressed the practical or production implications of these interventions in a commercial livestock environment, especially in beef cattle. Studies examining the health and performance effects of newer drugs with extended durations of activity are also needed. Regulatory approval of safe, cost-effective, and convenient analgesic compounds will support the implementation of practical pain management strategies as a part of standard industry practice at the time of castration.

ACKNOWLEDGMENTS

The author acknowledges the assistance of Dr Luciana Bergamasco and Mal Hoover in preparing the manuscript for publication.

REFERENCES

1. US Department of Agriculture National Agricultural Statistics Service. Agricultural statistics 2009. Available at: http://usda.mannlib.cornell.edu/usda/current/Catt/Catt-07-24-2009.pdf. Accessed August 19, 2009.
2. Stafford KJ, Mellor DJ. The welfare significance of the castration of cattle: a review. N Z Vet J 2005;53:271–8.

3. American Veterinary Medical Association. Welfare implications of castration of cattle (June 26, 2009). Available at: http://www.avma.org/reference/backgrounders/castration_cattle_bgnd.pdf. Accessed March 18, 2011.

4. Tarrant PV. The occurrence, cause and economic consequences of dark cutting in beef - a survey of current information. In: Hood DE, Tarrant PV, editors. Current topics in veterinary medicine and animal science, vol 10. The Hague (Netherlands): Martinus Nijhoff; 1981. p. 3–35.

5. Fisher AD, Crowe MA, Alonso de la Varga ME, et al. Effect of castration method and the provision of local anaesthesia on plasma cortisol, scrotal circumference, growth and feed intake of bull calves. J Anim Sci 1996;74:2336–43.

6. Pang WY, Earley B, Sweeney T, et al. Effect of carprofen administration during banding or burdizzo castration of bulls on plasma cortisol, in vitro interferon-gamma production, acute-phase proteins, feed intake, and growth. J Anim Sci 2006;84(2):351–9.

7. Pang WY, Earley B, Gath VP, et al. Effect of banding or burdizzo castration on plasma testosterone, acute-phase proteins, scrotal circumference, growth and health of bulls. Livest Sci 2008;117:79–87.

8. Stillwell G, Lima MS, Broom DM. Effects of nonsteroidal anti-inflammatory drugs on long-term pain in calves castrated by use of an external clamping technique following epidural anesthesia. Am J Vet Res 2008;69(6):744–50.

9. Currah JM, Hendrick SH, Stookey JM. The behavioral assessment and alleviation of pain associated with castration in beef calves treated with flunixin meglumine and caudal lidocaine epidural anesthesia with epinephrine. Can Vet J 2009;50(4):375–82.

10. González LA, Schwartzkopf-Genswein KS, Caulkett NA, et al. Pain mitigation after band castration of beef calves and its effects on performance, behavior, Escherichia coli, and salivary cortisol. J Anim Sci 2010;88:802–10.

11. Rollin BE. Annual meeting keynote address: animal agriculture and emerging social ethics for animals. J Anim Sci 2004;82:955–64.

12. Weary DM, Fraser D. Rethinking painful management practices. In: Benson GJ, Rollin BE, Ames IA, editors. The well-being of farm animals: challenges and solutions. 1st edition. Blackwell Publishing; 2004. p. 325–38.

13. Thurmon JC, Tranquilli WJ, Benson GJ. Preanesthetics and anesthetic adjuncts. In: Lumb and Jones veterinary anesthesia. 3rd edition. Baltimore (MD): Lippincott Williams & Wilkins; 1996. p. 183–209.

14. Coetzee JF, Nutsch A, Barbur LA, et al. A survey of castration methods and associated livestock management practices performed by bovine veterinarians in the United States. BMC Vet Res 2010;6:12. http://dx.doi.org/10.1186/1746-6148-6-12.

15. DEFRA. Code of recommendations for the welfare of livestock: cattle. London: DEFRA Publications; 2003. Available at: http://www.defra.gov.uk/foodfarm/farmanimal/welfare/onfarm/documents/cattcode.pdf. Accessed March 18, 2011.

16. Bayley AJ. Compendium of veterinary products. 13th edition. Port Huron (MI): North American Compendiums; 2010.

17. FDA-CVM. US Food and Drug Administration, Center for Veterinary Medicine. Guideline no. 123. Development of target animal safety and effectiveness data to support approval of non-steroidal anti-inflammatory drugs (NSAIDs) for use in animals. Available at: http://www.fda.gov/downloads/AnimalVeterinary/GuidanceComplianceEnforcement/GuidanceforIndustry/UCM052663.pdf. Accessed March 18, 2011.

18. Underwood WJ. Pain and distress in agriculture animals. J Am Vet Med Assoc 2002;221:208–11.

19. Molony V, Kent JE. Assessment of acute pain in farm animals using behavioral and physiological measurements. J Anim Sci 1997;75:266–72.
20. McMeekan CM, Stafford KJ, Mellor DJ, et al. Effects of a local anaesthetic and a non-steroidal anti-inflammatory analgesic on the behavioural responses of calves to dehorning. N Z Vet J 1999;47:92–6.
21. Coetzee JF, Lubbers BL, Toerber SE, et al. Plasma concentrations of substance P and cortisol in beef calves after castration or simulated castration. Am J Vet Res 2008;69(6):751–62.
22. Burrows HM, Dillon RD. Relationships between temperament and growth in a feedlot and commercial carcass traits of Bos indicus crossbreds. Aust J Exp Agr 1997;37:407–11.
23. Fell LR, Colditz IG, Walker KH, et al. Associations between temperament, performance, and immune function in cattle entering a commercial feedlot. Aust J Exp Agr 1999;39:795–802.
24. Baldridge SL, Coetzee JF, Dritz SS, et al. Pharmacokinetics and physiologic effects of xylazine-ketamine-butorphanol administered intramuscularly alone or in combination with orally administered sodium salicylate on biomarkers of pain in Holstein calves following concurrent castration and dehorning. Am J Vet Res 2011;72(10):1305–17.
25. White BJ, Coetzee JF, Renter DG, et al. Evaluation of two-dimensional accelerometers to monitor beef cattle behavior post-castration. Am J Vet Res 2008;69(8): 1005–12.
26. Schwartzkopf-Genswein KS, Booth-McLean ME, McAllister TA, et al. Physiological and behavioural changes in Holstein calves during and after dehorning or castration. Can J Anim Sci 2005;85:131–8.
27. Lents CA, White FJ, Floyd LN, et al. Method and timing of castration influences performance of bull calves. 2001 OSU animal science research report. 2010. Available at: http://www.ansi.okstate.edu/research/2001rr/48/48.htm. Accessed January 5, 2010.
28. Berry BA, Choat WT, Gill DR, et al. Effect of castration on health and performance of newly received stressed feedlot calves. 2001 OSU animal science research report. 2001. Available at: http://www.ansi.okstate.edu/research/research-reports-1/2001/2001%20Berry%20Research%20Report.pdf. Accessed March 18, 2011.
29. Stewart M, Stookey JM, Stafford KJ, et al. Effects of local anesthetic and nonsteroidal anti-inflammatory drug on pain responses of dairy calves to hot-iron dehorning. J Dairy Sci 2009;92(4):1512–9.
30. Stewart M, Verkerk GA, Stafford KJ, et al. Noninvasive assessment of autonomic activity for evaluation of pain in calves, using surgical castration as a model. J Dairy Sci 2010;93:3602–9.
31. von Borell E, Langbein J, Despres G, et al. Heart rate variability as a measure of autonomic regulation of cardiac activity for assessing stress and welfare in farm animals—a review. Physiol Behav 2007;92:293–316.
32. Kotschwar JL, Coetzee JF, Anderson DE, et al. Analgesic efficacy of sodium salicylate in an amphotericin B induced bovine synovitis-arthritis model. J Dairy Sci 2009;92(8):3731–43.
33. Gibson TJ, Johnson CB, Stafford KJ, et al. Validation of the acute electroencephalographic responses of calves to noxious stimulus with scoop dehorning. N Z Vet J 2007;55(4):152–7.
34. Bergamasco L, Coetzee JF, Gehring R, et al. Quantitative electroencephalographic findings associated with nociception following surgical castration in conscious calves. J Vet Pharmacol Ther 2011. http://dx.doi.org/10.1111/j.1365-2885.2011.01269.x.

35. Mellor DJ, Cook CJ, Stafford KJ. Quantifying some responses to pain as a stressor. In: Moberg GP, Mench JA, editors. The biology of animal stress: basic principals and implications for animal welfare. New York: CABI Publishing; 2000. p. 171–98.

36. Fell LR, Wells R, Shutt DA. Stress in calves castrated surgically or by the application of rubber rings. Aust Vet J 1986;63:16–8.

37. Macauley AS, Friend TH, LaBore JM. Behavioral and physiological responses of dairy calves to different methods of castration. J Anim Sci 1986;63:166.

38. Robertson IS, Kent JE, Molony V. Effects of different methods of castration on behavior and plasma cortisol in calves of 3 ages. Res Vet Sci 1994;56:8–17.

39. Fisher AD, Knight TW, Cosgrove GP, et al. Effects of surgical or banding castration on stress responses and behavior of bulls. Aust Vet J 2001;79(4):279–84.

40. Fisher AD, Crowe MA, O'Naullain EM, et al. Effects of cortisol on in vitro interferon-γ production, acute-phase proteins, growth and feed intake in a calf castration model. J Anim Sci 1997;75:1041–7.

41. Chase CC Jr, Larsen RE, Randel RD, et al. Plasma cortisol and white blood cell responses in different breeds of bulls: a comparison of two methods of castration. J Anim Sci 1995;73:975–80.

42. Earley B, Crowe MA. Effects of ketoprofen alone or in combination with local anesthesia during castration of bull calves on plasma cortisol, immunological, and inflammatory responses. J Anim Sci 2002;80:1044–52.

43. Stafford KJ, Mellor DJ, Todd SE, et al. Effects of local anaesthesia or local anaesthesia plus a non-steroidal anti-inflammatory drug on the acute cortisol response of calves to five different methods of castration. Res Vet Sci 2002;73(1):61–70.

44. Broom DM. The evolution of pain. In: Soulsby EJ, Morton D, editors. Pain: its nature and management in man and animals. London: The Royal Society of Medicine Press; 2000. p. 17–25.

45. Coetzee JF, Gehring R, Bettenhausen AC, et al. Mitigation of plasma cortisol response in bulls following intravenous sodium salicylate administration prior to castration. J Vet Pharmacol Ther 2007;30:305–13.

46. King BD, Cohen RD, Guenther CL, et al. The effect of age and method of castration on plasma cortisol in beef calves. Can J Anim Sci 1991;71:257–63.

47. Knight TW, Cosgrove GP, Lambert MG, et al. Effects of method and age at castration on growth rate and meat quality of bulls. New Zeal J Agr Res 1999;42:255–68.

48. ZoBell DR, Goonewardene LA, Ziegler K. Evaluation of the bloodless castration procedure for feedlot bulls. Can J Anim Sci 1993;73:967–70.

49. Onuoha GN, Alpar EK. Calcitonin gene-related peptide and other neuropeptides in the plasma of patients with soft tissue injury. Life Sci 1999;65(13):1351–8.

50. Benford SM, Dannemiller S. Use of electrodermal activity for assessment of pain/stress in laboratory animals. Animal Laboratory News 2004;1:13–23.

51. Richardson CA, Niel L, Leach MC, et al. Evaluation of the efficacy of a novel electronic pain assessment device, the Pain Gauge®, for measuring postoperative pain in rats. Lab Anim 2007;41:46–54.

52. Skarda RT. Techniques of local analgesia in ruminants and swine. Vet Clin North Am Food Anim Pract 1986;2:621–63.

53. Rust R, Thomson D, Loneragan G, et al. Effect of different castration methods on growth performance and behavioral responses of postpubertal beef bulls. Bov Pract 2007;41(2):116–8.

54. Valverde A, Doherty TJ. Anesthesia and analgesia of ruminants. In: Fish R, Danneman PJ, Brown M, et al, editors. Anesthesia and analgesia in laboratory animals. 2nd edition. Oxford (United Kingdom): Elsevier; 2008. p. 401.

55. Webb AI, Pablo LS. Injectable anaesthetic agents. In: Riviere JE, Papich MG, editors. Veterinary pharmacology and therapeutics. 9th edition. Ames (IA): Wiley-Blackwell; 2009. p. 383.

56. Boesch D, Steiner A, Gygax L, et al. Burdizzo castration of calves less than 1-week old with and without local anaesthesia: short-term behavioural responses and plasma cortisol levels. Appl Anim Behav Sci 2008;114(3–4):330–45.

57. Stafford KJ, Mellor DJ, McMeekan CM. A survey of the methods used by farmers to castrate calves in New Zealand. N Z Vet J 2000;48:16–9.

58. Kent JE, Thrusfield MV, Robertson IS, et al. Castration of calves: a study of methods used by farmers in the United Kingdom. Vet Rec 1996;138:384–7.

59. Ting ST, Earley B, Hughes JM, et al. Effect of ketoprofen, lidocaine local anesthesia, and combined xylazine and lidocaine caudal epidural anesthesia during castration of beef cattle on stress responses, immunity, performance and behavior. J Anim Sci 2003;81:1281–93.

60. Ting ST, Earley B, Crowe MA. Effect of repeated ketoprofen administration during surgical castration of bulls on cortisol, immunological function, performance and behavior. J Anim Sci 2003;81:1253–64.

61. Webster, H, Morin, D, Brown, L, et al. Effects of flunixin meglumine and local anesthetic on serum cortisol concentration and performance in dairy calves castrated at 2 to 3 months of age. Proceedings of the 43rd Annual Conference of the American Association of Bovine Practitioners, Albuquerque, August 18–21, 2010.

62. Coetzee JF, Edwards LN, Mosher RA, et al. Effect of oral meloxicam on health and performance of beef steers relative to bulls castrated on arrival at the feedlot. J Anim Sci 2012;90(3):1026–39.

63. Faulkner DB, Eurell T, Tranquilli WJ, et al. Performance and health of weanling bulls after butorphanol and xylazine administration at castration. J Anim Sci 1992;70:2970–4.

64. Caulkett NA, MacDonald DG, Janzen ED, et al. Xylazine hydrochloride epidural analgesia—a method of providing sedation and analgesia to facilitate castration of mature bulls. Compend Contin Educ Pract Vet 1993;15:1155–9.

65. Coetzee JF, Gehring R, Anderson DE, et al. Effect of sub-anaesthetic xylazine and ketamine ("ketamine stun") administered to calves prior to castration. Vet Anaesth Analg 2010;37(6):566–78.

66. Thüer S, Mellema S, Doherr MG, et al. Effect of local anaesthesia on short- and long-term pain induced by two bloodless castration methods in calves. Vet J 2007;173:333–42.

Bovine Dehorning
Assessing Pain and Providing Analgesic Management

Matthew L. Stock, VMD[a,d], Sarah L. Baldridge, DVM, MS[b],
Dee Griffin, DVM, MS[c], Johann F. Coetzee, BVSc, Cert CHP, PhD[a],*

KEYWORDS

- Dehorning • Cattle • Analgesia • Animal welfare

KEY POINTS

- Dehorning causes behavioral, physiologic, and neuroendocrine changes, indicating a stressful or painful response in cattle.
- Following dehorning, an acute painful response is observed within the first 30 minutes followed by a period of suggested inflammatory pain lasting up to 8 hours.
- Local anesthetics provide analgesia for the initial acute pain response; however, a delayed cortisol response is observed, presumably once sensitivity returns to the anesthetized area.
- Acute pain following dehorning is mitigated using local anesthetics, nonsteroidal anti-inflammatory drugs (NSAIDs), and sedatives providing analgesia.
- NSAIDs help to attenuate the inflammatory mediated pain response following dehorning.
- A multimodal approach using local anesthetics, NSAIDs and, when possible, sedative-analgesics, is recommended for the most effective reduction of pain response in cattle following dehorning.

INTRODUCTION

Dehorning is a commonly performed practice in both beef and dairy cattle industries. Dehorning or disbudding in cattle is performed for a variety of reasons, including safety for handling, decreased incidence of carcass wastage due to bruising, requirement of less feeding-trough space, decreased risk of injury to other cattle, increased

Dr Coetzee is supported by Agriculture and Food Research Initiative Competitive Grants #2008-35204-19238 and #2009-65120-05729 from the USDA National Institute of Food and Agriculture.
[a] Department of Biomedical Science, College of Veterinary Medicine, Iowa State University, 2008 Veterinary Medicine, Ames, IA 50011, USA; [b] Department of Clinical Sciences, College of Veterinary Medicine, Kansas State University, A-111 Mosier Hall, Manhattan, KS 66506-5606, USA; [c] Great Plains Veterinary Educational Center, Highway 18 Spur, PO Box 148, Clay Center, Nebraska 68933-0148, USA; [d] Department of Veterinary Diagnostic and Production Animal Medicine, College of Veterinary Medicine, Iowa State University, 2008 Veterinary Medicine, Ames, IA 50011, USA
* Corresponding author. Veterinary Diagnostic and Production Animal Medicine, College of Veterinary Medicine, Iowa State University, Ames, IA 50011.
E-mail address: hcoetzee@iastate.edu

value of the animal, and fewer aggressive behaviors.[1] Disbudding is a method of removing horns in calves up to around 8 weeks old, when horn buds are 5 to 10 mm long and can be removed via a heated disbudding iron.[2] Once horns grow longer, they become attached to the underlying frontal sinus and must be removed by amputation. For the purpose of clarity, throughout this article all disbudding and dehorning is collectively referred to as dehorning.

Although cattle are naturally horned for protective purposes, modern commercial industries decrease the necessity of these defenses. Within these production systems, for reasons listed above, cattle without horns can be more desirable. Horn growth is a genetically heritable autosomal recessive trait.[3] Polled cattle, which are hornless animals, result from an autosomal dominance pattern that has been shown recently to be a result of allelic heterogeneity of the polled locus.[3] Because the polled genetic inheritance reflects that of an autosomal dominant inheritable trait, artificial genetic selection could result in the decline of this undesirable characteristic of intensively raised cattle. This artificial selection for polled cattle has been observed in the beef industry, with a 58% reduction in beef calves born with horns from 1992 to 2007 as a result of breeding for polled animals.[4] However, this breeding selection has not been adopted by the dairy industry, with a reported 94% of dairy operations in the United States dehorning calves.[5]

Management practices have been adopted to dehorn animals to better fit within the production system. There are 3 primary methods of dehorning cattle: (1) amputation using scoop dehorners such as Barnes, Keystone, gauges, saws, and gigli wire; (2) cautery using a hot iron powered electrically, by gas, or battery; and (3) chemical application of caustic paste, usually consisting of a strong alkalotic agent such as sodium hydroxide or calcium hydroxide. Regardless of the dehorning method, following the procedure a behavior change is noted that is consistent with an acute stress response.[6–8] As a result, dehorning cattle can be a welfare issue if concerns of pain are not addressed during dehorning. For a more detailed discussion and review of assessing pain in food animals, refer to the article from Coetzee concerning castration elsewhere in this issue.

Recently, there has been increased social concern and awareness regarding the proper treatment of livestock.[9] Routine procedures in cattle such as dehorning can have a negative public perception. Subsequently, several countries including those belonging to the European Union, Australia, and New Zealand have created dehorning welfare legislation.[2] In North America, The Canadian Code of Practice for Dairy Cattle recommends the use of a local anesthetic combined with analgesia and sedation for dehorning calves; however, there are no current regulations in the United States for the use of analgesics.[10] Although it should be noted that the American Veterinary Medical Association "supports the use of procedures that reduce or eliminate the pain of dehorning and castrating of cattle" and proposes that "available methods of minimizing pain and stress include application of local anesthesia and the administration of analgesics."[11]

Survey evidence in the United States suggests that routine procedures such as dehorning and castration are performed together (92%) and are usually completed without the use of analgesics.[12] A survey of north-central and northeastern United States dairy producers indicated that 12.4% use a local anesthetic nerve block and only 1.8% use systemic analgesia at the time of dehorning.[13] In addition, another survey of United States veterinarians determined that 49% of beef calves and 63% of dairy calves younger than 6 months of age were administered an analgesic at the time of dehorning.[14] A Canadian survey indicated that approximately 72% of veterinarians provided analgesia at the time of dehorning calves.[15] Of note, additional positive influences for providing analgesia to calves at dehorning included geographic locations where significant public outreach for animal welfare has occurred.[15]

The use of analgesics following dehorning such as local anesthesia, systemic anti-inflammatories, and sedatives with analgesic properties has been investigated by several studies using behavioral, physiologic, and neuroendocrine biomarkers for assessment of pain.[16] In general, when using cortisol concentrations as an indicator of stress and pain, evidence exists of a rapid cortisol increase following dehorning that peaks within the first 30 minutes. Cortisol concentrations then plateau from 1 to 6 hours and then decline, returning to baseline 7 to 8 hours following dehorning (**Fig. 1**). Local anesthetics mitigate the cortisol response for their respective duration of action (ie, lidocaine: 2 hours; bupivacaine: 4 hours) following the procedure, but a delayed cortisol response is observed presumably once sensitivity returns to the anesthetized area.[17–19] Anti-inflammatories have aided in the reduction of this delayed cortisol response.[19–22] In addition, the use of sedatives with suggested analgesia can contribute to the reduction of the initial cortisol response, improving procedural success.[23,24] Most studies evaluating stress and pain changes in dehorned cattle investigate the acute response; however, few studies have examined chronic pain or stress responses following dehorning.

Within the United States there exist sufficient challenges to accurately assess and manage pain in food animals. This review assesses tools specifically used in the evaluation of the effectiveness of pain relief following dehorning. In addition, supportive evidence on using analgesia in dehorning to moderate changes associated with a pain response are detailed, using published literature in an evidence-based approach. Studies included in this analysis were identified as those that addressed the pain associated with dehorning using either analgesic-treated or placebo-treated controls. Pain biomarkers determined in these studies were used to determine a percent change associated with a drug treatment (**Tables 1–3**). The numerical values

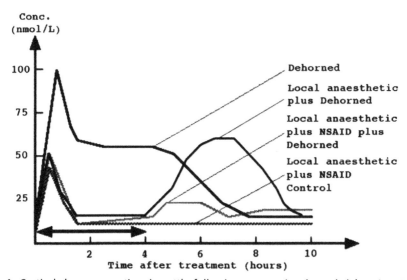

Fig. 1. Cortisol change over time in cattle following amputation (scoop) dehorning. Local anesthesia (bupivacaine) with administration of nonsteroidal anti-inflammatory drug (NSAID; ketoprofen) provides a reduction in measured cortisol concentrations, although a delayed cortisol response is evident without the addition of an anti-inflammatory. The double-headed arrow along the x-axis represents the duration of the local anesthesia provided by bupivacaine. (*Data from* Stafford KJ, Mellor DJ. Dehorning and disbudding distress and its alleviation in calves. Vet J 2005;169(3):337–49.)

Table 1
Summary of the scientific literature examining the effect of analgesic drug administration on plasma cortisol response in dehorned calves

Reference	Procedure	Study Population	Analgesic Regimen	Outcome Parameter	Change in Cortisol (%)	Significance (P Value)
Boandl et al,[36] 1989	Cautery (electric) dehorning	7–16 wk Dairy	Lidocaine local anesthesia (cornual nerve, 5 mL/horn), 5 min before dehorning	Cortisol (30 min)	−13.41	NS
Morisse et al,[26] 1995	Chemical paste dehorning	4 wk Dairy	Lidocaine local anesthesia (cornual nerve, 4 mL/horn), 15 min before dehorning	Cortisol (1 h)	−19.34	NR
				Cortisol (4 h)	−57.26	NR
				Cortisol (24 h)	−6.45	NR
	Cautery (electric) dehorning	8 wk Dairy	Lidocaine local anesthesia (cornual nerve, 4 mL/horn), 15 min before dehorning	Cortisol (1 h)	−18.03	NR
				Cortisol (4 h)	234.48	NR
				Cortisol (24 h)	101.56	NR
Petrie et al,[17] 1996	Amputation (scoop) dehorning	6–8 wk Dairy	Lidocaine local anesthesia (cornual nerve, 3 mL/horn), 20 min before dehorning	Cortisol (AUEC: 0–2 h)	−53.64	<.05
				Cortisol (AUEC: 2–9.5 h)	53.94	NS
				Cortisol (AUEC: 0–9.5 h)	10.92	NS
	Cautery (gas) dehorning		Lidocaine local anesthesia (cornual nerve, 3 mL/horn), 20 min before dehorning	Cortisol (AUEC:0–2 h)	−23.37	NS
				Cortisol (AUEC: 2–9.5 h)	22.78	NS
				Cortisol (AUEC: 0–9.5 h)	2.28	NS
McMeekan et al,[18] 1998	Amputation (scoop) dehorning	12–16 wk Dairy	Bupivacaine local anesthesia (cornual nerve, 6 mL/horn), 20 min before dehorning	Cortisol (AUEC: 0–3.83 h)	−61.00	<.05
				Cortisol (AUEC: 3.84–9.33 h)	109.71	NS
				Cortisol (AUEC: 0–9.33 h)	−10.24	NS
			Bupivacaine local anesthesia (cornual nerve, 6 mL/horn), immediately before dehorning	Cortisol (AUEC: 0–3.83 h)	−72.82	<.05
				Cortisol (AUEC: 3.84–9.33 h)	47.35	NS
				Cortisol (AUEC: 0–9.33 h)	−37.07	NS
			Bupivacaine local anesthesia (cornual nerve, 6 mL/horn), 20 min before dehorning and 4 h later	Cortisol (AUEC: 0–3.83 h)	−80.69	<.05
				Cortisol (AUEC: 3.84–9.33 h)	31.97	<.05
				Cortisol (AUEC: 0–9.33 h)	−47.18	<.05

Reference	Procedure	Age	Treatment	Measure	% Change	P
McMeekan et al,[20] 1998[a]	Amputation (scoop) dehorning	12–16 wk Dairy	Ketoprofen 3 mg/kg IV, 20 min before dehorning	Cortisol (C$_{max}$: 0–3.83 h)	−21.43	NS
				Cortisol (C$_{max}$: 3.83–9.33 h)	−93.33	<.05
			Bupivacaine local anesthesia (cornual nerve, 6 mL/horn), 20 min before dehorning	Cortisol (C$_{max}$: 0–3.83 h)	−46.43	NS
				Cortisol (C$_{max}$: 3.83–9.33 h)	3.33	NS
			Ketoprofen 3 mg/kg IV, bupivacaine local anesthesia (cornual nerve, 6 mL/horn), 20 min before dehorning	Cortisol (C$_{max}$: 0–3.83 h)	−50.00	<.01
				Cortisol (C$_{max}$: 3.83–9.33 h)	−46.67	NS
			Ketoprofen 3 mg/kg IV, lidocaine local anesthesia (cornual nerve, 6 mL/horn), 20 min before dehorning	Cortisol (C$_{max}$: 0–3.83 h)	−82.14	<.01
				Cortisol (C$_{max}$: 3.83–9.33 h)	−66.67	NS
Sylvester et al,[54] 1998	Amputation (scoop) dehorning	20–24 wk Dairy	Lidocaine local anesthesia (cornual nerve, 6 mL/horn), 30 min before dehorning	Cortisol AUEC	−50.48	<.05
			Lidocaine local anesthesia (cornual nerve, 6 mL/horn), 30 min before dehorning, cauterize wound following amputation	Cortisol AUEC	−75.24	<.05
Graf and Senn,[7] 1999[a]	Cautery (electric) dehorner	4–6 wk Dairy	Lidocaine local anesthesia (cornual nerve, 5 mL; caudal horn bud SQ, 5 mL; medial horn bud, 3 mL), 20 min	Cortisol (C$_{max}$: 0–4 h)	−38.78	<.05
			Saline injection (cornual nerve, 5 mL; caudal horn bud SQ, 5 mL; medial horn bud, 3 mL), 20 min	Cortisol (C$_{max}$: 0–4 h)	59.18	<.05
Grøndahl-Nielsen et al,[8] 1999[a]	Cautery (electric) dehorner	4–6 wk Dairy	Lidocaine local anesthesia (cornual nerve, unknown amount), 20 min before dehorning	Cortisol (C$_{max}$: 0–30 min)	−84.00	<.01
				Cortisol (C$_{max}$: 30–60 min)	−77.78	NS
				Cortisol (C$_{max}$: 60–150 min)	−90.91	NS
				Cortisol (C$_{max}$: 15–240 min)	−33.33	NS
			Xylazine 0.2 mg/kg and butorphanol 0.1 mg/kg, IM, 20 min before dehorning	Cortisol (C$_{max}$: 0–30 min)	−76.00	<.01
				Cortisol (C$_{max}$: 30–60 min)	−77.78	NS
				Cortisol (C$_{max}$: 60–150 min)	36.36	NS
				Cortisol (C$_{max}$: 150–240 min)	8.33	NS
			Xylazine 0.2 mg/kg and butorphanol 0.1 mg/kg, IM, 20 min before dehorning; lidocaine local anesthesia (cornual nerve, unknown amount), 15 min before dehorning	Cortisol (C$_{max}$: 0–30 min)	−60.00	<.05
				Cortisol (C$_{max}$: 30–60 min)	−92.59	NS
				Cortisol (C$_{max}$: 60–150 min)	−45.45	NS
				Cortisol (C$_{max}$: 150–240 min)	−91.67	NS

(continued on next page)

Table 1
(continued)

Reference	Procedure	Study Population	Analgesic Regimen	Outcome Parameter	Change in Cortisol (%)	Significance (P Value)
Sutherland et al,[55] 2002[a]	Amputation (scoop) dehorning	12–16 wk Dairy	Lidocaine local anesthesia (cornual nerve, 6 mL/horn) 15 min before dehorning; bupivacaine (cornual nerve, 6 mL/horn) 2 h following lidocaine injection	Cortisol (C_{max}: 0–5 h)	−70.06	<.05
				Cortisol (C_{max}: 5–10 h)	82.93	<.05
				Cortisol (C_{max}: 10–24 h)	10.00	NS
			Lidocaine local anesthesia (cornual nerve, 6 mL/horn) 15 min before dehorning followed by cautery; bupivacaine (cornual nerve, 6 mL/horn) 2 h following lidocaine injection	Cortisol (C_{max}: 0–5 h)	−56.69	<.05
				Cortisol (C_{max}: 5–10 h)	−12.20	NS
				Cortisol (C_{max}: 10–24 h)	10.00	NS
Sutherland et al,[19] 2002[a]	Amputation (scoop) dehorning	12–16 wk Dairy	Lidocaine local anesthesia (cornual nerve, 6 mL/horn) 15 min before dehorning; bupivacaine (cornual nerve, 6 mL/horn) 2 h following lidocaine injection	Cortisol AUEC (0–24 h)	−13.14	NS
				Cortisol (C_{max}: 0–5 h)	−70.06	<.05
				Cortisol (C_{max}: 5–10 h)	82.93	<.05
				Cortisol (C_{max}: 10–24 h)	10.00	NS
			Lidocaine local anesthesia (cornual nerve, 6 mL/horn), phenylbutazone 4.0–5.3 mg/kg, IV 15 min before dehorning; bupivacaine (cornual nerve, 6 mL/horn) 2 h following initial lidocaine injection	Cortisol AUEC (0–24 h)	−8.89	NS
				Cortisol (C_{max}: 0–5 h)	−54.74	<.05
				Cortisol (C_{max}: 5–10 h)	80.49	<.05
				Cortisol (C_{max}: 10–24 h)	2.50	NS
			Lidocaine local anesthesia (cornual nerve, 6 mL/horn), ketoprofen 3.0–3.75 mg/kg, IV 15 min before dehorning; bupivacaine (cornual nerve, 6 mL/horn) 2 h following initial lidocaine injection	Cortisol AUEC (0–24 h)	−21.41	NS
				Cortisol (C_{max}: 0–5 h)	−61.31	<.05
				Cortisol (C_{max}: 5–10 h)	−20.73	NS
				Cortisol (C_{max}: 10–24 h)	5.00	NS
Mellor et al,[45] 2002[a]	Amputation (scoop) dehorning	10 wk Dairy	Lidocaine local anesthesia (cornual nerve, 5 mL/horn) 20 min before dehorning	Cortisol (C_{max}: 0–2.5 h)	−47.83	<.05
				Cortisol (C_{max}: 2.5–8 h)	53.64	<.05

Study	Procedure	Age/Breed	Treatment	Measure	Value	Significance
Stafford et al,[23] 2003[a]	Amputation (scoop) dehorning	12 wk Dairy	Lidocaine local anesthesia (cornual nerve, 5 mL/horn) and ketoprofen 3 mg/kg IV, 15 min before dehorning	Cortisol AUEC	−55.17	NS
				Cortisol (C_{max}: 0–4 h)	−76.32	<.05
				Cortisol (C_{max}: 4–8 h)	−47.37	NS
			Xylazine 0.1 mg/kg IV, 20 min before castration	Cortisol AUEC	3.45	NS
				Cortisol (C_{max}: 0–4 h)	−44.74	<.05
				Cortisol (C_{max}: 4–8 h)	57.89	NS
			Xylazine 0.1 mg/kg IV, 20 min before dehorning and lidocaine local anesthesia (cornual nerve, 5 mL/horn) 15 min before dehorning	Cortisol AUEC	6.90	NS
				Cortisol (C_{max}: 0–4 h)	−73.68	<.05
				Cortisol (C_{max}: 4–8 h)	78.95	<.05
			Xylazine 0.1 mg/kg IV, 20 min before dehorning and lidocaine local anesthesia (cornual nerve, 5 mL/horn) 15 min before dehorning; tolazoline 2 mg/kg 5 min after dehorning	Cortisol AUEC	81.03	NS
				Cortisol (C_{max}: 0–4 h)	31.58	<.05
				Cortisol (C_{max}: 4–8 h)	136.84	<.05
Doherty et al,[30] 2007[a]	Cautery (electric) dehorning	10–12 wk Dairy	Lidocaine (2%) local anesthesia (cornual branch of zygomatic-temporal nerve, 3 mL/horn; cornual branch of infatrochlear nerve; 4 mL/horn rostral to horn base)	Cortisol (C_{max})	−25.00	<.05
			Lidocaine (5%) local anesthesia (cornual branch of zygomatic-temporal nerve, 3 mL/horn; cornual branch of infatrochlear nerve; 4 mL/ horn rostral to horn base)	Cortisol (C_{max})	−56.25	<.05
Stilwell et al,[37] 2008	Chemical paste dehorning	1.5–6 wk Dairy	Flunixin meglumine 2 mg/kg IV, 5 min before dehorning	Cortisol (1 h)	0.37	NS
				Cortisol (3 h)	−58.47	NS
				Cortisol (6 h)	−52.08	NS
				Cortisol (24 h)	37.70	NS
			Flunixin meglumine 2 mg/kg IV, 60 min before dehorning	Cortisol (1 h)	−8.08	NS
				Cortisol (3 h)	−2.18	NS
				Cortisol (6 h)	21.83	NS
				Cortisol (24 h)	96.48	NS

(continued on next page)

Table 1
(continued)

Reference	Procedure	Study Population	Analgesic Regimen	Outcome Parameter	Change in Cortisol (%)	Significance (P Value)
Stilwell et al,[21] 2009	Chemical paste dehorning	3–5 wk Dairy	Lidocaine local anesthesia (cornual nerve, 5 mL/horn) 5 min before dehorning	Cortisol (10 min)	−25.18	NS
				Cortisol (30 min)	−59.63	<.05
				Cortisol (50 min)	−65.19	<.05
				Cortisol (1 h)	−47.51	<.05
				Cortisol (3 h)	−5.50	NS
				Cortisol (6 h)	7.89	NS
				Cortisol (24 h)	34.68	NS
			Flunixin meglumine 2.2 mg/kg IV and lidocaine local anesthesia (cornual nerve, 5 mL/horn), 5 min before dehorning	Cortisol (10 min)	−9.40	NS
				Cortisol (30 min)	−50.06	<.05
				Cortisol (50 min)	−53.21	<.05
				Cortisol (1 h)	−77.68	<.05
				Cortisol (3 h)	−67.85	<.05
				Cortisol (6 h)	−24.64	NS
				Cortisol (24 h)	−25.61	NS
			Lidocaine local anesthesia (cornual nerve, 5 mL/horn) 5 min before dehorning	Cortisol (90 min)	−42.47	<.05
				Cortisol (120 min)	−51.26	NS
				Cortisol (150 min)	39.80	NS
				Cortisol (180 min)	59.19	<.05

First author, year	Procedure	Breed/age	Treatment	Measure	Percent change	Significance
Baldridge et al,[32] 2011	Amputation (scoop) dehorning followed by surgical castration	2–4 mo Dairy	Sodium salicylate at 2.5–5 mg/mL in the drinking water (13.62–151.99 mg of salicylate/kg body weight)	Cortisol (C_{max})	1.60	NS
				Cortisol AUEC (0–1 h)	−9.27	NS
				Cortisol AUEC (1–6 h)	−36.90	$P<.05$
				Cortisol AUEC (6–24 h)	−22.83	NS
			0.025 mg/kg butorphanol, 0.05 mg/kg xylazine, 0.1 mg/kg ketamine coadministered IM immediately before castration	Cortisol (C_{max})	−12.00	NS
				Cortisol AUEC (0–1 h)	−28.90	$P<.05$
				Cortisol AUEC (1–6 h)	−5.82	NS
				Cortisol AUEC (6–24 h)	−0.01	NS
			Sodium salicylate at 2.5–5 mg/mL in the drinking water (13.62–151.99 mg of salicylate/kg body weight) and 0.025 mg/kg butorphanol, 0.05 mg/kg xylazine, 0.1 mg/kg ketamine coadministered IM immediately before castration	Cortisol (C_{max})	−3.46	NS
				Cortisol AUEC (0–1 h)	−20.89	NS
				Cortisol AUEC (1–6 h)	−24.19	NS
				Cortisol AUEC (6–24 h)	−15.69	NS
Coetzee et al,[42] 2012	Amputation (scoop) followed by cautery (electric) dehorning	16–20 wk Dairy	Meloxicam 0.5 mg/kg IV immediately before dehorning	Cortisol AUEC	−7.95	NS
				Cortisol (C_{max})	3.66	NS

Percent change in cortisol was calculated using the formula [(Mean of analgesic group/Mean of dehorned control group) − 1] × 100.

Abbreviations: AUEC, area under the effect curve for cortisol; C_{max}, maximum plasma concentration; IM, intramuscular; IV, intravenous; NR, values not reported; NS, not significant; SQ, subcutaneous.

[a] Values were estimated from included published figures.

Table 2
Summary of the scientific literature examining the effect of analgesic drug administration on plasma cortisol response in dehorned calves using local anesthesia in the control group

Reference	Procedure	Study Population	Control Analgesic Regimen	Analgesic Regimen	Outcome Parameter	Change in Cortisol (%)	Significance (P Value)
Milligan et al,[22] 2004	Cautery (gas) dehorning	2 d–2 wk Dairy	Lidocaine local anesthesia (cornual nerve, 5 mL) 10 min before dehorning	Ketoprofen 3 mg/kg IM, 10 min before dehorning	Cortisol (3 h) Cortisol (0–3 h) Cortisol (6 h) Cortisol (3–6 h)	−24.91 −224.02 14.55 336.79	NS <.05 NS NS
Heinrich et al,[40] 2009	Cautery (electric) dehorning	6–12 wk Dairy	Lidocaine local anesthesia (cornual nerve, 5 mL) 10 min before dehorning	Meloxicam 0.5 mg/kg IM, 10 min before dehorning	Cortisol (0–6 h) Cortisol (24 h)	−80.88 0.86	<.01 NS
Duffield et al,[31] 2010	Cautery (electric) dehorning	4–8 wk Dairy	Lidocaine local anesthesia (cornual nerve, 5 mL) 10 min before dehorning	Ketoprofen 3 mg/kg IM, 10 min before dehorning	Cortisol (3 h) Cortisol (6 h)	4.62 10.45	NS NS
Stilwell et al,[24] 2010	Cautery (gas) dehorning	5–6 wk Dairy	Xylazine 0.2 mg/kg IM, 10 min before dehorning	Lidocaine local anesthesia (cornual nerve, 5 mL) 8 min before dehorning	Cortisol (10 min) Cortisol (25 min) Cortisol (40 min) Cortisol (60 min)	−8.94 5.07 17.41 53.65	NS NS NS NS

Percent change in cortisol was calculated using the formula [(Mean of analgesic group/Mean of dehorned control group) − 1] × 100.

Table 3
Summary of scientific literature examining the effect of analgesic drug administration on other outcomes in dehorned calves

Reference	Procedure	Study Population	Analgesic Regiment	Outcome Parameter	Percent Change (%)	Significance (P Value)
Morisse et al,[26] 1995	Chemical paste dehorning	4 wk Dairy	Lidocaine local anesthesia (cornual nerve, 4 mL/horn), 15 min before dehorning	Lying time	3.50	NS
	Cautery (electric) dehorning	8 wk Dairy	Lidocaine local anesthesia (cornual nerve, 4 mL/horn), 15 min before dehorning	Lying time	7.88	NS
Graf and Senn,[7] 1999[a]	Cautery (electric) dehorner	4–6 wk Dairy	Lidocaine local anesthesia (cornual nerve, 5 mL; caudal horn bud SQ, 5 mL; medial horn bud, 3 mL), 20 min	Vasopressin (C_{max})	−90.00	<.05
				ACTH (C_{max})	−72.50	<.05
			Saline injection (cornual nerve, 5 mL; caudal horn bud SQ, 5 mL; medial horn bud, 3 mL), 20 min	Vasopressin (C_{max})	125.00	NS
				ACTH (C_{max})	62.50	NS
Grondahl-Nielsen et al,[8] 1999[a]	Cautery (electric) dehorner	4–6 wk Dairy	Lidocaine local anesthesia (cornual nerve, unknown amount), 20 min before dehorning	ADG (0–7 d)	NR	NS
				Feed intake (0–4 h)	NR	NS
				Heart rate (0–4 h)	NR	NS
				Rumination (0–4 h)	NR	NS
				Rumination latency	−58.33	<.05
			Xylazine 0.2 mg/kg and butorphanol 0.1 mg/kg, IM, 20 min before dehorning	ADG (0–7 d)	NR	NS
				Feed intake (0–7 d)	NR	NS
				Heart rate (0–4 h)	NR	NS
				Rumination (0–4 h)	NR	NS
				Rumination latency	−37.50	<.05
			Xylazine 0.2 mg/kg and butorphanol 0.1 mg/kg, IM, 20 min before dehorning; lidocaine local anesthesia (cornual nerve, unknown amount), 15 min before dehorning	ADG (0–7 d)	NR	NS
				Feed intake (0–7 d)	NR	NS
				Heart rate (0–4 h)	NR	NS
				Rumination (0–4 h)	NR	NS
				Rumination latency	−46.67	<.05

(continued on next page)

Table 3
(continued)

Reference	Procedure	Study Population	Analgesic Regiment	Outcome Parameter	Percent Change (%)	Significance (P Value)
Faulkner and Weary,[27] 2000	Cautery (electric) dehorner	4–8 wk Dairy	Ketoprofen 3 mg/kg PO 2 h before dehorning, 2 h post dehorning, and 7 h after dehorning (Analgesic control: xylazine 0.2 mg/kg IM 20 min before dehorning and lidocaine local anesthesia [cornual nerve and ring block 4.5 mL/side] 10 min before dehorning)	Weight gain (0–24 h)	500.00	NS ($P = .07$)
Mellor et al,[45] 2002[a]	Amputation (scoop) dehorning	10 wk Dairy	Lidocaine local anesthesia (cornual nerve, 5 mL/horn) 20 min before dehorning	Noradrenaline (C_{max})	−16.00	NS
				Adrenaline (C_{max})	−9.09	NS
Doherty et al,[30] 2007	Cautery (electric) dehorning	10–12 wk Dairy	Lidocaine (2%) local anesthesia (cornual branch of zygomatic-temporal nerve, 3 mL/horn; cornual branch of infratrochlear nerve; 4 mL/horn rostral to horn base)	Neutrophil %	9.53	NS
				Lymphocyte %	−10.04	NS
				N:L %	−19.83	NS
				Fibrinogen	NA	NS
				α_1-acid glycoprotein	NA	NS
			Lidocaine (5%) local anesthesia (cornual branch of zygomatic-temporal nerve, 3 mL/horn; cornual branch of infratrochlear nerve; 4 mL/horn rostral to horn base)	Neutrophil %	0.23	NS
				Lymphocyte %	1.70	NS
				N:L %	−21.49	NS
				Fibrinogen	NA	NS
				α_1-acid glycoprotein	NA	NS

Study	Procedure	Age/Type	Treatment	Outcome Measure	Value	P
Heinrich et al,[40] 2009	Cautery (electric) dehorning	6–12 wk Dairy	Meloxicam 0.5 mg/kg IM given 10 min before dehorning; analgesic control: lidocaine local anesthesia (cornual nerve, 5 mL/horn)	Heart Rate	−20.43	<.05
				Respiratory rate	−100.00	<.05
Stewart et al,[41] 2009[a]	Cautery (gas) dehorning	4–5 wk Dairy	Lidocaine local anesthesia (cornual nerve, 5 mL/horn and ring block, 3–4 mL/horn) 10 min before dehorning	Eye temperature (2–3 h post dehorning difference)	−610.00	<.001
				Heart Rate (0–5 min)	−22.22	<.05
				HRV: LF Power (2–3 h)	13.16	<.05
				HRV: HF power (2–3 h)	−35.90	<.05
				HRV: LF:HF ratio (2–3 h)	500.00	<.05
			Meloxicam 0.5 mg/kg IV, 55 min before dehorning and lidocaine local anesthesia (cornual nerve, 5 mL/horn and ring block, 3–4 mL/horn) 10 min before dehorning		No change	NS
				Eye temperature (2–3 h post dehorning difference)	No change	NS
				Heart rate (0–5 min)	−26.98	<.05
				HRV: LF Power (2–3 h)	7.89	<.05
				HRV: HF power (2–3 h)	−15.38	<.05
				HRV: LF:HF ratio (2–3 h)	166.67	NS
Heinrich et al,[29] 2010	Cautery (electric) dehorning	6–12 wk Dairy	Meloxicam 0.5 mg/kg IM given 10 min before dehorning; analgesic control: lidocaine local anesthesia (cornual nerve, 5 mL/horn)	Accelerometer (0–5 h)	−10.26	<.05
				Pressure algometry	31.48	<.05
				Feed consumption	300.00	NS (P = .09)

(continued on next page)

Table 3
(continued)

Reference	Procedure	Study Population	Analgesic Regiment	Outcome Parameter	Percent Change (%)	Significance (P Value)
Baldridge et al,[32] 2011	Amputation (scoop) dehorning after surgical castration	2–4 mo Dairy	Sodium salicylate at 2.5–5 mg/mL in the drinking water (13.62–151.99 mg of salicylate/kg body weight)	ADG (0–13 d)	−1111.22	<.05
				Chute exit speed	0.97	NS
			0.025 mg/kg butorphanol, 0.05 mg/kg xylazine, 0.1 mg/kg ketamine coadministered IM immediately before castration	ADG (0–13 d)	−729.98	NS
				Chute exit speed	−77.81	<.05
			Sodium salicylate at 2.5–5 mg/mL in the drinking water (13.62–151.99 mg of salicylate/kg body weight) and 0.025 mg/kg butorphanol, 0.05 mg/kg xylazine, 0.1 mg/kg ketamine coadministered IM immediately before castration	ADG (0–13 d)	−1095.92	<.05
				Chute exit speed	−94.97	<.05
Theurer et al,[33] 2012[a]	Cautery (electric) dehorning	10 wk Dairy	Meloxicam 0.5 mg/kg PO immediately after dehorning	Lying down % (1–4 d)	20.13	<.05
				Hay feeder % (0–1 d)	−40.86	<.05
				Grain feeder % (0–1 d)	−50.00	<.05
				Grain feeder % (1–2 d)	80.00	<.05
Coetzee et al,[42] 2012	Amputation (scoop) followed by cautery (electric) dehorning	16–20 wk Dairy	Meloxicam 0.5 mg/kg IV, immediately before the start of dehorning	Substance P	−37.79	<.05
				Lying time %	−97.06	<.01
				Heart rate (8 and 10 h)	NR	<.05
				ADG (0–10 d)	162.50	<.05

Percent change in cortisol was calculated using the formula [((Mean of analgesic group/Mean of dehorned control group) − 1] × 100.
Abbreviations: ACTH, adrenocorticotropic hormone; ADG, average daily gain in body weight; HRV, heart-rate variability; LF, low frequency; HF, high frequency; NA, data not available; NR, values not reported; PO, by mouth.
[a] Values were estimated from included published figures.

of the biomarker used for comparison included: maximum concentration (C_{max}), area under the effect curve (AUEC), and concentration at specific time points. In addition, these values were further summarized following categorization by analgesic regimen when applicable (**Tables 4** and **5**). Following this summary analysis, a multimodal approach using local anesthetics, nonsteroidal anti-inflammatories and, when possible, sedative analgesics is recommended for the most effective reduction of pain response in cattle following dehorning. These recommendations are similar to those of other reviews concerning the management of pain in cattle following dehorning.[16]

This review on the pain associated with dehorning is meant to both be independent of and mirror the article assessing pain following castration. For a more detailed examination of similar themed topics including pain assessment, challenges associated with providing analgesia in food animals, and a pharmacology review, the reader is referred to the article on castration by Coetzee elsewhere in this issue.

ASSESSMENT TOOLS USED TO DETERMINE THE EFFICACY OF ANALGESIC DRUGS IN CATTLE FOLLOWING DEHORNING
Assessment of Behavioral Changes After Dehorning

Behavioral changes are often monitored and recorded in studies involving pain. The observed changes have been suggested as a more sensitive marker for pain in comparison with other physiologic markers such as cortisol.[25] Behavior indices have been recorded using videography,[7,22,26–31] chute behavior,[32] accelerometers,[33] and remote triangulation devices.[33] Head shaking, ear flicking, head rubbing, transition between standing and lying, inert lying, vocalization, and grooming are all behavioral changes frequently recorded in an ethological evaluation of cattle following dehorning.[8,21,26–28]

Behavioral responses are subject to interpretation. In the case of dehorning, reliable indicators of pain are difficult to assess in cattle following dehorning with and without analgesia.[27,29,31] For example, it has been suggested that head rubbing may be a result of increased nociception or may indicate irritation, itching, or healing.[31] However, correlation between behavioral responses and changes to cortisol concentrations has been reviewed.[2] For a more thorough evaluation of behavioral responses following dehorning, see the excellent reviews by Stafford and Mellor[2,16] detailing these behavioral changes.

Recently, Heinrich and colleagues[29] evaluated changes in behavior following cautery dehorning. Based on behavioral changes, the investigators determined that pain may be present for up to 44 hours following the procedure. Other studies have indicated a continuation of painful or decreased normal behaviors for up to 72 hours after dehorning.[16,27] The duration of pain observed in these studies beyond other physiologic or neuroendocrine parameters further supports the necessity to provide long-lasting effective analgesia for cattle during and after common procedures presumed to be painful, such as dehorning. Additional research is needed to investigate chronic pain responses associated with dehorning.

Assessment of Physiologic Changes After Dehorning

Changes to the physiology of cattle following dehorning are frequently observed biomarkers in pain assessment. Serum cortisol, heart rate, feed intake, and average daily weight gain (ADG) are often used in studies evaluating the efficacy of analgesics in painful or stressful procedures such as dehorning. Cortisol concentrations should be interpreted with caution because of the variations in cortisol response following a stressor, as well as a wide variety of inciting causes that can activate the

Table 4

Summary of the mean (range) percent change in peak plasma cortisol concentrations (C_{max}) and cortisol concentrations recorded at specific time points in analgesic-treated calves compared with untreated dehorned control calves in the published literature

Analgesia	Mean Percent Change in Cortisol (0–5 h)	Range (%)	Mean Percent Change in Cortisol (4–9.3 h)	Range (%)	Mean Percent Change in Cortisol (6–24 h)	Range (%)	Mean Percent Change in Cortisol (0–24 h)	Range (%)
Local	−25.98 (9)	−90.91–234.48	14.70 (5)	47.37–82.93	29.96 (4)	−6.45–101.56	−40.01 (2)	56.25 to −25.00
NSAID	−17.96 (2)	−58.47–0.37	−41.20 (2)	−93.33–21.83	67.09 (1)	NA	1.03 (2)	−1.60–3.66
NSAID + local	−63.40 (3)	−82.14–50.00	−15.64 (3)	−66.67–80.49	−6.04 (2)	−25.61–5.00	NA	NA
Sedative-analgesia	−28.12 (2)	−76.00–36.36	57.89 (1)	NA	NA	NA	−12.00 (1)	NA
Sedative-analgesia + NSAID	NA	NA	NA	NA	NA	NA	−3.46 (1)	NA
Sedative-analgesia + local	−59.71 (2)	−73.68 to −45.45	78.95 (1)	NA	NA	NA	NA	NA

Estimated cortisol concentrations were categorized according to the following time categories to best fit the pattern observed in the published literature. The number of treatment groups evaluated is indicated in parentheses. Percent change in cortisol was calculated using the formula [(Mean of analgesic group/Mean of dehorned control group) − 1] × 100.

Abbreviation: NSAID, nonsteroidal anti-inflammatory drug.

Table 5
Summary of the mean (range) percent change in area under the plasma cortisol concentration over time curve (AUEC) in analgesic-treated calves compared with untreated dehorned control calves in the published literature

Analgesia	Mean Percent Change in Cortisol (0–5 h)	Range (%)	Mean Percent Change in Cortisol (4–9.3 h)	Range (%)	Mean Percent Change in Cortisol (6–24 h)	Range (%)	Mean Percent Change in Cortisol (0–24 h)	Range (%)
Local	−58.30 (2)	−80.69–−23.37	53.15 (2)	22.78–109.71	NA	NA	−30.59 (5)	−75.24–−10.92
NSAID	−9.27 (1)	NA	36.90 (1)	NA	−22.83 (1)	NA	−7.95 (1)	NA
NSAID + Local	NA	NA	NA	NA	NA	NA	−15.15 (1)	NA
Sedative-analgesia	−28.90 (1)	NA	−5.82 (1)	NA	0.01 (1)	NA	3.45 (1)	NA
Sedative-analgesia + NSAID	−20.89 (1)	NA	24.19 (1)	NA	−15.69 (1)	NA	NA	NA
Sedative-analgesia + local	NA	NA	NA	NA	NA	NA	6.90 (1)	NA

Estimated cortisol concentrations were categorized according to the following times to best fit the pattern observed in the published literature. The number of treatment groups evaluated is indicated in parentheses. Percent change in cortisol was calculated using the formula [(Mean of analgesic group/Mean of dehorned control group) − 1] × 100.

hypothalamus-pituitary-adrenal (HPA) system responsible for cortisol release.[34,35] However, cortisol changes over time have been used frequently as a parameter assessing stress in cattle following dehorning.[7,17,19,36,37]

In cattle dehorned without analgesia, most studies indicate an initial peak in cortisol observed within the first 30 minutes that subsequently plateaus at an elevated concentration, until returning to baseline approximately 7 to 8 hours following the procedure.[16] It has been hypothesized that the initial peak in cortisol is a result of a significant noxious nociception owing to the removal of the horn tissue, whereas the observed plateau results from pain associated with inflammation.[20] The anti-inflammatory potential of cortisol has been suggested to result in the attenuation of the inflammatory-mediated pain response.[18,19]

Schwartzkopf-Genswein and colleagues[38] evaluated the cortisol response to dehorning over a period of 3 consecutive days in 26- to 59-day-old Holstein calves. Cortisol response was measured in calves that were not dehorned, sham dehorned, and then dehorned by hot iron without the addition of analgesia or anesthesia. The study found that elevations in cortisol were significantly higher from 0 to 30 minutes after dehorning, compared with between both 60 to 240 minutes and 24 to 48 hours. In addition, from 0 to 60 minutes the cortisol response was greater for calves dehorned in comparison with sham dehorning or no dehorning. Another study investigated the effects of electric dehorning on cortisol response in 18 Holstein calves at 8 weeks of age.[39] The study found calves dehorned at 8 weeks of age had significantly higher cortisol response at 5, 15, 30, and 60 minutes after dehorning compared with calves not dehorned.

In dehorning studies, cortisol responses can vary with age. As a covariate in one study, serum cortisol concentrations before dehorning and then at 3 and 6 hours after dehorning were adjusted based on calf age (range of 2 days to 2 weeks old).[22] It was determined that older calves had significantly lower serum cortisol concentrations immediately before ($P<.01$), 3 hours after ($P<.05$), and 6 hours after ($P<.01$) dehorning. These changes should be considered when evaluating different studies using subjects of different age.

Heart rate has been monitored and recorded in dehorning studies as an indicator of physiologic stress.[8,40–43] Compared with calves that were sham dehorned, heart rate remained elevated for up to 3 hours in dehorned calves receiving no analgesia.[8,41–43] Additional studies have indicated an acutely decreased heart rate following treatment with an analgesic, compared with placebo-treated controls.[40–42]

The cost of analgesics is often cited as one of the major influencing factors that motivate producers to not use analgesics in painful procedures.[12–15] If economic gains could balance the costs, the routine use of analgesic compounds at the time of dehorning might be adopted more readily by producers. The economics of pain management is reviewed by Newton and O'Connor elsewhere in this issue. Previous literature has not provided a reliable amount of supportive data for an increased ADG following dehorning with analgesia; however, more recent studies have indicated its beneficial use. Studies have indicated an increased time spent at the grain feeder and an increased ADG following the use of a nonsteroidal anti-inflammatory drug (NSAID) at the time of dehorning in comparison with cattle not treated with any analgesia.[27,32,33,42] Although Grøndahl-Nielsen and colleagues[8] did not observe any difference in ADG or feed intake in the 7 days following dehorning, there was a significant difference in animals treated with analgesics at the time of dehorning, initiating rumination more quickly than those without analgesics provided. This improved rumination has also been reported in other studies with extended observation periods.[16,44]

Other physiologic parameters have been evaluated in cattle following dehorning, indicating a pain response (see **Table 3**). Plasma adrenocorticotropic hormone,[7] vasopressin,[7] noradrenaline,[45] and adrenaline[45] concentrations increased acutely following dehorning and remained elevated for up to 1 hour.

Assessment of Neuroendocrine Changes After Dehorning

Neuroendocrine changes have been assessed in many studies evaluating nociception following dehorning, including substance P,[42] electrodermal activity,[32] infrared thermography,[41] heart-rate variability,[41] and electroencephalography (EEG).[46]

Substance P is a neuropeptide expressed within portions of the neuraxis, involved with pain, stress, and anxiety.[47] Increased concentrations are found in cattle following castration when compared with those sham castrated, thus potentially validating its use as biomarker of pain.[48] A recent study investigated concentrations of substance P following dehorning in 16- to 20-week-old calves treated with an anti-inflammatory at the time of dehorning.[42] Animals treated with meloxicam had a significant reduction in mean concentrations of substance P compared with the placebo-treated controls. In addition, there were no significant differences observed in cortisol concentrations between the 2 groups, thereby suggesting an improved sensitivity of using substance P as a biomarker of pain and determinant of drug efficacy in comparison with cortisol.

Heart-rate variability has been suggested to reflect a measurement of the autonomic nervous system through the assessment of sympathetic and parasympathetic activity, thus providing an evaluation of pain.[49] Using heart-rate variation, the control of the intervals between consecutive beats is increased through vagal tone (increased heart-rate variation, high-frequency power) or sympathetic (decreased heart-rate variation, low-frequency power). In 4- to 5-week-old calves dehorned using a cautery dehorning unit, changes in heart-rate variation illustrated a sympathovagal imbalance coinciding with reported pain associated with dehorning.[41]

In addition, a decreased eye temperature as determined by infrared thermography has been suggested as a neuroendocrine response mediated by sympathetic vasoconstriction on the induction of pain.[43] Stewart and colleagues[41] investigated eye temperature concurrently with heart-rate variability, and reported a decrease in eye temperature during the same time period as the changes in heart-rate variations, further supporting the sympathovagal imbalance.

Analysis of EEG following a painful procedure has been validated for the detection of acute pain in both dehorning and castration studies.[46,50] Acute noxious sensory stimuli produce changes within EEG frequencies, reflecting the cerebral cortical electrical activity perceiving the nociception.[46] A desynchronization occurs, which has been interpreted as perceived nociception. Mean EEG frequencies were evaluated in calves 24 to 36 weeks of age following amputation via scoop dehorning. EEG frequencies were recorded following the induction of minimal anesthesia in the calves using intravenous ketamine (3.4 mg/kg) and propofol (4.1 mg/kg). Although this minimal anesthesia model may have confounded the results, specific wavelengths were significantly altered following dehorning, indicating noxious nociception. Animals in which a local nerve block was administered had significantly fewer changes in EEG frequencies, providing supportive evidence of decreased nociception following dehorning in comparison with calves dehorned without analgesia.[46]

ANALGESIC STRATEGIES FOR DEHORNING AND THEIR EFFECTS ON PAIN BIOMARKERS
Dehorning Methods

Several studies have evaluated the different dehorning techniques on relative changes in biomarkers for pain. Sylvester and colleagues[6] compared the differences in cortisol concentrations in calves dehorned by 4 different methods of dehorning: Barnes scoop dehorning, guillotine shears, a butcher's saw, and embryotomy wire. This study found no differences among treatment groups during the 36 hours after dehorning for cortisol, except that calves dehorned by guillotine shears had a significantly lower cortisol at 2 to 2.5 hours after the procedure. The cortisol C_{max} and integrated cortisol response were not statistically different among treatment groups. Another study investigated differences in cortisol response to variations in performing the technique of scoop dehorning.[51] Shallow-scoop dehorning and deep-scoop dehorning were compared in 30 Friesian calves 14 to 16 weeks old, and no significant difference was found between increases in cortisol concentrations or the integrated cortisol response from 0.25 to 5 hours after dehorning. The only difference noted was that cortisol concentrations in calves undergoing shallow-scoop dehorning returned to control values by 8 hours, whereas deep-scoop dehorned calves returned to baseline by 6 hours.

Several studies have investigated cautery dehorning. In lambs, an attenuated cortisol response was observed following tail docking using a thermocautery device in comparison with a knife.[52] It was suggested that the tissue damage caused by the heat from the hot iron destroyed the nociceptors adjacent to the wound, thus mitigating the cortisol response.[2] This reported cortisol variation was also observed while comparing cautery dehorning with amputation. A study using scoop versus cautery dehorning by Petrie and colleagues[17] in 6- to 8-week-old Friesian calves found that scoop dehorning without the provision of anesthesia or analgesia produced a significantly higher cortisol area under the curve (AUC) from −70 minutes to 2 hours postprocedure, compared with cautery dehorning. The examination of 2 cautery dehorning methods using 3- to 4-week-old Holstein calves indicated no significant difference in C_{max} between Buddex (57.1 nmol/L) and cautery (60.4 nmol/L) methods.[53]

Chemical dehorning methods have also been recently evaluated.[26,28,37] Using behaviors such as head shaking, head rubbing, and lying to standing transitions, Vickers and colleagues[28] determined that caustic paste with a sedative was less painful than the use of a hot iron with a sedative and a local anesthetic in calves 10 to 35 days old. However, in an earlier study, 4-week-old calves dehorned with caustic paste had increased plasma cortisol concentrations in comparison with 8-week-old calves dehorned using a hot iron.[26] It is reported that the application of the caustic paste is not painful; however, within an hour both cortisol and behavioral changes indicate a pain or stress response, returning to pretreatment levels up to 24 hours following dehorning.

Without the provision of analgesics, it has been recommended to dehorn cattle using cautery rather than amputation or chemical methods.[16] This conclusion was reached as a result of an extensive review of the published literature indicating a decreased cortisol response in cautery dehorning; however, it was suggested that more research comparing the cautery and chemical dehorning methods should be completed.[16]

Local Anesthetics

Local anesthetics provided to cattle before dehorning have been shown to aid in the mitigation of the initial acute cortisol response.[7,17,18,21,30,54,55] Local anesthetics act at the sodium channel to prevent generation and propagation of nerve impulses or action potentials.[56] Most commonly, performed nerve blocks consist of infiltrating the perineural space surrounding the cornual nerve, a branch of the zygomaticotemporal portion of the ophthalmic division of the trigeminal nerve, with a local anesthetic; however, other local nerve blocks, such as ring blocks or caudal horn blocks, have been used in dehorning studies in efforts to increase the likelihood the effective anesthesia (**Fig. 2**).[7,27,30,57]

The cornual nerve block has been described by several studies and textbooks. In brief, a 2.5-cm 18- or 20-gauge needle is inserted lateral to the palpable temporal ridge of the frontal bone and 2.5 cm rostral to the base of the horn (see **Fig. 2**). Following a negative aspiration confirming the needle is placed subcutaneously, 5 to 10 mL of 2% lidocaine is injected, directing the needle toward the horn for desensitization of the area.[57] In cattle with larger horns, cutaneous branches of the second cervical nerve will need to be desensitized using a local anesthetic infiltration caudal to the horn.[57] Proper restraint is necessary to deliver the local anesthetic to the correct location for complete cessation of nociception (**Fig. 3**). This procedure can be performed using plastic disposable syringes or automatic syringes for multiple animals (see **Fig. 3**).

A recent study using 2-month-old dairy calves examined the efficacy of lidocaine with epinephrine using 4 local-anesthetic delivery techniques: cornual nerve block, ring block, percutaneous injection via a needle-free drug delivery system (JET), and a topical eutectic mixture of local anesthetics containing 2.5% lidocaine and 2.5% prilocaine (EMLA).[58] Although the calves in the study were not dehorned, a peripheral variable-output nerve stimulator was used to evaluate anesthetic efficacy. Consistent local anesthetic was achieved using the cornual nerve block (87.5%; 7 of 8 calves) and ring block (100%; 8 of 8 calves). In addition, there was no difference in onset time between the 2 techniques (cornual nerve: 2 minutes vs ring block: 3.25 minutes); however, the mean duration of the cornual nerve block was approximately 2.5 hours longer than that of the ring block (304 minutes vs 147 minutes, respectively). Both the JET delivery system and the EMLA cream failed to provide consistent, effective local anesthesia.

Sufficient evidence supports a delayed cortisol response that occurs following the return of sensitivity to an area once anesthetized.[17–19,54] As mentioned previously, local anesthetics mitigate the cortisol response for their respective duration of action (ie, lidocaine: 2 hours; bupivacaine: 4 hours) following the dehorning procedure, but a delayed cortisol response is observed, presumably once sensitivity returns to the anesthetized area. In addition, among dehorning studies with only local anesthesia provided, there is an initial reduction of the cortisol response; however, following this reduction an increased cortisol response is observed (see **Tables 4** and **5**).

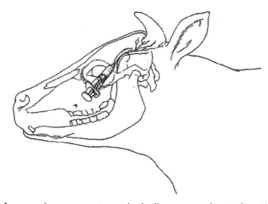

Fig. 2. Diagram of cornual nerve anatomy including approximate locations for local anesthetic injection. (*From* Skarda RT. Techniques of local analgesia in ruminants and swine. Vet Clin Food Anim Pract 1986;2:627; with permission.)

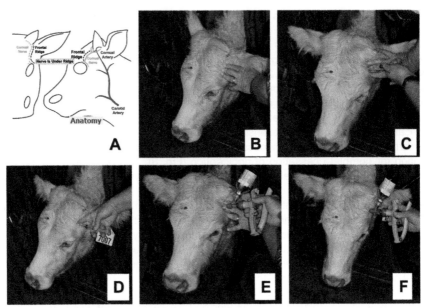

Fig. 3. Steps for providing local anesthetic for dehorning using a cornual nerve block. (*A*) Anatomy of the cornual innervation. (*B*) Palpation of the temporal ridge. (*C*) Insertion of the needle below the ridge and aspirate. (*D*) Injection of 5 to 10 mL of lidocaine. (*E*) Palpation of the frontal ridge and insertion of needle attached to automatic syringe. (*F*) Injection of 5 to 10 mL of lidocaine using an automatic syringe.

Lidocaine

Lidocaine 2% is the most commonly used analgesic in dehorning studies (see **Tables 1–3**). Pharmacokinetics studies following an inverted-L nerve block using a local lidocaine infusion in mature cattle indicated a serum elimination half-life of 4.19 ± 1.69 hours.[59] Clinically, studies assessing the analgesic duration of lidocaine report an approximate duration of 2 hours, based on both behavioral and physiologic changes.[2] Although integrated cortisol concentrations are typically not significantly different between cattle dehorned using local anesthesia and nontreated controls, consistent cortisol changes are significantly reduced or eliminated during the acute phase of the pain response.[7,17,18,54,55] In general, once the desensitization associated with local infusion of lidocaine has diminished, cortisol concentrations significantly increase in comparison with animals dehorned without lidocaine.[7,17,18,54,55]

Many studies look at the effects of nerve blocks on cortisol response to dehorning (see **Tables 1–3**). Although a few studies have indicated no difference in the pain or stress response following the provision of a local anesthetic before dehorning, most studies support its use because of a near elimination of the acute behavior and physiologic changes that are typically observed.[16,36] Graf and Senn[7] found that a cornual nerve block with 2% lidocaine significantly diminished the cortisol response in 4- to 6-week-old calves when compared with those injected with saline from 20 to 90 minutes after dehorning. A study investigated the use of cautery following amputation dehorning and local lidocaine anesthesia in 20- to 24-week-old calves.[54] The integrated cortisol response over a 9-hour period indicated a significant reduction using lidocaine local anesthesia before amputation dehorning. In addition to the use of lidocaine anesthesia, cautery following amputation dehorning significantly diminished the cortisol response by 75% (see **Table 1**).

The effects of scoop dehorning versus scoop dehorning with cautery, both with and without the addition of local anesthesia, have been evaluated.[55] This study found that calves undergoing dehorning had significant elevations in cortisol compared with control calves from 0.5 hours to 6 hours and then again at 13 to 15 hours. It is of interest that on administering local anesthesia with lidocaine and bupivacaine 15 minutes before the procedure and then again at 1 hour 45 minutes postprocedure, an increase in cortisol concentrations from 0 to 5 hours was abolished, and calves experienced a significant increase in cortisol response that was greater than that in calves dehorned without anesthesia at 6 and 7 hours. Calves receiving local anesthesia plus cautery in addition to scoop dehorning had almost no change in cortisol concentrations throughout the 24-hour period measured.

Doherty and colleagues[30] found that 10- to 12-week-old Holstein calves experienced a significantly lower cortisol response 30 and 60 minutes after dehorning after a cornual nerve block of either 10 mL of 5% lidocaine or 10 mL of 2% lidocaine administered 30 minutes before dehorning, compared with untreated, dehorned calves. No significant difference was noted between the 5% and 2% lidocaine solutions on cortisol response.

Of note, studies involving chemical dehorning indicated a decreased duration of analgesia efficacy using local lidocaine anesthesia alone.[21,28] Following dehorning using a caustic paste and local lidocaine anesthesia in 3- to 5-week-old calves, behavioral signs of distress were attenuated for the first hour but then became evident over the next 5 hours.[21] It was hypothesized that the alkalotic paste may have increased the pH of the surrounding tissue, thus affecting the equilibrium of the anesthetic solution and disrupting its function.[28]

Bupivacaine

In addition to lidocaine, bupivacaine has been used in several dehorning studies, mostly because of its prolonged clinical analgesic effect in comparison with lidocaine.[18,19,55] Clinical analgesic efficacy in one study was reported to be approximately 4 hours, as confirmed by a lack of behavioral reaction to a needle-prick of the skin adjacent to the horn.[18]

McMeekan and colleagues[18] evaluated the effect of timing of cornual nerve block administration using 0.25% bupivacaine on cortisol response in 3- to 4-month-old calves. Calves administered a cornual nerve block at 20 minutes before dehorning and then again 4 hours after dehorning experienced a significantly lower cortisol AUC than control calves dehorned without analgesia, calves administered the cornual nerve block only at 20 minutes prior, and calves administered the cornual nerve block immediately prior. Another study by McMeekan and colleagues[20] found that calves undergoing scoop dehorning with a cornual nerve block using bupivacaine administered 20 minutes prior and 4 hours after had a significantly lower AUC from 0 to 9.33 hours for cortisol, compared with the calves dehorned with only a cornual nerve block 20 minutes prior, immediately prior, or with no analgesia. However, for the first 3.83 hours, all calves receiving a cornual nerve block experienced a significantly lower AUC cortisol response than those undergoing scoop dehorning without treatment.

Nonsteroidal Anti-Inflammatory Drugs

As previously mentioned, following the acute pain associated with dehorning, a suggested inflammatory-mediated pain response exists,[20] which is evident in both continued distressful behaviors and increased cortisol concentrations following the initial cortisol response. In addition, among dehorning studies with only NSAIDs provided, there is a mild initial attenuation of the cortisol response, which continues past the initial acute phase and provides prolonged anesthesia (see **Tables 4** and **5**). The following NSAIDs have been studied for their role in the attenuation of the cortisol response both alone and in combination with a local anesthetic.

Ketoprofen

Several studies have evaluated the analgesic efficacy of ketoprofen following dehorning (see **Tables 1–3**).[19,20,22,23,27,31,60] Although the use of ketoprofen alone does not completely diminish the initial acute cortisol response following dehorning, evidence supports its use to aid in the decrease of the inflammatory component.[20] In combination with local anesthesia, cortisol AUC was significantly ameliorated for up to 5 hours after dehorning.[19,20] Another study in 4- to 8-week-old calves treated with local anesthesia, xylazine, and ketoprofen given 2 hours before and 2 and 7 hours after dehorning resulted in a tendency of weight gain over a 24-hour period following cautery dehorning ($P = .07$).[27] Because of the short elimination half-life of ketoprofen of 0.42 hours, administrations must be repeated to sustain analgesic concentrations.[61]

Calves treated with a cornual nerve block of 5 mL of 2% lidocaine and 0.03 mL/kg of 10% ketoprofen given intramuscularly 10 minutes before procedures experienced significantly lower cortisol concentrations from 0 to 3 hours compared with calves given only a cornual nerve block.[22] However, another study found there to be no difference in cortisol response at 3 and 6 hours after electrocautery dehorning in 4- to 8-week-old calves treated with 3 mg/kg ketoprofen intramuscularly plus a cornual nerve block in comparison with calves given an intramuscular injection of sterile saline plus a cornual nerve block.[31]

Phenylbutazone

Although phenylbutazone is not approved for cattle in the United States, historically it has been a commonly used analgesic in cattle.[62] One study has evaluated the benefit of phenylbutazone in providing analgesia to cattle following dehorning.[19] In combination with a 5-hour local anesthesia regimen using both lidocaine and bupivacaine, calves treated with phenylbutazone (4.0–5.3 mg/kg) did not show a significant attenuation of the delayed cortisol response following return of sensitivity to the anesthetized area. This finding is consistent with those of previous literature suggesting that phenylbutazone is known to have anti-inflammatory actions weaker than those of ketoprofen in calves.[63,64] Based on the lack of efficacy data and concerns regarding the potential toxicity to consumers of phenylbutazone tissue residues, the use of phenylbutazone at the time of dehorning is not recommended.

Meloxicam

The benefits of meloxicam, a potentially longer-acting NSAID, have been detailed in several dehorning studies.[29,33,40–42] A study by Heinrich and colleagues[40] found that 6- to 12-week-old calves treated with a cornual nerve block with 5 mL of 2% lidocaine given 10 minutes before cautery dehorning experienced significantly higher serum cortisol concentrations from 0 to 6 hours after dehorning when compared with calves administered the cornual nerve block plus a single intramuscular dose of 0.5 mg/kg meloxicam; however, no differences in cortisol concentrations were noted at 24 hours after dehorning. In addition, heart rate and respiratory rates were decreased for those animals treated with meloxicam. A decrease in heart rate was also observed in another study at 8 and 10 hours after administration of intravenous meloxicam (0.5 mg/kg) at the time of dehorning, indicating a continued reduction of stress without the effects of local anesthesia (**Fig. 4**).[42] Furthermore, pressure tolerance as measured by pressure algometry was significantly improved following meloxicam administration, indicating a reduced pain-associated nociception.[29]

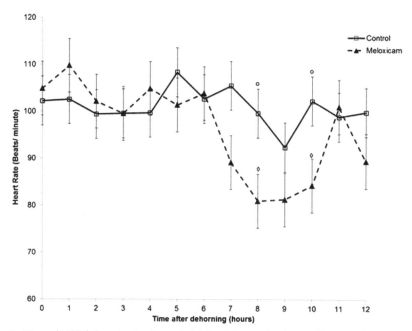

Fig. 4. Mean (±SEM) heart rate (beats/min) in dehorned calves collected after receiving 0.5 mg/kg intravenous meloxicam (*closed triangles*) or placebo (*open squares*) immediately before dehorning. Columns not connected by a symbol of the same shape and color are significantly different (*P*<.05). Heart rate was collected every 15 seconds over 12 hours. Significant reduction in heart rate is observed at 8 and 10 hours for meloxicam-treated calves compared with placebo-treated controls, indicating a prolonged effect of meloxicam administered at the time of dehorning without the effects of a local anesthetic. (*From* Coetzee JF, Mosher RA, KuKanich B, et al. Pharmacokinetics and effect of intravenous meloxicam in weaned Holstein calves following scoop dehorning without local anesthesia. BMC Vet Res 2012;8:153. http://dx.doi.org/10.1186/1746-6148-8-153; with permission.)

Theurer and colleagues[33] determined that 10-week-old calves treated with oral meloxicam (0.5 mg/kg) at the time of dehorning spent more time at the grain feeder on days 2 and 6 than those without treatment. In addition, Coetzee and colleagues[42] treated 16- to 20-week-old calves with intravenous meloxicam (0.5 mg/kg) at the time of dehorning, which resulted in a significant weight gain over a 10-day period compared with those dehorned without analgesia. The difference in ADG observed in this study was suggested to have been a result of the increased time at the grain feeder.

Flunixin meglumine
The analgesic effects of flunixin meglumine following dehorning are not well studied in the literature. Only 2 studies have investigated the use of flunixin meglumine and its effects on cortisol response in calves following only chemical dehorning (see **Tables 1** and **3**).[21,37] The effects of flunixin meglumine (2.2 mg/kg) administered intravenously and injected either 1 hour or 5 minutes before chemical dehorning were investigated in 10- to 40-day-old calves.[37] This study determined that no acute treatment effect was observed by providing preemptive analgesia, as all groups experienced significantly higher cortisol concentrations 1 hour after dehorning procedures; however, by 3 hours calves treated with flunixin meglumine were not significantly different from non-dehorned animals, whereas cortisol concentrations

in placebo-treated animals were significantly higher. Cortisol concentrations in placebo-treated calves and calves treated with flunixin meglumine were not significantly different from each other, and by 6 to 24 hours all groups experienced similar cortisol concentrations.

In another study, local anesthesia was used during chemical dehorning procedures in a study of 3- to 5-week-old calves.[21] Calves administered 2.2 mg/kg intravenous flunixin in combination with a cornual nerve block had decreased cortisol concentrations at 3 hours postprocedure, compared with those calves administered only a cornual nerve block and untreated control calves. However, by 6 hours and beyond, no significant difference in cortisol concentrations among treatment groups were observed.

Salicylic acid derivatives

Baldridge and colleagues[32] investigated the effects of 2.5 to 5 mg/mL sodium salicylate administered in water 72 hours prior and 48 hours following a simultaneous surgical castration and amputation dehorning. An increased ADG was observed for 13 days in calves treated with an analgesic perioperatively. In addition, calves receiving sodium salicylate also had a significantly lower AUEC for cortisol 1 to 6 hours after dehorning-castration.

Sedative-Analgesic Drugs

Pharmaceutical agents such as α2-agonists, opioids, and N-methyl-D-aspartate (NMDA) receptor antagonists have all been investigated to determine the potential effects on pain biomarkers following dehorning. Potential benefits of these analgesics include the attenuation of the acute cortisol response, which can aid in the reduction of prolonged handling stress associated with dehorning; however, there is no evidence of continued analgesia following this initial period (see **Tables 4** and **5**).[8,23,24]

α2-Adrenergic agonists and opioids

Xylazine, a common α2-agonist, has been studied alone and in combination with opioids such as butorphanol, NMDA receptor antagonists (ketamine), and local anesthesia.[8,23,24,32] Grøndahl-Nielsen and colleagues[8] evaluated the effects of treatment with a cornual nerve block, xylazine (0.2 mg/kg), and butorphanol (0.1 mg/kg) intramuscularly, or no treatment on cortisol response in 4- to 6-week-old calves. This study found that cortisol increased significantly for calves in the untreated and dehorned group immediately after dehorning in comparison with the other treatment groups. However, after 10 minutes there was no significant difference among treatment groups.

The use of an α2-antagonist to reverse the sedative effects of an α2-agonist was studied to determine the effect on cortisol response following dehorning.[23] Tolazoline given to calves 5 minutes following dehorning resulted in a significant increase in cortisol concentrations greater than concentrations of those animals dehorned without analgesia. This effect was significantly prolonged for the 8 hours during which cortisol concentrations were measured; however, the AUEC was not significantly different.

Another study by Stilwell and colleagues[24] examined the effects of 0.2 mg/kg xylazine administered intramuscularly 10 minutes before dehorning, alone or in combination with 5 mL 2% lidocaine administered as a cornual nerve block on the cortisol response of calves dehorned by a hot iron. These treatments did not mitigate the cortisol response to dehorning, as both treatment groups had values significantly higher than those of control calves from 10 to 60 minutes after dehorning.

Tramadol

Tramadol ((1RS,2RS)-2[(dimethylamino-methyl]-1-(3-methoxyphenyl)-cyclohexanol) is a centrally acting analgesic primarily used in humans and companion animals to treat mild to moderate pain.[65,66] Analgesia is suggested to be a result of a dual mechanism involving both opioid-receptor activation and increased serotonin and norepinephrine transmission.[65] Although pharmacokinetic and pharmacodynamics values have not been determined in cattle, one study evaluated its antinociceptive potential following chemical dehorning in 3-week-old dairy calves using an intravenous dose of 4 mg/kg or a rectal dose of 200 mg.[67] Following an evaluation of pain-associated behaviors while using a numerical rating scale to determine pain levels, tramadol administered at the investigated doses and routes did not provide adequate analgesia for controlling pain related to chemical dehorning.

FUTURE PROSPECTS FOR TREATING PAIN ASSOCIATED WITH DEHORNING

A multimodal approach is necessary for the continued treatment and management of pain associated with dehorning. Education is paramount to the successful delivery of analgesia to cattle following common noxious procedures. This aspect is best evidenced in a Canadian survey concerning analgesia associated with dehorning, which found that clinicians in geographic areas with aggressive education in pain management were more likely to provide analgesia at the time of noxious procedures.[15] In addition, research needs to continue to determine better biomarkers of pain to improve the assessment of an appropriate analgesic therapy. Finally, artificial selection by breeding polled sires will aid in decreasing the population of horned animals.

SUMMARY

The literature focusing on pain management in cattle during dehorning is plentiful. As demonstrated, there have been several studies looking at the effects of dehorning on concentrations of plasma cortisol. In addition, several analgesic regimens have been used in efforts to relieve pain during these procedures, with varying results. Following this review, the authors suggest a multimodal approach using local anesthetics, NSAIDs and, when possible, sedatives with analgesic properties to best provide analgesia to cattle following dehorning (see **Tables 4** and **5**). Local anesthetics and sedative-analgesics aid in the attenuation of the acute cortisol response, and NSAIDs mitigate the observed inflammation-associated pain. As with all pharmaceutical agents administered to food-producing species, especially for the treatment of pain, valid veterinary client-patient relationships must be maintained and appropriate withdrawal times must be followed. Further research should be implemented to determine safe, long-lasting, and cost-effective analgesics for food animals following noxious procedures.

REFERENCES

1. American Veterinary Medical Association. Welfare implications of dehorning and disbudding of cattle; 2012. Available at: https://www.avma.org/KB/Resources/Backgrounders/Documents/dehorning_cattle_bgnd.pdf. Accessed September 1, 2012.
2. Stafford KJ, Mellor DJ. Dehorning and disbudding distress and its alleviation in calves. Vet J 2005;169(3):337–49.
3. Medugorac I, Seichter D, Graf A, et al. Bovine polledness—an autosomal dominant trait with allelic heterogeneity. PLoS One 2012;7:11.

4. USDA. Beef 2007-08. Part III: changes in the U.S. beef cow-calf industry, 1993-2008. USDA-APHIS National Animal Health Monitoring System; 2009. 79.
5. USDA. Dairy 2007: part V: changes in dairy cattle health and management practices in the United States, 1996-2007. USDA-APHIS National Animal Health Monitoring System; 2009. 91.
6. Sylvester SP, Stafford KJ, Mellor DJ, et al. Acute cortisol responses of calves to four methods of dehorning by amputation. Aust Vet J 1998;76:123–6.
7. Graf B, Senn M. Behavioural and physiological responses of calves to dehorning by heat cauterization with or without local anaesthesia. Appl Anim Behav Sci 1999;62:153–71.
8. Grøndahl-Nielsen C, Simonsen HB, Lund JD, et al. Behavioural, endocrine and cardiac responses in young calves undergoing dehorning without and with use of sedation and analgesia. Vet J 1999;158:14–20.
9. Rollin BE. Veterinary medical ethics. Can Vet J 2012;53:223–4.
10. Bradley A, MacRae R. Legitimacy and Canadian farm animal welfare standards development: the case of the National Farm Animal Care Council. J Agr Environ Ethics 2011;24:19–47.
11. American Veterinary Medical Association. AVMA Policy: castration and dehorning of cattle; 2008. Available at: https://www.avma.org/KB/Policies/Pages/Castration-and-Dehorning-of-Cattle.aspx. Accessed September 1, 2012.
12. Coetzee JF, Nutsch AL, Barbur LA, et al. A survey of castration methods and associated livestock management practices performed by bovine veterinarians in the United States. BMC Vet Res 2010;6:19.
13. Fulwider WK, Grandin T, Rollin BE, et al. Survey of dairy management practices on one hundred thirteen north central and northeastern united states dairies. J Dairy Sci 2008;91:1686–92.
14. Fajt VR, Wagner SA, Norby B. Analgesic drug administration and attitudes about analgesia in cattle among bovine practitioners in the United States. J Am Vet Med Assoc 2011;238:755–67.
15. Hewson CJ, Dohoo IR, Lemke KA, et al. Factors affecting Canadian veterinarians' use of analgesics when dehorning beef and dairy calves. Can Vet J 2007;48: 1129–36.
16. Stafford KJ, Mellor DJ. Addressing the pain associated with disbudding and dehorning in cattle. Appl Anim Behav Sci 2011;135:226–31.
17. Petrie NJ, Mellor DJ, Stafford KJ, et al. Cortisol responses of calves to two methods of disbudding used with or without local anaesthetic. N Z Vet J 1996; 44(1):9–14.
18. McMeekan CM, Mellor DJ, Stafford KJ, et al. Effects of local anaesthesia of 4 to 8 hours' duration on the acute cortisol response to scoop dehorning in calves. Aust Vet J 1998;76(4):281–5.
19. Sutherland MA, Mellow DJ, Stafford KJ, et al. Cortisol responses to dehorning of calves given a 5-h local anaesthetic regimen plus phenylbutazone, ketoprofen, or adrenocorticotropic hormone prior to dehorning. Res Vet Sci 2002;73(2):115–23.
20. McMeekan CM, Stafford KJ, Mellor DJ, et al. Effects of regional analgesia and/or a non-steroidal anti-inflammatory analgesic on the acute cortisol response to dehorning in calves. Res Vet Sci 1998;64(2):147–50.
21. Stilwell G, de Carvalho RC, Lima MS, et al. Effect of caustic paste disbudding, using local anaesthesia with and without analgesia, on behaviour and cortisol of calves. Appl Anim Behav Sci 2009;116:35–44.
22. Milligan BN, Duffield T, Lissemore K. The utility of ketoprofen for alleviating pain following dehorning in young dairy calves. Can Vet J 2004;45(2):140–3.

23. Stafford KJ, Mellor DJ, Todd SE, et al. The effect of different combinations of lignocaine, ketoprofen, xylazine and tolazoline on the acute cortisol response to dehorning in calves. N Z Vet J 2003;51(5):219–26.

24. Stilwell G, Carvalho RC, Carolino N, et al. Effect of hot-iron disbudding on behaviour and plasma cortisol of calves sedated with xylazine. Res Vet Sci 2010;88(1): 188–93.

25. Anil SS, Anil L, Deen J. Challenges of pain assessment in domestic animals. J Am Vet Med Assoc 2002;220:313–9.

26. Morisse JP, Cotte JP, Huonnic D. Effect of dehorning on behavior and plasma cortisol responses in young calves. Appl Anim Behav Sci 1995;43:239–47.

27. Faulkner PM, Weary DM. Reducing pain after dehorning in dairy calves. J Dairy Sci 2000;83(9):2037–41.

28. Vickers KJ, Niel L, Kiehlbauch LM, et al. Calf response to caustic paste and hot-iron dehorning using sedation with and without local anesthetic. J Dairy Sci 2005; 88(4):1454–9.

29. Heinrich A, Duffield TF, Lissemore KD, et al. The effect of meloxicam on behavior and pain sensitivity of dairy calves following cautery dehorning with a local anesthetic. J Dairy Sci 2010;93:2450–7.

30. Doherty TJ, Kattesh HG, Adcock RJ, et al. Effects of a concentrated lidocaine solution on the acute phase stress response to dehorning in dairy calves. J Dairy Sci 2007;90:4232–9.

31. Duffield TF, Heinrich A, Millman ST, et al. Reduction in pain response by combined use of local lidocaine anesthesia and systemic ketoprofen in dairy calves dehorned by heat cauterization. Can Vet J 2010;51:283–8.

32. Baldridge SL, Coetzee JE, Dritz SS, et al. Pharmacokinetics and physiologic effects of intramuscularly administered xylazine hydrochloride-ketamine hydrochloride-butorphanol tartrate alone or in combination with orally administered sodium salicylate on biomarkers of pain in Holstein calves following castration and dehorning. Am J Vet Res 2011;72:1305–17.

33. Theurer ME, White BJ, Coetzee JF, et al. Assessment of behavioral changes associated with oral meloxicam administration at time of dehorning in calves using a remote triangulation device and accelerometers. BMC Vet Res 2012; 8:48.

34. Molony V, Kent JE. Assessment of acute pain in farm animals using behavioral and physiological measurements. J Anim Sci 1997;75:266–72.

35. Mellor DJ, Stafford KJ. Interpretation of cortisol responses in calf disbudding studies. N Z Vet J 1997;45(3):126–7.

36. Boandl KE, Wohlt JE, Carsia RV. Effects of handling, administration of a local anesthetic, and electrical dehorning on plasma cortisol in Holstein calves. J Dairy Sci 1989;72(8):2193–7.

37. Stilwell G, Lima MS, Broom DM. Comparing plasma cortisol and behaviour of calves dehorned with caustic paste after non-steroidal-anti-inflammatory analgesia. Livest Sci 2008;119:63–9.

38. Schwartzkopf-Genswein KS, Booth-McLean ME, McAllister TA, et al. Physiological and behavioural changes in Holstein calves during and after dehorning or castration. Can J Anim Sci 2005;85:131–8.

39. Laden SA, Wohlt JE, Zajac PK, et al. Effects of stress from electrical dehorning on feed-intake, growth, and blood constituents of Holstein heifer calves. J Dairy Sci 1985;68:3062–6.

40. Heinrich A, Duffield TF, Lissemore KD, et al. The impact of meloxicam on postsurgical stress associated with cautery dehorning. J Dairy Sci 2009;92:540–7.

41. Stewart M, Stookey JM, Stafford KJ, et al. Effects of local anesthetic and a nonsteroidal antiinflammatory drug on pain responses of dairy calves to hot-iron dehorning. J Dairy Sci 2009;92:1512–9.

42. Coetzee JF, Mosher RA, KuKanich B, et al. Pharmacokinetics and effect of intravenous meloxicam in weaned Holstein calves following scoop dehorning without local anesthesia. BMC Vet Res 2012;8:153. http://dx.doi.org/10.1186/1746-6148-8-153.

43. Stewart M, Stafford KJ, Dowling SK, et al. Eye temperature and heart rate variability of calves disbudded with or without local anaesthetic. Physiol Behav 2008;93:789–97.

44. Sylvester SP, Stafford KJ, Mellor DJ, et al. Behavioural responses of calves to amputation dehorning with and without local anaesthesia. Aust Vet J 2004;82:697–700.

45. Mellor DJ, Stafford KJ, Todd SE, et al. A comparison of catecholamine and cortisol responses of young lambs and calves to painful husbandry procedures. Aust Vet J 2002;80(4):228–33.

46. Gibson TJ, Johnson CB, Stafford KJ, et al. Validation of the acute electroencephalographic responses of calves to noxious stimulus with scoop dehorning. N Z Vet J 2007;55:152–7.

47. Coetzee JF. A review of pain assessment techniques and pharmacological approaches to pain relief after bovine castration: practical implications for cattle production within the United States. Appl Anim Behav Sci 2011;135:192–213.

48. Coetzee JF, Lubbers BV, Toerber SE, et al. Plasma concentrations of substance P and cortisol in beef calves after castration or simulated castration. Am J Vet Res 2008;69:751–62.

49. von Borell E, Langbein J, Despres G, et al. Heart rate variability as a measure of autonomic regulation of cardiac activity for assessing stress and welfare in farm animals—a review. Physiol Behav 2007;92:293–316.

50. Bergamasco L, Coetzee JF, Gehring R, et al. Quantitative electroencephalographic findings associated with nociception following surgical castration in conscious calves. J Vet Pharmacol Ther 2011. http://dx.doi.org/10.1111/j.1365-2885.2011.01269.x.

51. McMeekan CM, Mellor DJ, Stafford KJ, et al. Effects of shallow scoop and deep scoop dehorning on plasma cortisol concentrations in calves. N Z Vet J 1997; 45(2):72–4.

52. Lester SJ, Mellor DJ, Ward RN, et al. Cortisol response of young lambs to castration and tailing using different methods. N Z Vet J 1991;39:134–8.

53. Wohlt JE, Allyn ME, Zajac PK, et al. Cortisol increases in plasma of Holstein heifer calves from handling and method of electrical dehorning. J Dairy Sci 1994; 77(12):3725–9.

54. Sylvester SP, Mellor DJ, Stafford KJ, et al. Acute cortisol responses of calves to scoop dehorning using local anaesthesia and/or cautery of the wound. Aust Vet J 1998;76:118–22.

55. Sutherland MA, Mellor DJ, Stafford KJ, et al. Effect of local anaesthetic combined with wound cauterisation on the cortisol response to dehorning in calves. Aust Vet J 2002;80(3):165–7.

56. Webb AI, Pablo LS. Local anesthetics. In: Riviere JE, Papich MG, editors. Veterinary pharmacology and therapeutics. 9th edition. Ames (IA): Wiley-Blackwell; 2009. p. 382.

57. Skarda RT. Techniques of local analgesia in ruminants and swine. Vet Clin North Am Food Anim Pract 1986;2:621–63.

58. Fierheller EE, Caulkett NA, Haley DB, et al. Onset, duration and efficacy of four methods of local anesthesia of the horn bud in calves. Vet Anaesth Analg 2012;39:431–5.

59. Sellers G, Lin HC, Riddell MG, et al. Pharmacokinetics of lidocaine in serum and milk of mature Holstein cows. J Vet Pharmacol Ther 2009;32(5):446–50.

60. McMeekan C, Stafford KJ, Mellor DJ, et al. Effects of a local anaesthetic and a non-steroidal anti-inflammatory analgesic on the behavioural responses of calves to dehorning. N Z Vet J 1999;47(3):92–6.

61. Landoni MF, Cunningham FM, Lees P. Pharmacokinetics and pharmacodynamics of ketoprofen in calves applying PK/PD modeling. J Vet Pharmacol Ther 1995;18: 315–24.

62. Smith GW, Davis JL, Tell LA, et al. FARAD digest—Extralabel use of nonsteroidal anti-inflammatory drugs in cattle. J Am Vet Med Assoc 2008;232(5):697–701.

63. Lees P, Landoni MF, Giraudel J, et al. Pharmacodynamics and pharmacokinetics of nonsteroidal anti-inflammatory drugs in species of veterinary interest. J Vet Pharmacol Ther 2004;27:479–90.

64. Lees P, Giraudel J, Landoni MF, et al. PK-PD integration and PK-PD modelling of nonsteroidal anti-inflammatory drugs: principles and applications in veterinary pharmacology. J Vet Pharmacol Ther 2004;27:491–502.

65. Reeves RR, Burke RS. Tramadol: basic pharmacology and emerging concepts. Drugs Today 2008;44:827–36.

66. KuKanich B, Papich MG. Pharmacokinetics and antinociceptive effects of oral tramadol hydrochloride administration in Greyhounds. Am J Vet Res 2011;72: 256–62.

67. Braz M, Carreira M, Carolino N, et al. Effect of rectal or intravenous tramadol on the incidence of pain-related behaviour after disbudding calves with caustic paste. Appl Anim Behav Sci 2012;136:20–5.

Assessment and Management of Pain Associated with Lameness in Cattle

Jan K. Shearer, DVM, MS[a],*, Matthew L. Stock, VMD[b],
Sarel R. Van Amstel, BVSc, M MED VET[c],
Johann F. Coetzee, BVSc, Cert CHP, PhD[b,d]

KEYWORDS

- Lameness • Locomotion scoring systems • Pain management • Cattle

KEY POINTS

- Lameness impacts the cattle industry in economic losses and welfare considerations.
- To improve earlier detection and treatment of lameness, locomotion scoring systems have been developed for routine use by farm employees.
- Earlier analgesia treatment may aid in the alleviation of acute pain perception or in the mitigation of wind-up that can lead to central sensitization.
- In lame cattle, pain can best be alleviated by implementing a multimodal approach including corrective claw trimming and placement of foot blocks combined with additional benefits provided by analgesic compounds.

Lameness impacts the cattle industry in economic losses and welfare considerations. In addition to production deficits, pain and distress associated with lameness have been documented.[1] Furthermore, the evaluation and prevalence of lame cattle is one of the primary factors in third-party welfare audit programs including National Dairy Farmers Assuring Responsible Management Program, Validus, New York State Cattle Health Assurance Program, and others.[2–4] Involuntary culling of lame cattle continues to be an important reason for losses in the dairy and beef industries.[5,6] Mean lameness prevalence in herds has been reported as 33.7% and 36.8% in Wisconsin and the United Kingdom, respectively; however, in other survey studies a less than 10% prevalence of lame cattle was reported by producers.[7–9] It should be noted

[a] Dairy Production Medicine, Lameness, Animal Welfare, Iowa State University, Ames, IA 50011, USA; [b] Department of Biomedical Science, College of Veterinary Medicine, Iowa State University, Ames, IA 50011, USA; [c] Department of Large Animal Clinical Sciences, College of Veterinary Medicine, The University of Tennessee, Knoxville, TN 37996, USA; [d] Department of Veterinary Diagnostic and Production Medicine, College of Veterinary Medicine, Iowa State University, Ames, IA 50011, USA
* Corresponding author. Department of Veterinary Diagnostic and Production Animal Medicine, College of Veterinary Medicine, Iowa State University, Ames, IA 50011, USA.
E-mail address: jks@iastate.edu

Vet Clin Food Anim 29 (2013) 135–156
http://dx.doi.org/10.1016/j.cvfa.2012.11.012
0749-0720/13/$ – see front matter © 2013 Published by Elsevier Inc.
vetfood.theclinics.com

that lameness is usually underreported by producers compared with independent observers potentially because of a decreased objectivity or diagnostic sensitivity in detecting lame cattle.[10,11]

To improve earlier detection and treatment of lameness, locomotion scoring systems have been developed for routine use by farm employees.[12,13] It has been suggested that earlier analgesia treatment may aid in the alleviation of acute pain perception or in the mitigation of wind-up that can lead to central sensitization.[14] Central sensitization is responsible for the observed pain-related behavioral changes through increased sensitivity of pain (hyperalgesia) and pain from nonpainful stimuli (allodynia).[14] Whay and colleagues[1] reported hyperalgesia in lame cattle compared with sound animals through significant decreases in nociceptive thresholds at the time of lameness detection and 28 days later suggesting prolonged chronicity. Analgesic treatment difficulties in chronic lame cattle may be best explained through the aforementioned central sensitization based on current pain models. As a result, preemptive analgesia that is usually advocated is difficult, if not impossible, to implement in lame cattle.[14] Recommendations for pain management typically include the use of a multimodal therapeutic approach (discussed by Coetzee JF and colleagues, elsewhere in this issue). Similarly, in lame cattle, pain can best be alleviated by implementing a multimodal approach including corrective claw trimming and placement of foot blocks combined with additional benefits provided by analgesic compounds.

ASSESSMENT OF PAIN IN LAME CATTLE
Locomotion or Lameness Scoring Systems

Behavioral changes associated with lameness indicate attempts by the animal to protect the affected limb from further injury.[15] Although these may vary between individual animals, such signs as head bobbing, an arching of the spine, or changes in stride length allow rapid identification of lame individuals.[15] Changes in posture associated with lameness have been summarized in an excellent review article by Whay[15] and form the basis of most locomotion scoring systems. An arched back is frequently associated with lameness and is the key behavioral change evaluated in the Sprecher lameness scoring system (**Table 1**).[12] Other behavioral changes associated with lameness that can be visually scored include the following[15]:

1. Hanging or "bobbing" of the head during locomotion
2. Shortening or lengthening of the stride

Table 1	
Sprecher lameness scoring system	
Lameness Score	**Clinical Description**
1	Normal-Stands and walks normally, with all feet placed with purpose
2	Mildly lame-Stands with flat back, but arches when walks, gait is slightly abnormal
3	Moderately lame-Stands and walks with an arched back, and short strides with one or more legs
4	Lame-Arched back standing and walking, with one or more limbs favored but at least partially weight bearing
5	Severely lame-Arched back, refuses to bear weight on one limb, may refuse or have great difficulty moving from lying position

From Sprecher DJ, Hostetler DE, Kaneene JB. A lameness scoring system that uses posture and gait to predict dairy cattle reproductive performance. Theriogenology 1997;47:1179; with permission.

3. Changes in the degree of abduction or adduction of the limbs with an increased deviation from the vertical seen in one hindlimb
4. Changes in claw placement (overextension or underextension of the stride) resulting in the hind claw not being placed in the same location as the front claw after initiation of the stride
5. Changes in the alignment of the pin bones (tuber coxae) when walking, which results in deviations from a hypothetical horizontal line when viewed from behind
6. Changes in the animal's willingness to walk with a reluctance to move being frequently associated with lameness affecting multiple claws
7. Changes in the stance phase of the stride resulting in the animal maintaining its weight on the sound limb for as long as possible to minimize weight-bearing time on the lame limb

The extent to which the aforementioned changes occur can be assigned a score ranging from a simple binomial score (present or absent) to an ordinal scale based on the presence and perceived severity of one or more of these behavioral signs in the same animal. Ordinal data should be analyzed using appropriate statistical methods and should not be subjected to analysis using such methods as paired t tests that are reserved for continuous data.

In the future, visual analog scales (VAS) may become more widely used as an alternative to ordinal locomotion scoring methods in a research setting because these generate continuous data. This information is considered to provide more robust outcomes when analyzed statistically because traditional methods of assessment for continuous data, such as t tests, can be used. The VAS is a 100-mm (10 cm) line anchored at either end by descriptors, typically "normal" or "lame," or in humans "no pain" or "worst pain imaginable."[13,16] The scorer marks the line between the two descriptors to indicate the lameness or pain intensity. A millimeter scale is used to measure the score from the zero anchor point to the scorer's mark. This system potentially provides 101 levels of intensity that are considered more sensitive for assessing the effects of an analgesic compound than an ordinal scale. Lame cattle have been successfully identified using overall VAS scores with VAS assessment possessing reasonable intraobserver and interobserver reliability; however, a five-point numeric rating system provided a better estimate of hoof lesions.[13] Additional research is necessary for further evaluation and its potential application.

A deficiency of locomotion scoring systems is the potential for a lack of reproducibility between scorers. This has restricted the use of locomotion scoring as a validated outcome measure for assessing analgesic efficacy during the drug approval process. In the authors experience (JFC), there is typically a 70% to 80% agreement between two masked scorers evaluating lameness simultaneously using the Sprecher system. Furthermore, male scorers tend to assign lower pain scores compared with female scorers. These factors have necessitated the development of more objective methods of pain assessment involving the use of force plates or pressure mats.

Pressure Mats

A commercially available floor mat–based pressure or force measurement system (MatScan; Tekscan, South Boston, MA) can be used to record and analyze naturally occurring or experimentally induced lameness. The pressure mat is calibrated daily and each time the computer software is engaged using a known mass to ensure accuracy of the measurements at each time point. Another benefit of this system is that video synchronization can be used to ensure consistent gait between and within calves for each time point and to correlate lameness scores with pressure mat data. Research-grade software (HUGEMAT Research 5.83; Tekscan) is used to determine the contact pressure, contact area, and stance phase duration in the affected claws. Surface area is calculated by area only of the loaded or "contact" sensing elements inside a measurement box. Contact pressure is calculated as force on the loaded sensing elements inside a measurement box divided by the contact area.[17]

Kotschwar and coworkers[17] found that contact surface area by Sprecher lameness score (LS) was different ($P = .018$) in calves subjected to induced lameness using amphotericin B. Calves with LS 1 had a greater surface area compared with LS 3 and 4 calves (**Fig. 1**). Furthermore, contact pressure was found to be different across Sprecher LS ($P = .02$) with calves classified as LS 3 exerting greater ground contact pressure compared with that of LS 1 calves (**Fig. 2**). This was likely caused by the calf weight being applied to a smaller contact surface area in calves with higher LS.

Weighing Platform

Much like the difference detected in pressure mats for lame cattle, weight distributions of individual limbs have also been calculated using a weighing platform (Pacific Industrial Scale, Richmond, British Columbia, Canada) containing four stainless steel load cells (3 mV Shear Beam Load cells; Anyload LLC, Santa Rosa, CA [maximum capacity = 454 kg/load cell]).[18–22] Neveus and colleagues[18] first described the use of this weight platform to measure the redistributions of weight to cattle limbs that occurs in response to pain associated with lameness. These platforms indicate cattle redistribute weight to avoid uncomfortable surfaces and distribute weight away from a limb with discomfort primarily toward the contralateral limb.[18] After studies involving the use of this assessment technique, variations in weight distributions in lame animals

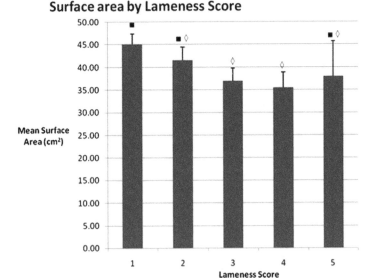

Fig. 1. Mean surface area ± SEM by lameness score for all treatment groups. Data points with different symbols indicate $P<.05$. (*From* Kotschwar JL, Coetzee JF, Anderson DE, et al. Analgesic efficacy of sodium salicylate in an amphotericin B-induced bovine synovitis-arthritis model. J Dairy Sci 2009;92:3731–43; with permission.)

Contact Pressure by Lameness Score

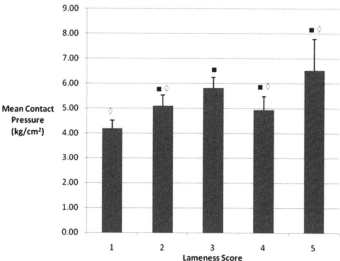

Fig. 2. Mean contact pressure ± SEM by lameness score for all treatment groups. Data points with different symbols indicate *P*<.05. (*From* Kotschwar JL, Coetzee JF, Anderson DE, et al. Analgesic efficacy of sodium salicylate in an amphotericin B-induced bovine synovitis-arthritis model. J Dairy Sci 2009;92:3731–43; with permission.)

were mildly attenuated through the use of analgesia, such as nonsteroidal anti-inflammatory drugs (NSAIDs) or a local anesthetic.[20–22]

Nociceptive Threshold

Because of a hyperalgesic state, it has been suggested lame cattle have a more sensitive and exaggerated reaction to noxious stimuli compared with sound animals.[1] Using a mechanical pneumatic blunt pin (2 mm in diameter) pressed on the dorsal aspect of the metatarsus with gradually increasing pressure, a reaction from the animal can be observed.[23,24] The pressure in which the reaction occurs has been recorded as the nociceptive threshold, thus presumably quantifying regional sensitivity and potentially pain. The results of this test may be related to other sensory perception rather than pain but Whay and colleagues[24] described the use of nociceptive threshold as a more sensitive measure of pain associated with lameness compared with a visual locomotion scoring technique. Increased nociceptive thresholds have been reported in cattle over a 28-day period after 3 days of ketoprofen administered at the detection of lameness[24]; however, this suggested long-term attenuation of the hyperalgesic state caused by the administration of NSAIDs was not observed in another study using nociceptive thresholds.[25]

Heart Rate

Heart rate data can be recorded and analyzed using commercially available heart rate monitors and the associated research software (RS800 and Polar Pro Trainer Equine Edition; Polar Electro, Lake Success, NY). The heart rate monitor consists of a transmitter placed over the heart in the left foreflank attached to a girth strap placed around the heart girth of the calves. A wrist unit attached to the elastic strap receives and records the signal from the transmitter. Appropriate conductance for the electrodes on the strap, one positioned on the sternum and one over the right scapula, is facilitated by use of ultrasound gel. The transmitter measures the electric signal (electrocardiogram) of the heart every 15 seconds. Kotschwar and coworkers[17] found that mean heart rate was less in LS 1 calves compared with that of LS 2, 3, and 4 calves (**Fig. 3**).

Cortisol Response

Serum cortisol can be determined using a solid-phase competitive chemiluminescent enzyme immunoassay and an automated analyzer system (Immulite 1000 Cortisol; Siemens Medical Solutions Diagnostics, Los Angeles, CA) or a radiolabeled immunoassay. Kotschwar and coworkers[17] reported that mean serum cortisol concentrations were less in LS 1 calves compared with that of LS 3 calves ($P = .004$) (**Fig. 4**).

Accelerometers

Accelerometers are devices that continuously measure gravitational force in multiple axes, and these values can be processed to determine activity and postural behaviors (discussed by Theurer ME and colleagues, elsewhere in this issue). Schulz and coworkers[26] reported that flunixin-treated steers spent a significantly greater percentage of time standing after lameness induction with amphotericin B than the control calves in the initial postinduction period.

PAIN MANAGEMENT USING CORRECTIVE CLAW TRIMMING AND FOOT BLOCKS

Most assume that the management of pain associated with lameness requires the use of some form of anti-inflammatory therapy. However, the discomfort caused by claw lesions can be dramatically reduced by corrective trimming techniques and the application of a foot block to the healthy claw. Beyond corrective trimming and the relief of

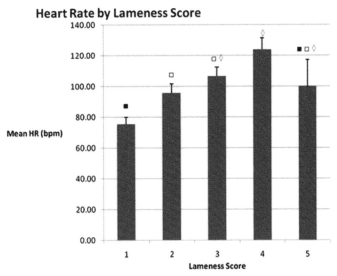

Fig. 3. Mean heart rate ± SEM by lameness score for all treatment groups. Data points with different symbols indicate $P<.05$. (*From* Kotschwar JL, Coetzee JF, Anderson DE, et al. Analgesic efficacy of sodium salicylate in an amphotericin B-induced bovine synovitis-arthritis model. J Dairy Sci 2009;92:3731–43; with permission.)

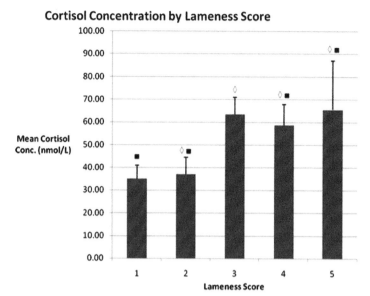

Fig. 4. Mean cortisol concentration ± SEM by lameness score for all treatment groups. Data points with different symbols indicate P<.05. (*From* Kotschwar JL, Coetzee JF, Anderson DE, et al. Analgesic efficacy of sodium salicylate in an amphotericin B-induced bovine synovitis-arthritis model. J Dairy Sci 2009;92:3731–43; with permission.)

weight bearing on injured claws are housing considerations, whereby moving animals to pastures or special needs areas can increase the comfort of uncomfortable cows.

Pathogenesis of Claw Lesions

Ulcers and white line disease are largely a consequence of metabolic disorders and mechanical loading that contributes to injury of the solar and perioplic (corium of the heel) corium.[27] The metabolic conditions predisposing to claw lesions include rumen acidosis and laminitis, activation of metalloproteinases, and hormonal changes, specifically relaxin and estrogen in the peripartum period.[28–31] The mechanical loading occurs from the overgrowth of claw horn that leads to unbalanced weight bearing whereby the damage associated with metabolic disease disorders is compounded by excessive weight load.[32]

Traumatic lesions of the sole associated with penetration of the sole by foreign bodies, such as a nail, stone, or other sharp object, are a common cause of subsolar abscess formation. Depending on the depth of penetration, these types of lesions can have serious consequences. For example, when the foreign body is able to penetrate sufficiently deep to make contact with the third phalanx, a severe osteitis is likely to develop. In cases where the foreign object penetrates only the more superficial tissues of the corium and digital cushion, the prognosis is more favorable.

Complicated lesions of the claw or foot that result in deep digital sepsis cause severe lameness and extreme discomfort for affected animals. The options for management of deep digital sepsis conditions include surgery and euthanasia. The key to minimizing pain is early recognition of the condition and prompt application of the most appropriate of these options taking into consideration the likely prognosis, cost, and welfare of the animal.

Corrective Trimming to Relieve Pain and Promote Recovery from Claw Lesions

Cows with lameness disorders involving the claw capsule of the digit or claw generally require some degree of corrective trimming. This consists of the removal of all necrotic and loose or undermined horn to create an aerobic microenvironment that reduces the possibility of further complication associated with abscess formation. When these procedures are conducted carefully to avoid damage to peripheral tissues of the corium, postprocedural pain is minimized and the rate of recovery more rapid.[32–35]

A second step in the corrective trimming of claw lesions is to adjust weight bearing on diseased or damaged claws. This may be accomplished by trimming the weight-bearing surface of the injured claw lower and further by applying a foot block to the healthy claw.[32–35] By adjusting weight bearing on injured claws, pain is relieved and healing may proceed without interruption.

Although frequently used, topical treatment and the application of a bandage or wrap are generally not advised.[32–35] Exceptions to this include conditions in which corrective trimming has resulted in severe bleeding (should occur rarely) or the exposure of a large area of the corium for which protection of these delicate tissues is desired. Good restraint, local anesthesia as needed, and a sharp knife are the primary tools required for corrective trimming procedures.

Anesthesia of the Lower Limb and Foot

Whenever it is necessary to perform procedures that may be uncomfortable, anesthesia is indicated. There are at least two methods: intravenous regional anesthesia and ring block. Both procedures are easy to perform under field conditions. In addition to alleviating discomfort for the cow, anesthesia lessens movement of the foot associated with corrective trimming adjacent to sensitive tissues of the corium. This eases trimming procedures and reduces the potential for inadvertent movement by the cow that might lead to accidental damage of healthy tissues.

Anesthesia of the foot is indicated for corrective trimming and surgical conditions that are likely to be uncomfortable. All that is required is a tourniquet, 20 to 30 mL of 2% lidocaine, and a 1-in 19-gauge butterfly catheter. Veins used most commonly are those on the medial or lateral aspect of the digits (ie, medial and lateral digital veins, respectively) approximately 1-in anterior to the dewclaws or the common digital vein, which lies on the dorsal aspect on the midline below the fetlock and between the digits.[33,35]

Intravenous regional anesthesia

For anesthesia of the foot, begin by applying a tourniquet approximately 3 to 4 in above the fetlock joint. Next, prepare the injection site by doing a light surgical scrub to clean the injection site areas. Some prefer to shave these areas to improve asepsis. It is a good idea to prepare two sites (eg, the front and lateral or medial aspects) in case a second site is needed. After the site is prepared, remove the butterfly catheter from its package, along with the needle guard and end cap on the extension tube. Pick the desired site for introduction of the needle (note that the vein may not be visible, so placement of the needle is often where the vein is likely to be). The needle is inserted rapidly and straight into the desired area (perpendicular to the skin, do not try to thread the needle into the vein) (**Fig. 5**). The cow may jerk or move her leg slightly as the needle is inserted. Next, slowly remove the needle outward until blood flows into the catheter. As soon as there is a good flow of blood into the catheter, attach the syringe of lidocaine to the extension tube and administer it into the vein. It is best to inject the lidocaine over a period of 30 to 60 seconds to avoid damage to the vein. Complete anesthesia is usually accomplished within 3 to 5 minutes. In chronic cases where there is extreme inflammation anesthesia may require a larger dose of lidocaine (30 mL) and

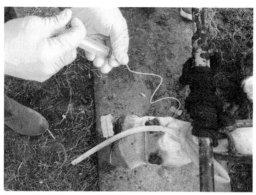

Fig. 5. Intravenous regional anesthesia with a tourniquet and 20 mL of lidocaine administered using 19-gauge butterfly catheter.

a little longer for complete anesthesia. The tourniquet should not be left in place longer than 45 minutes and certainly less if at all possible. Anesthesia is relatively short-lived after the tourniquet is removed.

On release from the trimming chute the cow has immediate use of the foot and walks noticeably better (ie, without lameness assuming the problem was in the foot) tempting one to think the problem has been remedied by the treatment just performed. Although some of the improvement may be a result of the treatment, anesthesia masks much of the discomfort until its effects have worn off, which usually occurs over a period of 30 to 60 minutes beyond removal of the tourniquet.

Ring block anesthesia
The ring block generally requires more lidocaine and a little more time for complete anesthesia. There are four sites for injection of the lidocaine. First, on the midline of the dorsal aspect of the digit below the fetlock joint place a 1.5-in needle directly (anterior to posterior) into this region to the hub and inject approximately 15 to 20 mL as the needle is withdrawn being sure to deposit approximately 2 mL subcutaneously. Do the same on the posterior or ventral aspect by placement of a 1.5-in needle into the skin fold or crease (between the digits) and inject 15 to 20 mL of lidocaine as the needle is withdrawn. The final two injections are on the medial and lateral aspects of the lower leg just above the dewclaws; inject 10 to 15 mL of lidocaine subcutaneously going from anterior to posterior, beginning approximately 2 in dorsal to the dewclaws.[33,35] Complete anesthesia may require a little longer than that achieved by the intravenous route depending on how much the blood supply to affected areas has been compromised by the inflammatory response. A tourniquet is unnecessary for this procedure.

APPLICATION OF CORRECTIVE TRIMMING PROCEDURES

Raven[32] describes the principles of corrective hoof trimming as removal of all loose or undermined, necrotic horn tissue without causing damage to adjacent healthy tissues; and adjustment of weight bearing within and between the claws by raising the affected area of the injured or diseased claw so that it does not bear weight.

The primary claw lesions are ulcers, white line disease, and traumatic lesions of the sole. Regardless of cause, they are all treated by the application of these principles of corrective trimming.

Removal of Loose and Undermined Claw Horn

Whenever claw horn lesions are encountered, the first step is removal of all loose horn irrespective of how extensive it might be. Pare away hard ridges to create smooth surfaces so that there is less of a tendency for the collection or entrapment of organic matter in horn lesions. Only healthy hoof horn should be left in place.

Always slope horn away from the lesion. Never dig holes in the sole, because these are quickly filled by organic matter that prevents or delays healing. For example, trim the area around sole ulcers and slope the sole axially. When trimming white line lesions slope the lesion abaxially and remove portions of the lateral wall, white line, and sole that are defective. Trim carefully and try not to damage new healthy horn. In all cases, avoid damage to the corium (ie, stop when trimming leads to bleeding of the corium).

Adjust Weight Bearing on Damaged Claws

When confronted with claw lesions, pare the damaged claw lower to increase weight bearing on the healthy claw. In most cases the diseased claw is the outside claw of the rear and medial claw of the front feet. Specific indications for this trimming procedure include conditions in which overgrowth has led to overloading or excessive weight bearing on the claw. Lowering the damaged claw reduces weight-bearing and thus pain, and permits recovery and eventual return to normal function and health. In many cases it is necessary to apply a claw block to the healthy claw to achieve reduced weight bearing in the damaged claw. The details of claw block application are described next.

FOOT BLOCKS FOR RELIEF OF WEIGHT-BEARING IN DISEASED OR INJURED CLAWS

The application of corrective trimming procedures often provide a sufficient difference in height between the two claws to relieve weight bearing and promote recovery of claw lesions. However, when pain is severe or one is unable to create sufficient difference in height between the two claws, additional elevation of the diseased claw can be achieved by means of a block attached to the sound claw. Proper application of claw blocks requires attention to the following[32–35]:

1. Before attaching a block to the healthy claw, the claw must be pared flat and in the same plane as the corresponding injured claw. When claws have been trimmed by the functional trimming method, claws are already flat ready (or near ready) for the application of a foot block. This provides a bearing surface that is perpendicular to the long axis of the leg.
2. Prepare the claw with a rasp or angle grinder fitted with a grinding wheel or sand paper–type disk so that the block adhesive properly adheres to the wall and sole of the claw.
3. Mix the adhesive to the proper consistency and apply to the block and claw as needed. Follow the manufacturer's directions for proper use of adhesives.
4. Apply the block and position it so that it lies flat on the sole and provides proper support of the heel. This is one of the most common mistakes made in applying blocks. Blocks should be even with the back of the heel bulb to provide sufficient support.
5. Always ensure that adhesive is cleared away from the area between the block and the heel. Heel horn is very soft and can easily be damaged by the hard and sometimes very sharp edges of fully cured adhesive material.
6. Remove blocks after a period of 3 to 4 weeks. Blocks that are wearing abnormally or cause discomfort before then should be removed sooner. Encourage owners,

managers, and employees to pull cows that are not walking correctly on blocked claws. Note that foot blocks generally wear faster at the heel. Furthermore, as the claw grows, the block tends to gradually move forward. Wear at the heel and continued claw horn growth results in upward rotation of the toe of the blocked claw. Excess weight bearing and continued trauma to the heel may lead to the formation of a sole or heel ulcer. It is for this reason that readers are advised to monitor claw blocks and recheck no later than 30 days after application (sooner in conditions where block wear is more rapid).

7. After removing a block, always retrim the foot and adjust weight bearing as needed. Foot blocks are a critical adjunct to the therapy for claw lesions; however, they do require management by observation and changing as necessary. One scenario might be to use a foot block to treat acute claw lesions that result in lameness during the first 30 days. After this time, recheck the foot and remove the claw block, retrim the claws, and adjust weight bearing in the damaged claw by lowering the damaged portion.

THE APPLICATION OF BANDAGES OR WRAPS TO LESIONS OF THE CLAW CAPSULE

Correction of horn lesions often results in small to moderate exposure of the corium. In general, minor lesions or injuries to the corium are best left untreated and without a bandage. Severe lesions in which large areas of the corium may be exposed may benefit from topical treatment with a mild antiseptic or nonirritating antibiotic under a bandage with the proviso that it be removed within 3 to 5 days. If it is the practice of the dairy to allow bandages to fall off on their own, they should probably be left off from the start. Indeed, results from a Cornell study comparing cows with claw lesions with a wrap verses no wrap indicate no advantage to the application of bandage.[36]

The environment of most dairy cows is such that bandages become very contaminated within a day or so of application. It is doubtful that they offer significant therapeutic benefit beyond this point. A second problem with bandages in herds using footbaths is that after one or two trips through the footbath, the bandage becomes soaked with footbath solutions. These are generally very irritating types of formulations (eg, formaldehyde and copper sulfate) and prone to cause increased irritation to raw corium tissues.

However, antibiotics under a loose wrap are very effective for treatment of infectious skin disorders, such as digital dermatitis.[33–35] Lesions treated with topical oxytetracycline under a bandage seem to respond rapidly with cows demonstrating improved gait and pain relief within 24 hours of treatment. The improvement after treatment of digital dermatitis with topical antibiotics demonstrates the value of properly directed therapy whereby antibiotics are used to treat an infectious skin disease. Claw lesions in cows are unlikely to respond to topical antibiotic therapy because their pathogenesis is related to metabolic and mechanical factors rather than infectious agents.

TOPICAL THERAPY OF CLAW LESIONS: WHY OR WHY NOT?

Claw lesions are indeed very painful conditions that generally cause one to conclude that surely some form of topical treatment and a bandage would be an essential part of therapy. In reality, it is quite likely that treatment beyond corrective trimming and a foot block is counterproductive.

The best way to understand why it may not be beneficial to aggressively treat claw lesions is to consider their pathogenesis. Sole ulcers, for example, are lesions that develop as a consequence of the sinking of the third phalanx (P3) within the claw horn capsule subsequent to laminitis, activated metalloproteinase enzymes, or hormonal changes. Regardless of cause, the sinking of P3 results in compression of the solar corium and digital cushion immediately beneath P3 that is exacerbated by claw horn overgrowth, particularly of the outside claw of the rear foot. After a period of time and with continued trauma to these tissues, the formation horn at the heel-sole junction (described as the "typical site" for sole ulcers) is interrupted. This is the start of the development of a sole ulcer. Eventually, the ulcer becomes sufficiently inflamed to cause pain and lameness, which prompts the evaluation and discovery of the lesion during the course of trimming. The point is this: ulcers are not caused by infectious organisms, but rather by conditions (eg, laminitis) that predispose to the sinking of P3 and physical trauma to the corium complicated by excessive weight bearing.

White line disease frequently results in abscess formation, so one might ask why antibiotics are not an essential part of therapy in this instance. There are essentially two types of bacteria responsible for lesions in dairy cows: anerobic (bacteria that require little or no oxygen for life) and aerobic (bacteria that require oxygen for life). The bacteria that commonly cause abscesses in cattle claw disorders are anerobes. They require, in fact thrive, in those conditions (inside the abscess) where they become sealed off from exposure to air, and particularly oxygen. As long as they are able to maintain themselves within this microenvironment they continue to multiply and in the process expand the size of their environment (continue to undermine claw horn). The abscess capsule in which they reside continues to enlarge and in the process does more and more damage as long as they remain enclosed. The point is this: the single most important factor in managing abscesses caused by white line disease or sole ulcers is to remove all loose and damaged horn, which changes the microenvironment from an oxygen-deprived to an oxygen-rich environment thereby eliminating anaerobic bacteria and preventing further abscess development.

When topical treatment under a wrap is deemed necessary readers are encouraged to read label directions on guidance for such applications. Avoid using topical medications that are not intended for use under a bandage or wrap. If necessary, only nonirritating types of antibiotics or other compounds should be used. In summary, when considering treatment of claw lesions, the best rule of thumb is quite logically, "do not do anything to a cow's foot that you would not do to your own foot."

HOUSING CONSIDERATIONS FOR COWS WITH LAMENESS DISORDERS

In deciding on follow-up care for a lame animal it is important to consider the severity of the animal's condition, its mobility, distance from the trim chute and hospital, and possible complications for the animal if returned to its pen of origin. For example, for a lactating cow it is important to consider the distance and number of times per day it must walk to and from the milking parlor. If returned to the pen of origin, will the animal be able to comfortably use a stall? Will it be able to lie down and rise without complication? Is it likely to become the victim of bullying by others within the group? Care during the convalescence period has a significant influence on treatment outcome.

Some of the obstacles presented by stalls can be overcome by moving animals to such areas as pasture, dry lot, or a bedded pack where natural behaviors associated with lying down and rising are unrestricted. Canadian researchers found that lame cows offered a 4-week period on pasture had improved gait scores, despite spending less time lying down.[37] These results indicate that moving lame cows to pasture can help lame cattle recover in part because it provides them a more comfortable surface for recovery from hoof and leg injuries. Barberg and colleagues[38] reported improved foot and leg health whereby the prevalence of lameness in compost barns was 7.8% (locomotion score $\geq$3), with two herds having no lame cows.

Behavioral observations by Endres and Barberg[39] of 147 cows in 12 compost barns found that cows moved freely on the bedded pack and were observed to assume all natural lying positions. Observations of social interactions from a total of 96 continuous hourly observations found that chasing and pushing behaviors occurred 0.94 and head butting 1.4 times per hour. Positive interactions, such as grooming and social licking, occurred 2.3 times per hour. Researchers concluded that these interactions were very similar to the kind of behaviors one would expect to observe on pasture.

In either case, lame cow areas or pens should be within close proximity to the milking parlor to reduce the distance animals are required to walk each day. Flooring surfaces should be clean and secure to prevent slipping. Properly textured surfaces or rubber flooring may improve comfort and also footing. It is also advantageous to house lame cows near the hospital where animals can be observed and treated more conveniently by health and foot care personnel. A trim chute should also be located near these areas so that animals may be examined or re-treated as needed.

PAIN MANAGEMENT OF LAMENESS USING ANALGESIA

In addition to the management of pain associated with lameness through corrective trimming and foot blocks, a multimodal approach using analgesics, such as local anesthetics, NSAIDs, and sedative-analgesics, may be beneficial to lame cattle. As observed in other painful procedures detailed by Stock ML and colleagues elsewhere in this issue, such as castration and dehorning, a multimodal approach provides the greatest pain management strategy. In the case of lame cattle, this approach includes the use of pharmaceuticals together with the use of corrective foot trimming with foot blocks, as discussed previously.

A review of publications revealed a scant amount of controlled studies investigating the effects of analgesic compounds on cattle lameness. The literature was identified on PubMed or Web of Knowledge databases using the search terms "Lame," "Bovine," and "Analgesia." Two types of studies emerged after examination of the published material. The first type of study involved mostly field trials with animal recruitment occurring by lameness detected by the use of a visual locomotion scoring system (numeric rating score) in lactating adult dairy cattle (**Table 2**).[20–22,24,25,40,41] Additional studies induced lameness in cattle by an intra-articular injection of amphotericin B in the distal interphalangeal joint resulting in a transient lameness (**Table 3**).[17,26] Amphotericin B is a polyene antimicrobial that is primarily used as an antifungal but after an intra-articular injection causes an aseptic synovitis as a result of disrupting lysosomes and release of inflammatory mediators within the synovial tissue.[42] This model for lameness has historical reference in studies involving equine lameness.[42]

Behavioral, physiologic, and neuroendocrine changes have been reported in the studies evaluating the pain associated with lameness. Generally, anti-inflammatories, such as flunixin meglumine, have demonstrated substantial acute analgesia in induced lameness models illustrated through modifications of gait and improved pressures placed on the affected foot and claw; however, in field trials, anti-inflammatories have yielded variable results with mild improvement to locomotion score and nociceptive thresholds. An inconsistent translation from lameness induced models to clinical field trials may be a result of clinical heterogeneity present in

Table 2
Summary of the scientific literature examining the effect of analgesic drug administration on cattle lameness detected by a visual locomotion score

References	Lameness Recruitment	Study Population	Analgesic Regiment	Outcome Parameter	Percent Change (%)	Significance
Whay et al,[24] 2005	Detected by a visual locomotion score	Adult cattle dairy	Ketoprofen, 3 mg/kg IM administered for 3 d, 1 h before locomotion score and nociception threshold testing	Locomotion score (1 d)	−14.29	NS
				Locomotion score (3 d)	−20	NS
				Locomotion score (8 d)	100	NS
				Locomotion score (28 d)	50	NS
				Nociceptive threshold (1 d)	0	NS
				Nociceptive threshold (3 d)	13.64	NS
				Nociceptive threshold (8 d)	14.44	NS
				Nociceptive threshold (28 d)	15.22	NS
Rushen et al,[22] 2006	Detected by a visual locomotion score	Adult cattle dairy	Lidocaine local anesthetic (palmar digital nerves medial and lateral; 2 mL each site)	Locomotion score	−7.75	NR
				Weight distribution (SD)	−55.56	<0.05
Flower et al,[40] 2008	Detected by a visual locomotion score	Adult cattle dairy	Ketoprofen, 0.3 mg/kg IM administered 1 h before gait assessment	Locomotion score	−128.57	NS
				Gait attributes (VAS) (ie, back arch, tracking up, joint flexion, asymmetric steps, head bob, reluctance to bear weight)	3	NS
			Ketoprofen, 1.5 mg/kg administered 1 h (IM) or 15 min (IV) before gait assessment	Locomotion score	−185.71	NS
				Gait attributes (VAS) (ie, back arch, tracking up, joint flexion, asymmetric steps, head bob, reluctance to bear weight)	−17.98	NS
			Ketoprofen, 3 mg/kg IM administered 1 h (IM) and 15 min (IV) before gait assessment	Locomotion score	−357.14	<0.05
				Gait attributes (VAS) (ie, back arch, tracking up, joint flexion, asymmetric steps, head bob, reluctance to bear weight)	149.86	NS

Study	Lameness detection	Animal	Intervention	Outcome measure	Value	Significance
Laven et al,[25] 2008	Detected by a visual locomotion score and confirmed by veterinarian to have only noninfectious foot disease	Adult cattle dairy	Corrective trimming and tolfenamic acid, 2 mg/kg	Nociceptive threshold (3 d)	25	NS
				Nociceptive threshold (8 d)	0	NS
				Nociceptive threshold (28 d)	0	NS
				Nociceptive threshold (100 d)	0	NS
				Locomotion score (3 d)	20	NS
				Locomotion score (8 d)	0	NS
				Locomotion score (28 d)	0	NS
				Locomotion score (100 d)	-11.11	NS
			Corrective trimming and tolfenamic acid, 2 mg/kg, and plastic shoe placed on the contralateral claw of the affected foot to elevate foot to elevate lesion from weight bearing	Nociceptive threshold (3 d)	0	NS
				Nociceptive threshold (8 d)	0	NS
				Nociceptive threshold (28 d)	0	NS
				Nociceptive threshold (100 d)	0	NS
				Locomotion score (3 d)	20	NS
				Locomotion score (8 d)	0	NS
				Locomotion score (28 d)	0	NS
				Locomotion score (100 d)	0	NS
Chapinal et al,[20] 2010	Detected by a visual locomotion score	Adult cattle dairy	Ketoprofen, 3 mg/kg IM once daily for 2 d administered 2 h before gait scoring and measures of weight distributions	Locomotion score	NR	NS
				Weight distribution (SD)	18	<0.01
				Activity (ie, lying %, frequency of lying bouts, frequency of steps)	NR	NS
Chapinal et al,[21] 2010	Detected by a visual locomotion score	Adult cattle dairy	Flunixin meglumine, 2.2 mg/kg IV once daily for 2 d administered immediately before hoof trimming on the first day and 2 h before gait scoring and measures of weight distributions	Locomotion score (VAS) (analgesia: 24 h)	1030	NS
				Locomotion score (VAS) (analgesia: 48 h)	-167.28	NS
				Weight distribution of rear legs (SD) (analgesia: 24 h)	47200	<0.10
				Weight distribution of rear legs (SD) (analgesia: 48 h)	215.46	NS
				Rear leg weight ratio (analgesia: 24 h)	-166.67	NS
				Rear leg weight ratio (analgesia: 48 h)	1030	NS
				Daily lying time (analgesia: 48 h)	2.09	NS
				Daily lying time (24 h postanalgesia)	-113.69	<0.10
				Frequency of steps (analgesia: 48 h)	-80.30	NS
				Frequency of steps (24 h postanalgesia)	-140.62	NS

(continued on next page)

Table 2
(continued)

References	Lameness Recruitment	Study Population	Analgesic Regiment	Outcome Parameter	Percent Change (%)	Significance
Rizk et al,[41] 2012	Lame cattle diagnosed with a sole ulcer referred to tertiary referral hospital for surgical claw treatment	Adult cattle dairy	Xylazine, 0.05 mg/kg IM 15 min before placement in lateral recumbency and 20 min before local anesthesia of 20 mL of 2% procaine at the start of claw surgery	Heart rate (15 min)	−27.91	<0.001
				Heart rate (lateral recumbency)	−20	<0.001
				Heart rate (1 h postoperative)	−2.50	NS
				Heart rate (3 h postoperative)	3.75	NS
				Respiratory rate (15 min)	−57.45	<0.01
				Respiratory rate (lateral recumbency)	−38	0.01
				Respiratory rate (1 h postoperative)	−21.43	NS
				Respiratory rate (3 h postoperative)	−26.53	NS
				Cortisol (15 min)	−57.72	<0.01
				Cortisol (lateral recumbency)	4.16	NS
				Cortisol (1 h postoperative)	6.40	NS
				Cortisol (3 h postoperative)	11.76	NS
				Locomotion score (1 h)	−25	<0.05
				Locomotion score (2 h)	−6.25	NS
				Locomotion score (3 h)	−3.23	NS
				Pedometer standing (1 h)	106.78	<0.01
				Pedometer standing (2 h)	63.52	NS
				Pedometer standing (3 h)	34.45	NS

Percent change was calculated using the formula [(Mean of analgesic group/Mean of control group)−1]*100.

The outcome parameter "locomotion score" was determined by a five-point numerical rating system unless otherwise noted as "VAS" indicating the use of a 100-unit visual analog scale.

Abbreviations: IM, intramuscularly; IV, intravenously; NR, values were not reported; VAS, visual analog scale.

Table 3
Summary of the scientific literature examining the effect of analgesic drug administration after an amphotericin B-induced lameness model

References	Lameness Recruitment	Study Population	Analgesic Regiment	Outcome Parameter	Percent Change (%)	Significance
Kotschwar et al,[17] 2009	Induced: amphotericin B (20 mg) injected lateral distal interphalangeal joint of hindlimb	4–6 mo Beef	Sodium salicylate, 50 mg/kg, IV administered 4 min after arthritis induction model	Cortisol (AUEC)	9.35	NS
				Surface area (cm²) (AUEC)	3.51	NS
				Contact pressure (AUEC)	−1.17	NS
				Stance phase duration (AUEC)	−0.88	NS
				Heart rate (AUEC)	20.30	NS
				Electrodermal activity (AUEC)	0.53	NS
			Sodium salicylate, 50 mg/kg, IV administered 4 min and 24 h after arthritis induction model	Cortisol (AUEC)	3.93	NS
				Surface area (cm²) (AUEC)	8.67	NS
				Contact pressure (AUEC)	−5.47	NS
				Stance phase duration (AUEC)	4.07	NS
				Heart rate (AUEC)	11.25	NS
				Electrodermal activity (AUEC)	−1.23	NS
Schulz et al,[26] 2011	Induced: amphotericin B (20 mg) injected lateral distal interphalangeal joint of hindlimb	Adult cattle beef	Flunixin meglumine, 1 mg/kg IV administered immediately and 12 h after synovitis-arthritis induction	Cortisol	NR	P = .13
				Visual lameness score (probability of having a score >0)	−55.86	<0.05
				Lying % (d 0 and 1)[a]	−18.42	<0.01
				Lying % (d 2 and 3)[a]	−0.79	NS
				Pressure mat analysis		
				Arthritis-synovitis induced limb: max force	24.54	P = .03
				Arthritis-synovitis induced limb: mean force	28.38	P = .05
				Arthritis-synovitis induced limb: mean area	25.42	P = .04
				Arthritis-synovitis induced limb: impulse	51.28	P = .06
				Arthritis-synovitis induced claw: max force	26.27	P = .02
				Arthritis-synovitis induced claw: mean force	48.51	P = .01
				Arthritis-synovitis induced claw: mean area	39.41	P = .01
				Arthritis-synovitis induced claw: impulse	73.66	P = .03

Percent change was calculated using the formula [(Mean of analgesic group/Mean of control group)−1]*100.
Abbreviations: AUEC, area under the effect curve; IV, intravenously; NR, values were not reported.

different cases of clinical lameness, the sensitivity of experiments to detect differences in analgesic-treated animals, or the potential for the central sensitization from pain noted to occur in lame cattle resulting in animals being more refractory to pain management.[1,14] Additional studies are necessary to further evaluate pharmacologic analgesia in mitigating the pain associated with lameness using induced lameness models and field studies. The evaluation of additional analgesic compounds and developing methods with improved sensitivity to detecting changes associated with the provision of analgesia are paramount to further pain management in lame cattle.

Local Anesthetics

Rushen and colleagues[22] evaluated the analgesic effects of lidocaine in adult lactating cattle after lameness detection by a five-point locomotion score. After the administration of local anesthesia, gait scores were reduced (0.3) but significance was not reported. Interestingly, the variance (standard deviation) observed in weight bearing between the affected limb and the contralateral limb was significantly reduced after the administration of lidocaine. Therefore, the use of a local anesthetic, such as lidocaine, reduces gait scores and effects distribution of weight acutely.

Nonsteroidal Anti-inflammatory Drugs

Ketoprofen
The NSAID ketoprofen has been evaluated in multiple clinical field trials to determine its analgesia effectiveness on the pain mitigation of lameness in cattle.[20,24,40] In all studies, adult lactating dairy cattle were detected as lame using a locomotion scoring technique before enrollment into the study.[13] After ketoprofen administration of a gradually increasing dose with a maximum dose of 3 mg/kg, mild improvements were observed in gait attributes including an increased number of symmetric steps and a more even weight distribution among all four limbs.[40] Moreover, a reduced variation in weight distribution has also been reported after administration of ketoprofen analgesia.[20] Based on the results of a numerical rating scale, locomotion score mildly improved (0.25 ± 0.05); however, this improvement should be interpreted with caution because this value is similar to the reported resolution of the scoring system used.[40] Nociceptive threshold was tested four times over 28 days indicating acute and chronic improvements after ketoprofen administration for the first 3 days; however, this increase was not significantly different than placebo-treated controls on each nociceptive threshold test day.[24]

Flunixin meglumine
The analgesic efficacy of intravenously administered flunixin meglumine (1 mg/kg) in an amphotericin B–induced lameness model was evaluated.[26] Compared with untreated control subjects, animals receiving flunixin meglumine at the time of lameness induction and 12 hours after were less likely to be lame as determined by a locomotion score, placed more pressure and surface area contact on pressure mats with their affected foot and the contralateral claw of the affected foot. Additionally, treated cattle were recumbent less than untreated control subjects on the day of induction and the following day; however, lying percentage was not different after the first day. Although cortisol levels were not significantly different ($P = .13$), the authors state that untreated control cattle generally had elevated cortisol concentrations compared with those treated with flunixin meglumine. Results from this study suggest the acute analgesic properties of flunixin meglumine in a lameness model in cattle.

Additionally, analgesic properties of flunixin meglumine were evaluated in a clinical trial using lame cattle detected by locomotion scoring.[21] In this study, lame cattle were administered flunixin meglumine (2.2 mg/kg) immediately before corrective hoof trimming and 24 hours after the first treatment. Gait scores as determined by a VAS and weight distribution were not significantly affected by the provision of analgesia; however, a prolonged increase in daily lying time was observed in untreated control subjects compared with those administered flunixin meglumine. Additionally, a mild significant reduction in variation (SD) of weight distribution of the rear legs was observed after analgesia administration as observed acutely with lidocaine or ketoprofen administration.[20,22]

Salicylic acid derivatives

In an amphotericin B–induced lameness model of 4- to 6-month-old steers, sodium salicylate (50 mg/kg) administered intravenously was investigated for its potential analgesic efficacy.[17] After analgesic treatment at the time of lameness induction and 24 hours postinduction, cortisol concentrations, pressure mat measurements including contact pressure and surface area, percent standing, heart rate, electrodermal activity, and LS were examined for analgesic effects. Analyses of the data indicate no overall differences between salicylate- and placebo-treated animals indicating its ineffectiveness at providing analgesia to a lameness model in cattle.

Tolfenamic acid

Although not approved for use in the United States, tolfenamic acid, an NSAID in the anthracilic acid class, was evaluated for analgesic potential in lame cattle in a New Zealand field study.[25] Cattle were enrolled into the study by farm staff detection of lameness and confirmation by a veterinarian. Only animals with noninfectious foot disease were included (ie, white line disease and sole penetration) and corrective trimming was performed on all cattle. Evaluations of nociceptive threshold and gait scores were recorded on Days 1, 3, 8, 28, and 100 with treated cows receiving tolfenamic acid (2 mg/kg) or a foot block. All cows showed improvement over time in nociceptive threshold and gait scores; however, no significant differences were reported in the acute or chronic period after treatment with tolfenamic acid compared with the untreated control animals. All cattle had access to pasture after treatment, which may have resulted in an improved response in the control cattle.

Sedative-Analgesic Drugs

Xylazine

The analgesic effects of xylazine were examined in one study evaluating adult cattle referred to a university hospital for claw surgery.[41] Animals were administered either xylazine (0.05 mg/kg, intramuscular) or a placebo treatment. After placement into lateral recumbency on a surgery tipping table, regional anesthesia was performed of the affected limb using procaine 2%, and surgery of the affected claw was initiated. As expected with administration of α_2-adrenergic agonist, heart rate and respiratory rate were reduced in the acute period. Additionally, cortisol was significantly decreased for xylazine-treated cattle compared with placebo-treated during the initial 15 minutes after xylazine administration; however, no differences were observed at later time points. Modifications were observed acutely to gait and behavior. Xylazine-treated animals stood longer and had reduced gait scores in the first hour compared with placebo-treated animals suggesting the provision of acute analgesia. This change was not observed after 2 or more hours.

Gabapentin

Gabapentin (1-[aminomethyl] cyclohexane acetic acid) is a γ-aminobutyric acid analog originally developed for the treatment of spastic disorders and epilepsy.[43]

Studies have reported that gabapentin is also effective for the management of chronic pain of inflammatory of neuropathic origin.[44] It has also been reported that gabapentin can interact synergistically with NSAIDs to produce antihyperalgesic effects.[44] The pharmacokinetics of gabapentin suggest that this compound may be useful in mitigating chronic neuropathic and inflammatory pain in ruminant cattle.[45] In a study conducted by the authors' research group it was found that administration of gabapentin at 15 mg/kg combined with meloxicam at 0.5 mg/kg once daily for 4 days increased the amount of force applied on the lame claw in calves subjected to an experimental lameness model. Stride length was also improved in calves that received gabapentin combined with meloxicam compared with placebo-treated controls. Further studies are needed to investigate the utility of gabapentin as an adjunctive therapy in the treatment of pain associated with lameness.

REFERENCES

1. Whay HR, Waterman AE, Webster AJ, et al. The influence of lesions type on the duration of hyperalgesia associated with hindlimb lameness in dairy cattle. Vet J 1998;156:23–9.
2. National Dairy FARM Program. Farmers assuring responsible management. 2012. Available at: http://www.nationaldairyfarm.com/. Accessed September 13, 2012.
3. Validus Ventures, LLC, 2012. Available at: http://www.validusservices.com/. Accessed September 13, 2012.
4. NYS Department of Agriculture and Markets, New York State Cattle Health Assurance Program (NYSCHAP), 2002. Available at: http://nyschap.vet.cornell.edu/. Accessed September 13, 2012.
5. Cattle and calves non-predator death loss in the United States, 2010. USDA-APHIS National Animal Health Monitoring System. 2011.
6. Dairy 2007. Facility characteristics and cow comfort on U.S. dairy operations, 2007. USDA-APHIS National Animal Health Monitoring System. 2010.
7. Cook NB. Prevalence of lameness among dairy cattle in Wisconsin as a function of housing type and stall surface. J Am Vet Med Assoc 2003;223:1324–8.
8. Barker ZE, Leach KA, Whay HR, et al. Assessment of lameness prevalence and associated risk factors in dairy herds in England and Wales. J Dairy Sci 2010;93:932–41.
9. Fulwider WK, Grandin T, Rollin BE, et al. Survey of dairy management practices on one hundred thirteen North Central and Northeastern United States dairies. J Dairy Sci 2008;91:1686–92.
10. Wells SJ, Trent AM, Marsh WE, et al. Prevalence and severity of lameness in lactating dairy cows in a sample of Minnesota and Wisconsin herds. J Am Vet Med Assoc 1993;202:78–82.
11. Whay HR, Main DC, Green LE, et al. Assessment of the welfare of dairy cattle using animal-based measurements: direct observations and investigation of farm records. Vet Rec 2003;153:197–202.
12. Sprecher DJ, Hostetler DE, Kaneene JB. A lameness scoring system that uses posture and gait to predict dairy cattle reproductive performance. Theriogenology 1997;47:1179–87.
13. Flower FC, Weary DM. Effect of hoof pathologies on subjective assessments of dairy cow gait. J Dairy Sci 2006;89:139–46.
14. Anderson DE, Muir WM. Pain management in cattle. Vet Clin North Am Food Anim Pract 2005;21:623–35.
15. Whay HR. Locomotion scoring and lameness detection in dairy cattle. Practice 2002;24:444–9.

16. Williamson A, Hoggart B. Pain: a review of three commonly used pain rating scales. J Clin Nurs 2005;14:798–804.

17. Kotschwar JL, Coetzee JF, Anderson DE, et al. Analgesic efficacy of sodium salicylate in an amphotericin B-induced bovine synovitis-arthritis model. J Dairy Sci 2009;92:3731–43.

18. Neveus S, Weary DM, Rushen J, et al. Hoof discomfort changes how dairy cattle distribute their body weight. J Dairy Sci 2006;89:2503–9.

19. Chapinal N, de Passillé AM, Rushen J. Weight distribution and gait in dairy cattle are affected by milking and late pregnancy. J Dairy Sci 2009;92:581–8.

20. Chapinal N, de Passillé AM, Rushen J, et al. Automated methods for detecting lameness and measuring analgesia in dairy cattle. J Dairy Sci 2010;93:2007–13.

21. Chapinal N, de Passillé AM, Rushen J, et al. Effect of analgesia during hoof trimming on gait, weight distribution, and activity of dairy cattle. J Dairy Sci 2010;93:3039–46.

22. Rushen J, Pombourcq E, de Passillé AM. Validation of two measures of lameness in dairy cows. Appl Anim Behav Sci 2006;106:173–7.

23. Chambers JP, Waterman AE, Livingston A. Further development of equipment to measure nociceptive thresholds in large animals. J Vet Anaesth 1994;21:66–72.

24. Whay HR, Webster AJ, Waterman-Pearson AE. Role of ketoprofen in the modulation of hyperalgesia associated with lameness in dairy cattle. Vet Rec 2005;157:729–33.

25. Laven RA, Lawrence KE, Weston JF, et al. Assessment of the duration of the pain response associated with lameness in dairy cows, and the influence of treatment. N Z Vet J 2008;56:210–7.

26. Schulz KL, Anderson DE, Coetzee JF, et al. Effect of flunixin meglumine on the amelioration of lameness in dairy steers with amphotericin B-induced transient synovitis-arthritis. Am J Vet Res 2011;72:1431–8.

27. Ossent P, Lischer CJ. Bovine laminitis: the lesions and their pathogenesis. In practice 1998;20:415–27.

28. Lischer CJ, Ossent P, Raber M, et al. The suspensory structures and supporting tissues of the bovine 3rd phalanx and their relevance in the development of sole ulcers at the typical site. Vet Rec 2002;151(23):694–8.

29. Mulling CK, Lischer CJ. New aspects on etiology and pathogenesis of laminitis in cattle. In: Proc of the XXII World Buiatrics Congress (keynote lectures). Hanover (Germany); 2002. p. 236–47.

30. Tarleton JF, Holah DE, Evans KM, et al. Biomechanical and histopathological changes in the support structures of bovine hooves around the time of first calving. Vet J 2002;163:196–204.

31. Webster J. Effect of environment and management on the development of claw and leg diseases. In: Proc of the XXII World Buiatrics Congress (keynote lectures). Hanover (Germany); 2002. p. 248–56.

32. Raven T. Cattle footcare and claw trimming. Ipswich (IP): Farming Press; 1989.

33. Shearer JK, van Amstel SR. Functional and corrective claw trimming. Vet Clin North Am Food Anim Pract 2001;17(1):53–72.

34. Shearer JK, van Amstel SR. Manual of foot care in cattle. Fort Atkinson (WI): WD Hoard's & Sons; 2005.

35. Van Amstel SR, Shearer JK. Manual for the treatment and control of lameness in cattle. Ames (IA): Blackwell Publishing Professional; 2006.

36. White EM, Glickman LT, Embree IC. A randomized field trial for evaluation of bandaging sole abscesses in cattle. J Am Vet Med Assoc 1981;178:375–7.

37. Hernandez-Mendo O, von Keyserlingk MA, Veira DM, et al. Effects of pasture on lameness in dairy cows. J Dairy Sci 2007;90(3):1209–14.

38. Barberg AE, Endres MI, Salfer JA, et al. Performance, health and well-being of dairy cows in an alternative housing system in Minnesota. J Dairy Sci 2007;90: 1575–83.

39. Endres MI, Barberg AE. Behavior of dairy cows in an alternative bedded-pack housing system. J Dairy Sci 2007;90:4192–200.

40. Flower FC, Sedlbauer M, Carter E, et al. Analgesics improve the gait of lame dairy cattle. J Dairy Sci 2008;91:3010–4.

41. Rizk A, Herdtweck S, Offinger J, et al. The use of xylazine hydrochloride in an analgesic protocol for claw treatment of lame dairy cows in lateral recumbency on a surgical tipping table. Vet J 2012;192:193–8.

42. McIlwraith CW, Fessler JF, Blevins WE, et al. Experimentally induced arthritis of the equine carpus: clinical determinations. Am J Vet Res 1979;40:11–20.

43. Cheng JK, Chiou LC. Mechanisms of the antinociceptive action of gabapentin. J Pharm Sci 2006;100:471–86.

44. Hurley RW, Chatterjea D, Rose Feng M, et al. Gabapentin and pregabalin can interact synergistically with naproxen to produce antihyperalgesia. Anesthesiology 2002;97:1263–73.

45. Coetzee JF, Mosher RA, Kohake LE, et al. Pharmacokinetics of oral gabapentin alone or co-administered with meloxicam in ruminant beef calves. Vet J 2011; 190:98–102.

Prevention and Management of Surgical Pain in Cattle

David E. Anderson, DVM, MS[a],*, Misty A. Edmondson, DVM, MS[b]

KEYWORDS

- Surgery • Pain • Cattle • Prevention

KEY POINTS

- Management of pain continues to be an important consideration in livestock on which surgical procedures are performed.
- A balance must be achieved between the need to mitigate discomfort and the economic constraints of the production enterprise.
- Moral and ethical dilemmas have increased among consumers and these concerns have stimulated interest to reexamine the methods used to achieve the shared goals of humane production of safe, affordable animal products for human consumption.

Management of pain continues to be an important consideration in livestock on which surgical procedures are performed.[1,2] In these animals, a balance must be achieved between the need to mitigate discomfort and the economic constraints of the production enterprise. Moral and ethical dilemmas have increased among consumers and these concerns have stimulated interest to reexamine the methods used to achieve the shared goals of humane production of safe, affordable animal products for human consumption. Administration of drugs to mitigate pain is variable among veterinarians. In a survey of Canadian veterinarians' practices regarding the use of analgesics in livestock, piglets received analgesics for castration in less than 0.001% of procedures compared with 6.9% for beef calves and 18.7% of dairy calves less than 6 months old.[3] In another survey, the surgical procedure least likely to be done after administration of analgesia was castration of calves less than 6 months old (<34%); the procedure most likely to be done after administration of analgesia was cesarean section (C-section; >99%).[4] In that study, the drugs most commonly used for mitigation of pain associated with surgery were nonsteroidal antiinflammatory drugs (NSAIDs; eg, flunixin meglumine), local anesthetics (eg, lidocaine HCl), and α-2 agonists (eg, xylazine HCl). Similar results were reported for opinions of veterinarians in New Zealand who considered surgery for claw amputation, C-section, and displacement of the

[a] Large Animal Clinical Sciences, College of Veterinary Medicine, University of Tennessee, 2407 River Road, Knoxville, TN 37996, USA; [b] Department of Clinical Sciences, College of Veterinary Medicine, Auburn University, 1500 Wire Road, Auburn, AL 36849, USA
* Corresponding author.
E-mail address: david.anderson@utk.edu

Vet Clin Food Anim 29 (2013) 157–184
http://dx.doi.org/10.1016/j.cvfa.2012.11.006
0749-0720/13/$ – see front matter © 2013 Elsevier Inc. All rights reserved.

abomasum to be the most painful procedures.[5] In that study, both gender and age bias regarding pain in cattle was revealed, with female respondents and recent graduates assigning higher pain scores to various procedures compared with older and male respondents. These results were similar to those of a previous survey of veterinarians in the United Kingdom.[6] Pain management for performance of on-farm surgical procedures needs more education and research to define optimal guidelines for veterinarians and producers.

In field settings, surgical procedures are performed both on an elective and emergency basis. These surgeries are expected to cause variable degrees of pain or distress. Pain and the biological responses to it are part of a highly integrated multidimensional system that causes animals to react to protect themselves from the noxious stimulus.[7–9] Pain perception (nociception) is not considered to fully represent the pain experience and may help to explain the relationship between painful experiences and pain behaviors in animals. In this context, pain can be broadly categorized as either adaptive or maladaptive.[10] Adaptive pain increases the potential for survival by protecting the animal from injury and by promoting healing. Adaptive pain is expected with surgical procedures performed in healthy tissue, such as castration, dehorning, and laparotomy. By contrast, maladaptive pain is a disease created by pathologic processes that result in the persistence of pain long after the initiating cause(s) have been removed. Examples of maladaptive pain include septic arthritis, claw amputation for deep digital infections, tendon and muscle laceration, and fractures with tissue destruction. With prolonged, intense stimuli, the recognition of pain by the patient can transform into pathologic pain (**Fig. 1**).[11] Tissue damage and the associated inflammatory response lead to the production and release of nociceptor activators and/or sensitizers including hydrogen and potassium ions, prostaglandins, histamine,

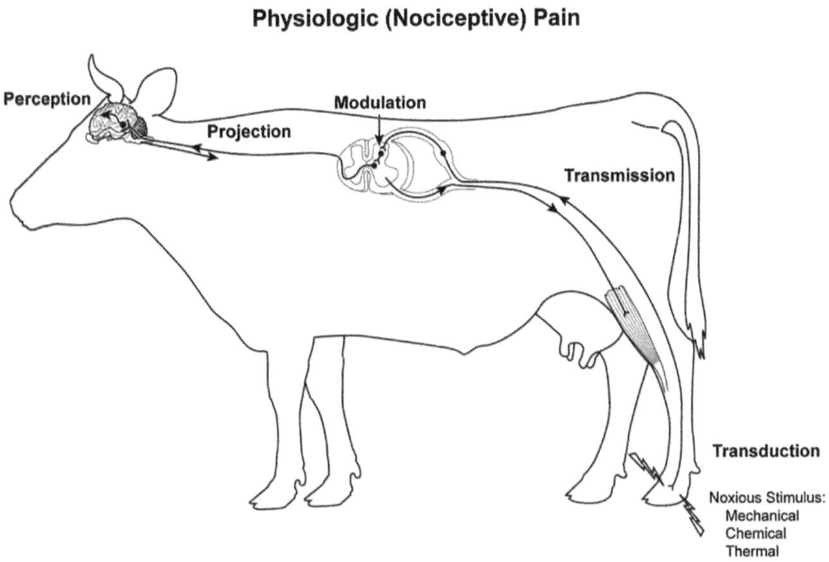

Physiologic (Nociceptive) Pain

Fig. 1. The neurophysiology of acute, physiologic pain. A noxious stimulus is transduced, transmitted, modulated, projected, and perceived, resulting in the brain generating a response that travels via descending nerve pathways that facilitate or inhibit (modulate) sensory input to the spinal cord. (*From* Anderson DE, Muir WW. Pain management in ruminants. Vet Clin North Am 2005;21:19–31; with permission.)

bradykinin, nerve growth factor, cytokines, and chemokines. Together these factors convert high-threshold nociceptors into low-threshold nociceptors and activate quiescent nocireceptors, resulting in a zone of primary hyperalgesia (**Fig. 2**).[11,12] Local vasodilation and plasma extravasation result in a further amplification of the inflammatory response and the spread of hypersensitivity to surrounding tissues (secondary hyperalgesia). Central sensitization occurs when the cumulative effects of frequent or severe peripheral nociceptor input release excessive quantities of central nervous system neurotransmitters (substance P, neurokinin A, brain-derived neurotrophic factor [BDNF]), including glutamate, which remove the normally present magnesium (Mg^{-2}) block of N-methyl-D-aspartate (NMDA), thereby activating these and other receptors in the superficial layers of the dorsal horn of the spinal cord and resulting in an increase in their sensitivity (see **Fig. 2**).[12] Activation of NMDA receptors leads to an increase in calcium (Ca^{+2}) in dorsal horn neurons, resulting in increased excitability and spontaneous ectopic discharge. Sensitization of dorsal horn neurons can last for hours and is thought to be responsible for pain outside the area of tissue injury (secondary hyperalgesia) and allodynia. Central sensitization is different from peripheral sensitization in that it enables low-intensity stimuli to produce pain sensations when pain is chronic and enables sensory fibers that normally transmit no painful stimuli (low threshold Aβ fibers) to produce pain as a result of changes in sensory processing in the spinal cord. Together, the development of peripheral sensitization, wind-up, and central sensitization represent a continuum of the pain process that exists as consequence of continuous, unrelenting, and untreated pain.

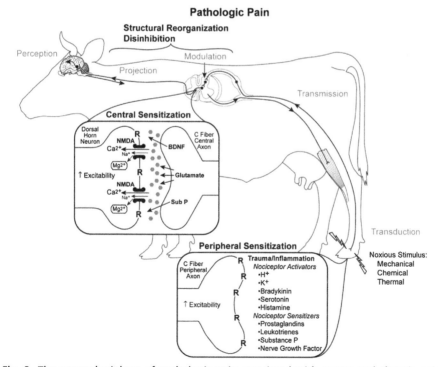

Fig. 2. The neurophysiology of pathologic pain associated with severe and chronic pain conditions. BDNF, brain-derived neurotrophic factor; NMDA, N-methyl-D-aspartate; R, receptor. (*From* Anderson DE, Muir WW. Pain management in ruminants. Vet Clin North Am 2005;21:19–31; with permission.)

The pain system includes sensors, neural pathways, and processing centers that are responsible for detecting, transmitting, and actualizing biological and behavioral responses to noxious events (see **Fig. 1**).[11,13,14] Understanding these pathways allows selection of specific strategies (eg, peripheral nerve blockade, central nerve blockade, systemic analgesia or anesthesia) and selection of appropriate drugs or drug combinations to prevent or treat the perception of pain. Drug selection and strategy should be tailored to minimize or prevent unwanted side effects such as changes in distribution of blood flow. Drug therapy for pain or distress should be chosen in combination with the overall management of the case to optimize patient comfort, restore function, and minimize adverse events. Pain is responsible for stress and can lead to distress.[15,16] Stress is an adaptive pattern of behavioral, neural, endocrine, immune, hematological, and metabolic changes directed toward the restoration of homeostasis. The stress response prepares the animal for an emergency reaction and fosters survival in circumstances of immediate threats (fight or flight). Acute pain is capable of producing a significant stress response by initiating activation of the sympathetic nervous system, secretion of glucocorticoids (primarily cortisol), hypermetabolism, sodium and water retention, and altered carbohydrate and protein metabolism.[17–19] The maintenance of normal homeostatic balance to an acute stress-producing event (pain) is maintained by negative feedback controls that act at multiple levels within the brain (amygdala) and sympathoadrenal and hypothalamic-pituitary-adrenal (HPA) axes, thereby increasing catecholamines and glucocorticoids and leading to enhanced arousal, appraisal, and cardiorespiratory and cognitive performance in order to deal with the immediate threat. Increases in corticotrophin-releasing hormone (CRH), plasma cortisol, and vasopressin often directly correlate with the stressful or painful event(s) and help to restore homeostasis. However, severe or prolonged pain resulting in severe stress eventually becomes maladaptive, producing depression and immunosuppression (sickness syndrome), which, if not controlled, can lead to distress and the activation of self-sustaining cascades of neural and endocrine responses that derail physiologic homeostasis.[20] Prolonged stress impairs the animal's ability to interact and learn and changes the animal's behavioral phenotype.[7] Severe pain produces behavioral, autonomic, neuroendocrine, and immunologic responses that can result in self-mutilation, immune incompetence, and a poor quality of life, potentially leading to gradual deterioration and death.

Apparent anxiety may be observed in ruminants.[21,22] This form of pain-free distress may adversely affect the animal's response to therapy. Anxiety states are most commonly observed in cattle with limited human contact or having had adverse human contact, such as beef heifers in dystocia that have not been handled since calfhood. Another example is beef neonates abruptly separated from the dam. Anxiety states can be observed from isolation in stalls or hospital environments. Social isolation is common among species with intense herd instincts (eg, sheep, llamas, alpacas) but also has been observed among dairy cattle and goats. Use of drugs for anxiolytic effects may result in improved efficacy and duration of effect compared with analgesic drug therapy alone. A recent study regarding behavior of dairy cows in isolation and restraint is noteworthy.[23] In this study, dairy cows were subjected to isolation, head restrain, exposure to new herdmates, and compared with the control group of resident cows in response to adverse stimuli. Dairy cows subjected to social stress showed hypoalgesia, decreased response to stimuli, decreased ruminations, and increased serum cortisol. Thus, some behavioral observations classically used to assess pain in ruminants may lead to errors in judgment. Instead of pain, these cows may be suffering psychological stress and changes in clinical management will likely be more successful than drug therapy. This possibility is supported by our clinical observations that some cows do not return to normal in an expected time frame after surgery until they have been returned to the herd setting. However, anxiolytic drugs must be administered with caution. The most clinically available anxiolytic is acepromazine. Although acepromazine may be administered in low dosages (0.02–0.04 mg/kg), this drug is contraindicated when the potential for profound hypotension is present (eg, abomasal volvulus, hypovolemia, hemorrhagic shock).

Although drug therapy is a useful tool for mitigation of pain or distress, this must be done with consideration for violative drug residues in meat and milk. Observation of appropriate withholding times in accordance with the Animal Medical Drug Use and Clarification Act (AMDUCA) is vital to the veterinary-client-patient relationship, to the preservation of a safe and wholesome food supply, and to the preservation of consumer trust. The Food Animal Residue Avoidance Database should be consulted for current withholding guidelines for anesthetic and analgesic drugs when used in food animals (www.farad.org).

RECOGNITION OF PAIN

Ruminants, especially cattle, differ in behaviors associated with pain.[21,23] Ruminants often become subdued, spend more time lying down, spend less time eating and ruminating, fail to clean the nostrils as frequently, and so forth when in pain or stressed. Galindo and Broom[24] observed that lame cows had more lying time, less eating time, more lying time outside of cubicles, and performed fewer aggressive behavior actions despite having the same frequency of aggressive behavior interactions. These lame cows licked other cows less, and were themselves licked more. Many social and environmental factors influence pain perception and responses in cattle. Rushen and colleagues[25] showed that cows subjected to social isolation, alone, had increased vocalization, heart rate, and cortisol. Strategies for recognizing pain in ruminants are described by Millman ST and colleagues elsewhere in this issue.

TREATMENT AND PREVENTION OF PAIN

The easiest type of pain to prevent is that which is induced.[1,2,26] The magnitude of surgical pain is influenced by the procedure, the methods used, and the experience and skill of the practitioner. Some strategies to inhibit or minimize pain before it occurs (eg, preemptive) are obvious: local anesthesia, general anesthesia, sedation, and tranquilization. Careful assessment of cardiovascular status and hemodynamic balance must be done during the drug selection process. Drugs that adversely affect homeostasis or may be counterproductive in the management of shock should not be used to address pain. A detailed discussion of the drugs used in sedation and general anesthesia protocols for cattle are presented by Theurer ME and colleagues elsewhere in this issue. The current article focuses on antiinflammatory drugs and various forms of selective (eg, local, regional, epidural) anesthesia. Some thought should be given to the physiologic processes that are induced by tissue injury and that may lead to pathologic pain after surgery. Sedatives, tranquilizers, narcotics, anesthetics, and so forth inhibit detection or perception of pain by interfering with pain pathways, but these drugs should not be considered therapeutic beyond the clinical benefit of lessening the distress caused by the pain stimulus,[26] because these drugs do not treat the disease or processes (eg, inflammation) causing the noxious stimuli. Multimodal therapy refers to the simultaneous treatment of the disease, physiologic side effects of the disease or treatment used, and pain. Multimodal pain management often refers to administration of a combination of drugs of different pharmacologic classes and or different routes of administration to achieve more effective analgesia and return to normal. NSAIDs can be a critical link to multimodal therapy for pain (**Table 1**). The clinician should not have elimination of all pain as the end point for therapy. Rather, the goal is to minimize pain such that the patient can return to more normal self-care activities such as eating, drinking, urination, defecation, grooming, physical activity, and milk production. However, the clinician should recognize that reactive pain management (eg, administration of analgesic drugs only after pain is recognized) is less effective and likely impedes the recovery of the patient. Preemptive pain management is more successful and optimizes animal well-being. Preemptive therapy should be done with the intention of controlling pain throughout the stimulus, which may last for hours, days, or weeks. Unwanted side effects of NSAIDs are related to nonselective prostaglandin inhibition. This inhibition may increase the risk of abomasal ulcers and renal failure, and may adversely affect healing. Prostaglandins are vital to abomasal mucosal integrity (eg, prostaglandin E-2), vascular regulation (eg, prostaglandin I), and homeostasis. The clinically beneficial effects of NSAID therapy are usually thought to be more helpful than the risks, but adjunct therapy must be instituted to minimize complications. Adjunct therapy may include the use of these drugs at the minimum required dose and frequency of administration, but may also include administration of intravenous (IV) fluids or gastrointestinal protectants during the course of therapy.

PERIOPERATIVE USE OF ANTIINFLAMMATORY DRUGS

A variety of antiinflammatory drugs are available for clinical use.[1,2,26] Steroids and NSAIDs may have benefits to the patient such as mitigation of pain, lessening of swelling, diminishing inflammation at the incision site and/or damaged tissues, and more rapid patient recovery after the procedure. Pain, uncontrolled inflammation, excessive swelling, local ischemia, and tissue injury can suppress immune system function and allow the establishment of infection or slow the rate of wound healing by prolongation of the phases of wound response and repair.

Glucocorticoids have profound inhibition of the inflammatory cascade (**Fig. 3**). The use of steroids for management of pain and inflammation associated with surgery is discouraged because of concerns for increased risk of infection either at the site of the surgical wound or associated with the disease process necessitating surgery. Although steroids can have inhibitory effects on the migration and function of white blood cells, many clinicians think that the benefits of a single dose of steroid with

Table 1			
NSAIDs used to alleviate surgical pain in ruminants			
Drug	**Dose (mg/kg)**	**Route**	**Frequency**
Na-salicylate	50–100	Oral	Every 12 h
Flunixin meglumine	1–2	IV	Every 12–24 h
Ketoprofen	1.5	IV or IM	Every 24–48 h
Carprofen	1.4	IV or SC	
Phenylbutazone	5	Oral	Every 24–48 h
	10	Oral	Every 48–72 h
Meloxicam	0.5–1.0	Oral	Every 24 to 72 h

Except for flunixin meglumine, none of these NSAIDs are approved for use in cattle in the United States. Meat and milk withholding times must be cautiously estimated. Phenylbutazone is prohibited for use in lactating dairy cows.

Abbreviations: IM, intramuscular; IV, intravenous; SC, subcutaneous.

Data from Refs.[1,2,63]

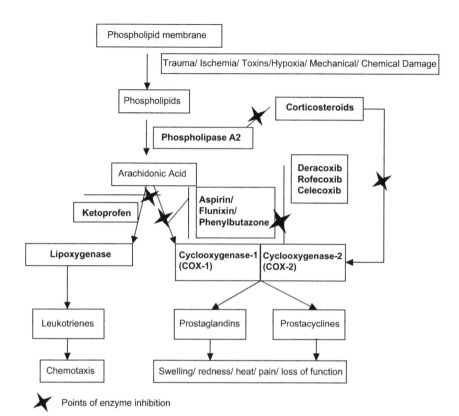

Fig. 3. Inflammatory cascade and points of enzyme inhibition of antiinflammatory drugs. (*Courtesy of* Johann F. Coetzee, BVSc, PhD, Ames, IA.)

a short to moderate duration of action (eg, dexamethasone at 0.1 mg/kg body weight) outweigh the potential adverse effects. The authors caution against the routine use of steroids perioperatively unless needed as part of the management of shock or severe, progressive deterioration of the tissues or the patient.

NSAIDs have been shown to have a beneficial effect on mitigation of pain and maintenance of normal behavioral activities in livestock. The bulk of this research has focused on routine husbandry surgical procedures such as castration and dehorning. Little research has been done to document the effects of NSAIDs administered perioperatively in livestock having surgical procedures for disease conditions such as displacement of the abomasum or C-section.

NSAIDs inhibit cyclooxygenase enzymes (COX) (see **Fig. 3**).[1,2,26] COX acts on arachidonic acids to liberate prostaglandins and other mediators of inflammation. Multiple isoforms of COX enzyme exist, with COX-1 recognized as primarily involved with normal homeostatic mechanisms and COX-2 as an enzyme induced in response to injury. COX inhibitors prevent production of these factors. Nonspecific COX inhibitors include aspirin, flunixin, and phenylbutazone. More selective COX-2 inhibitors are rapidly being developed and include etodolac, carprofen, and meloxicam. NSAIDs have differential activity because of the presence of variable receptors and variable drug effects. Our clinical experience suggests that, although these drugs may be safer for long-term use (eg, COX-2 inhibition is less likely to interfere with homeostasis of abomasal mucosa or renal perfusion), COX-2 inhibitors provide less potent analgesia.

Much of the pain research that has been performed has shown benefits of preemptive analgesia. There is a less marked effect of the administration of analgesic medication after the noxious stimulus has become established. In a study in which flunixin meglumine was administered before laparotomy for correction of abomasal displacement, cows receiving flunixin (2.2 mg/kg IV) had significantly greater rumen contracts during the first 24 hours after surgery compared with control cows.[27] This administration of flunixin may not represent preemptive analgesia because of the prior abomasal displacement. Another study was designed to investigate the effect of preoperative and 24-hour postoperative administration of flunixin meglumine (1.25 g IV) on postoperative recovery of cows having surgical correction of left displaced abomasum.[28] In that study, cows receiving flunixin meglumine immediately before and 24 hours after surgery had significantly better appetite, defecation, and milk production compared with cows that were not given flunixin. A risk-benefit analysis should be done on a case-by-case basis to determine whether an NSAID should be administerd.[29] Meloxicam has been used recently for pain management in cattle for a variety of conditions. This NSAID has been shown to be effective in mitigating the pain of castration and dehorning and the pharmacokinetics suggest that meloxicam should be effective for perioperative pain management as well.[30] Clinical experience has been positive with this drug when (0.5–1 mg/kg body weight) given orally, every 24 to 48 hours. Future research is needed to more fully elucidate the clinical indication for the use of meloxicam. Based on AMDUCA guidelines, the authors only use meloxicam when sustained effect is needed (>3 days), because the more selective COX-2 inhibition should be safe for prolonged administration compared with flunixin. In cases of severe, prolonged pain when a pathologic pain state has become established, gabapentin can be administered as a complimentary drug to meloxicam as a multimodal therapy.[31] The use of gabapentin (10 mg/kg, orally, every 12 hours) has been useful in cases of deep digital sepsis and septic arthritis as a tool to dampen the exaggerated central nervous response to the limb pain.

OPIOIDS

Opioids are useful in a wide variety of settings because there are limited cardiovascular side effects (**Table 2**). Economic constraints have limited the use of these drugs in ruminant practice.[1,2,26] The most common narcotic drug used in cattle is butorphanol tartrate (0.02–0.04 mg/kg, IV or subcutaneous [SC] every 4–6 hours). Morphine (0.05–0.1 mg/kg, SC every 4–12 hours) and buprenorphine (0.005–0.01 mg/kg, SC

Table 2
Opioids used for analgesia during surgery in ruminants

Drug	Dose	Route	Frequency
Morphine	0.5–1 mg/kg	IV	Every 12 h
	0.05–0.1 mg/kg	Epidural	Every 24 h
Fentanyl	0.05–0.5 µg/kg	Transdermal patch	Every 72 h
Meperidine	3.3–4.4 mg/kg	SC or IM	—
Buprenorphine	0.005–0.01 mg/kg (sheep and goats)	IM	Every 6–12 h
Butorphanol	0.02–0.05 mg/kg	IV	Every 2–4 h
		SC	Every 6–8 h

None of these drugs are approved for use in cattle in the United States. Meat and milk withholding times must be cautiously estimated.
Data from Refs.[1,2,63]

every 6–12 hours) have been used in cattle to variable effect. Although typically used at greater dosage rates in other species, fentanyl transdermal patches applied at a rate of 0.05 to 0.1 μg/kg have shown clinical benefit for up to 72 hours duration. A combination of butorphanol, xylazine, and ketamine (also known as ketamine stun) has recently been shown to provide analgesia, chemical restraint, and disassociation from the procedure.[32,33] The combination of an opioid (butorphanol at 0.025 mg/kg), α-2 agonist (xylazine at 0.05 mg/kg), and neuroleptic (ketamine at 0.1 mg/kg) seems to create an altered state of consciousness that has been very beneficial when performing surgical procedures on fractious cattle or cattle suffering extreme pain as a result of the disease condition.

LOCAL ANESTHESIA

Local anesthetics are the most common preemptive and emptive analgesic drugs used for surgery in food animal practice.[34] These drugs, especially lidocaine 2% HCl, are used to prevent pain during surgery. These drugs act locally or regionally when perineural anesthesia is performed, but have no systemic or behavioral effect except when given intravenously or at extremely high dosages. Local anesthetics block nerve fibers (B-fibers for motor/touch >C-fibers, which are nonmyelinated and are pain and temperature sensitive >A-fibers, which are primarily associated with motor function and proprioception).[35] The acuteness or severity of the perception of pain is influenced by the stimulus. Intensity of perception diminishes in the order of pain → cold → warmth → touch → deep pressure. Local anesthetic drugs act primarily by inhibiting Na channels to impede nerve conduction by preventing depolarization of the nerve fiber. These drugs must disassociate in an alkaline environment for this to occur. In infected, ischemic, or injured tissues, quality of local anesthesia is often poor because the relatively more acidic environment prevents disassociation of drug. An example of this effect is septic cellulitis associated with complicated sole ulcer complex in dairy cows. The acidic environment associated with the bacterial cellulitis may cause local administration of lidocaine to be ineffectual with continued pain sensation. One solution to this problem is to administer the block remote to infected tissues. Another consideration with local anesthetic drugs is the adverse stimuli associated with the caustic nature of the acid stable drug. Lidocaine 2% HCL has been observed and reported to be painful during administration. This noxious characteristic can be eliminated by adding Na-bicarbonate to neutralize the solution. The lidocaine can be buffered by adding 5 mL of 8.5% sodium bicarbonate with 50 mL of 2% lidocaine HCl. This practice may diminish or eliminate the sting of injection.

Local anesthetics vary in their potency, duration, toxicity, and cost.[7] Practitioners are challenged with balancing the immediate needs for anesthesia to complete the surgical procedure and the desire to have postoperative analgesia while maintaining safety and cost-effectiveness. Lidocaine hydrochloride (2%) is the most commonly used local anesthetic drug in cattle because of its consistent time of onset, efficacy, low cost, and low risk of toxicity. Lidocaine is considered to be more potent than procaine and diffuses more widely into the tissues. However, lidocaine has an intermediate duration of action of 60 to 90 minutes.[8] In cattle, procaine (1%–2%) is expected to have a longer time to onset of anesthesia compared with lidocaine and a shorter duration of action, lasting no more than 60 minutes. As an alternative, mepivacaine (1%–2%) is expected to have a similar time to onset of anesthesia but longer duration of activity (range 120–180 minutes) than lidocaine. Bupivacaine (0.25%–0.5%) is a long-acting local anesthetic (range up to 360 minutes),[36] but this drug can be toxic to cattle if given intravenously. For this reason, bupivacaine is not recommended for routine clinical use because of the risk of inadvertent intravenous injection. The duration of action of lidocaine can be extended by adding a vasoconstrictor, such as epinephrine (5 μg/mL), to the local anesthetic solution (0.1 mL of epinephrine [1:1000] to 20 mL of local anesthetic), which increases the potency and duration of activity. Caution should be observed when using local anesthetics containing epinephrine (1:200,000) because vasoconstriction could affect revascularization of the wound edges when used peripherally or could increase the risk of producing tissue necrosis and spinal cord ischemia if used epidurally.[9,37] In a study of skin lesions occurring in cattle after the use of a combination of lidocaine and epinephrine, skin lesions were hypothesized to be caused by the low pH of the injected solution, the total volume of injection, and the effects of the epinephrine. Based on previous research in sheep, the maximum concentration of epinephrine combined with lidocaine is 12.5 μg/mL total solution.[38]

Local anesthetics can be used in a variety of techniques including local block, inverted L block, ring block, selected perineural block, regional blocks (eg, paravertebral, epidural), and intravenous regional blocks distal to a tourniquet. In our experience, topical products for inducing local anesthesia have limited efficacy in cattle. The failure of these products may be associated with the characteristics of bovine skin. Bovine skin, especially flank and dorsal skin, may be too thick or resistant to absorption of the anesthetic to induce clinically useful anesthesia. However, 5% lidocaine gel has been beneficial when applied to the skin surface of injured teats to facilitate palpation and cannulation of the teat. Clinical analgesia is expected within 10 minutes after application of the gel to dry skin.

In all patients, the toxic dose for lidocaine should be considered and preventive measures taken to ensure that overdosage does not occur. This precaution is most critical when local anesthesia is being performed in a large area, such as for C-section. In cattle, 10 mg/kg body weight may be used to estimate the maximum safe dose of lidocaine HCl. Using this threshold, the maximum safe dose of 2% (20 mg/mL) lidocaine HCl for a 700-kg cow would be 350 mL. The maximum safe dose in a 70-kg calf would be 35 mL. In small ruminants, a maximum safe dose estimate of 4 mg/kg may be used. Thus, a 70-kg goat would receive no more than 14 mL of 2% lidocaine HCl.

LOCAL INFILTRATION AND LINE BLOCK

The simplest form of anesthesia/analgesia to a specific site is the local infiltration of the drug. In North America, 2% lidocaine HCl is most commonly used for this purpose. The length and gauge of needle used is based on the skin thickness and tissue depth desired for infiltration. Most commonly, an 18-gauge needle is used because the bore diameter is small enough not to cause excessive discomfort and strong enough to minimize the risk of the needle bending or breaking during insertion or infusion. For flank laparotomy, a 3.8-cm (1.5-inch) needle is sufficient to allow subcutaneous infiltration as well as intramuscular infiltration. Although lidocaine efficiently diffuses for short distances within a tissue plane, the user must be aware that diffusion across fascial planes is less effective. This difference may account for instances of incomplete blockade of the site despite administration of an ample volume. The distance between needle insertion points should not exceed twice the length of the needle (eg, 2 insertion points of a 3.8-cm needle would be no further than 7.6 cm apart) to ensure that gaps in the area of anesthesia do not remain. Pain of successive injections may be alleviated by placing the edge of the needle into the edge of the previously desensitized area. Dissociation of lidocaine must occur to optimize Na channel blockade, which occurs efficiently at neutral pH but does not occur consistently in acidic pH fluids. This difference may explain the absence of expected anesthesia in infected, ischemic, traumatized, and anaerobic tissues.

The initial point of insertion should be intended to achieve subcutaneous infiltration. The needle and syringe are held at a 60° angle to the skin and then advanced until resistance abruptly diminishes. The skin tenting technique can be used as an alternative, whereby the skin is pulled away from the body to form a tent and the needle directed parallel to the body and along the long axis of the tent. The syringe is used to aspirate to ensure that a vessel has not been entered before infusion of the anesthetic. Then, the needle is advanced along the plane of the proposed incision line for the full length of the needle and in both directions along the anticipated incision. In this way, the smallest number of skin insertion points can be made by maximizing the length of the needle for infusion. A sufficient volume of lidocaine should be infused to create a bleb or noticeable swelling underneath the skin (usually 1–5 mL). After the subcutaneous space has been infiltrated, a similar procedure is done to infiltrate the muscles in the plane of the anticipated incision. Lidocaine is infused as the needle is advanced into and retracted from the muscles to ensure that lidocaine is distributed among the separate muscle planes. In the case of flank laparotomy, the external abdominal oblique muscle, internal abdominal oblique muscle, and transversus abdominis muscle must be anesthetized. Line blocks are not expected to anesthetize the peritoneum and the surgeon must anticipate adverse reaction to this tissue being penetrated. The zone of anesthesia is expected to extend 2 to 3 cm on either side of the line of infiltration. Injection of large volumes of lidocaine may increase the zone of anesthesia, but the presence of large quantities of lidocaine may increase the potential for tissue toxicity and incisional morbidity.

INVERTED L BLOCK

The inverted L block is a nonspecific regional block that locally blocks the tissue bordering the caudal aspect of the 13th rib and the ventral aspect of the transverse processes of the lumbar vertebrae.[39] An 18-gauge 3.8-cm needle is used to inject up to a total of 100 mL of local anesthetic solution in multiple small injection sites into the tissues bordering the dorsocaudal aspect of the 13th rib and ventrolateral aspect of the transverse processes of the lumbar vertebrae (**Fig. 4**). This technique creates an area of anesthesia under the inverted L block. Advantages of the inverted L block include that the block is simple to perform and does not interfere with ambulation, and deposition of anesthetic away from the incision site minimizes incisional edema and hematoma.[40] Disadvantages include incomplete analgesia and muscle relaxation of the deeper layers of the abdominal wall (particularly in obese animals), possible toxicity after larger doses of anesthetic, and increased cost because of larger doses of local anesthetic.

PROXIMAL PARAVERTEBRAL BLOCK

The proximal paravertebral nerve block desensitizes the dorsal and ventral nerve roots of the last thoracic (T13) and first and second lumbar (L1 and L2) spinal nerves as they emerge from the intervertebral foramina (**Fig. 5**). To facilitate proper needle placement of anesthetic, the skin at the cranial edges of the transverse processes of L1, L2, and L3 and at a point 2.5 to 5 cm off the dorsal midline can desensitized by injecting 2 to 3 mL of local anesthetic using an 18-gauge 2.5-cm needle. A 14-gauge 2.5-cm needle is used as a cannula or guide needle to minimize skin resistance during insertion of an 18-gauge 10-cm to 15-cm spinal needle (see **Fig. 5**). Approximately 5 mL of local

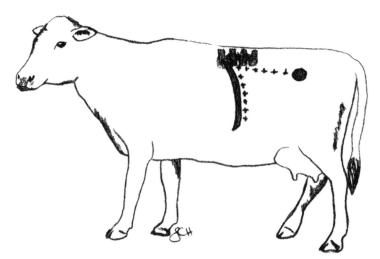

Fig. 4. Inverted L block for paralumbar anesthesia, showing multiple infusion sites (*asterisks*), the last rib, the lumbar vertebra, and tuber coxae.

anesthetic may be placed through the cannula to further anesthetize the tract for needle placement.

To desensitize T13, the cannula needle is placed through the skin at the anterior edge of the transverse process of L1 approximately 4 to 5 cm lateral to the dorsal

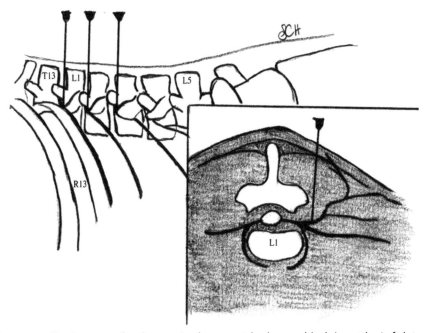

Fig. 5. Needle placement for the proximal paravertebral nerve block in cattle. Left lateral view and cranial view at the thoracolumbar junction. R13, last rib; T13, last thoracic vertebra; L1, first lumbar vertebra; L5, fifth lumbar vertebra.

midline. The 18-gauge 10-cm to 15-cm spinal needle is passed ventrally until it contacts the transverse process of L1. The needle is then walked off the cranial edge of the transverse process of L1 and advanced approximately 1 cm to pass slightly ventral to the process and into the transverse ligament. Between 6 and 8 mL of local anesthetic are injected with little resistance to desensitize the ventral branch of T13. The needle is then withdrawn 1 to 2.5 cm above the fascia or just dorsal to the transverse process and 6 to 8 mL of local anesthetic are infused to desensitize the dorsal branch of the nerve.

To desensitize L1 and L2, the needle is inserted just caudal to the transverse processes of L1 and L2. The needle is walked off the caudal edges of the transverse processes of L1 and L2, at a depth similar to the injection site for T13, and advanced approximately 1 cm to pass slightly ventral to the process and into the transverse ligament. Between 6 and 8 mL of local anesthetic are injected with little resistance to desensitize the ventral branches of the nerves. The needle is then withdrawn 1 to 2.5 cm above the fascia or just dorsal to the transverse processes and 6 to 8 mL of local anesthetic are infused to desensitize the dorsal branch of the nerves.

Ina study designed to compare proximal paravertebral anesthetic block and a combination line block plus inverted L block for flank laparotomy in cattle, the proximal paravertebral block provided significantly better clinical analgesia during the creation of the incision into the abdomen.[41] Evidence of a successful proximal paravertebral nerve block includes increased temperature of the skin; analgesia of the skin, muscles, and peritoneum of the abdominal wall of the paralumbar fossa; and scoliosis of the spine toward the desensitized side. Advantages of the proximal paravertebral nerve block include small doses of anesthetic, wide and uniform area of analgesia and muscle relaxation, decreased intra-abdominal pressure, and absence of local anesthetic at the margins of the surgical site. Disadvantages of the proximal paravertebral nerve block include scoliosis of the spine, which may make closure of the incision more difficult; difficulty in identifying landmarks in obese and heavily muscled animals; and more skill or practice required for consistent results.[39,40,42]

DISTAL PARAVERTEBRAL BLOCK

The distal paravertebral nerve block desensitizes the dorsal and ventral rami of the spinal nerves T13, L1, and L2 at the distal ends of the transverse processes of L1, L2, and L4, respectively (**Fig. 6**). An 18-gauge 3.5-cm to 5.5-cm needle is inserted ventral to the transverse process and 10 mL of local anesthetic are infused in a fan-shaped pattern. The needle can then be removed and reinserted or redirected dorsally, in a caudal direction, where 10 mL of local anesthetic are again infused in a fan-shaped pattern. This procedure is repeated for the transverse processes of the second and fourth lumbar vertebrae. Advantages of the distal paravertebral nerve block compared with the proximal paravertebral nerve block include lack of scoliosis, arguably being easier to perform, and offering more consistent results. Disadvantages of the distal paravertebral nerve block compared with the proximal paravertebral nerve block include that larger doses of anesthetic are required and variations in efficiency caused by variation in the anatomic pathways of the nerves.[39,40,42]

EPIDURAL ANESTHESIA

Epidural anesthesia has been the focus of attention of many research projects in cattle in an attempt to minimize pelvic and perineal pain (**Table 3**).[43-49] Caudal epidural anesthesia is easily applied in cattle and a variety of drugs have been shown to be beneficial. A high caudal epidural at the sacrococcygeal space (S5–Co1) desensitizes

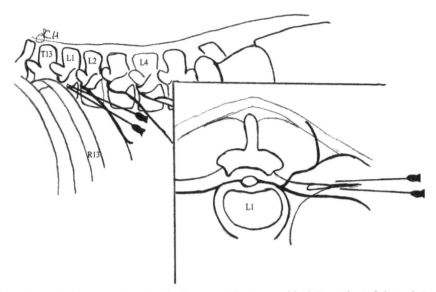

Fig. 6. Needle placement for the distal paravertebral nerve block in cattle. Left lateral view and cranial view at the thoracolumbar junction. L2, second lumbar vertebra; L4, fourth lumbar vertebra.

sacral nerves S2, S3, S4, and S5. The low caudal epidural at the first coccygeal space (Co1–Co2) desensitizes sacral nerves S3, S4, and S5; as the anesthetic dose increases, nerves cranial to S2 may also become affected.[50] If possible, the hair should be clipped and the skin scrubbed and disinfected. Standing alongside the cow, the tail should be moved up and down to locate the fossa between the last sacral vertebra and the first coccygeal vertebra or between the first and second coccygeal

Table 3 Usage of epidural anesthesia for standing paralumbar analgesia or laparotomy in cattle			
Drug	**Dosage**	**Onset of Analgesia (min)**	**Duration of Analgesia**
Lidocaine 2%	0.2 mg/kg (5 mL)	5	10–115 min
Xylazine	0.05 mg/kg (5 mL in saline)	20–40	2–3 h
Clonidine	2–3 µg/kg diluted to 8 mL in saline	2 µg dose: 19 3 µg dose: 9	2 µg dose: 192 min 3 µg dose: 311 min Peak effect during 60–180 min
Ketamine 5%	5 mL (250 mg) 10 mL (500 mg) 20 mL (1000 mg)	5 mL: 6.5 10 mL: 5 20 mL: 5	5 mL: 17 min 10 mL: 34 min 20 mL: 62 min
Procaine HCl 5%	300 mg (6 mL)	8–20	45–127 min Mean, 83 min
Medetomidine	15 µg/kg (5 mL)	5	412 min
Detomidine	40 µg/kg	—	—
Romifidine + morphine	Romifidine: 50 µg/kg Morphine: 0.1 mg/kg	—	12 h maximum

vertebrae. An 18-gauge 3.8-cm needle (with no syringe attached) is directed perpendicular to the skin surface (**Fig. 7**). Once the skin is penetrated, place a drop of local anesthetic solution in the hub of the needle (hanging drop technique). The needle should then be advanced slowly until the anesthetic solution is drawn into the epidural space by negative pressure. The syringe may then be attached to the needle and anesthetic solution slowly injected with no resistance. Lidocaine HCl 2% can be used for perineal analgesia (low-volume: <1 mL/50 kg body weight) or pelvic and abdominal analgesia (high volume: 1 mL/5 kg). The duration of clinically apparent analgesia after low-volume caudal epidural anesthesia is expected to be 60 to 90 minutes. Ropivacaine 0.75% is administered via caudal epidural injection at a rate of 0.11 mg/kg body weight.[51] In that study, the time of onset for analgesia of the perineum ranged from 9 to 15 minutes but the duration of analgesia was 359 (±90) minutes. Although slight ataxia was observed in some cows, adverse events were not noted.

High-volume caudal epidural anesthesia refers to the infusion of large volumes of drugs via the standard caudal epidural site as per perineal anesthesia. The standard low-volume caudal epidural uses lidocaine 2% HCl with or without α-2 agonists (recommended volume 0.5 mL/50 kg body weight; maximum volume 1 mL per 50 kg body weight with mild ataxia). This volume is sufficient for procedures involving the tail, perineum, and vagina (eg, rectovaginal fistula repair, urethral extension surgery, tail amputation). High-volume epidurals use injection volumes of 1 mL per 5 kg body weight, but volumes up to 0.5 mL/kg body weight have been used in calves without adverse events noted.[52] When high-volume epidurals use local anesthetics such as lidocaine, recumbency is required because of loss of motor control of the rear limbs. High-volume epidural anesthesia is advantageous because surgical anesthesia is attained with little to no adverse cardiovascular effect when given within the safe dosage range. This technique has been described for surgery of the rear limbs and umbilicus in calves.[52–54] One of the authors (DEA) has used high-volume epidural anesthesia with lidocaine HCl 2% at a dose of 1 mL per 5 kg body weight (eg, a 500-kg cow would receive 100 mL lidocaine HCl 2%) to facilitate ventral midline C-section, preputial

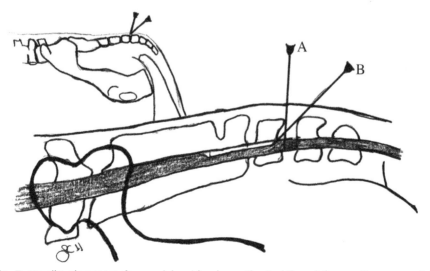

Fig. 7. Needle placement for caudal epidural anesthesia (*A*) and for continuous caudal epidural anesthesia (*B*) located between the first and second coccygeal vertebrae.

translocation for teaser bull preparation, and for placement of transfixation pin-casts for tibia fractures. The patient is nonambulatory for 4 to 6 hours after administration of the epidural. Therefore, postoperative management is crucial to minimize the risks of self-trauma during the period of ataxia. The patient should be placed in a small area with excellent footing (eg, sand bedded stall or small grass pen) and remain undisturbed until standing unassisted. Hobbles are placed on the rear limbs to prevent splaying of the rear limbs, which could cause hip luxation or muscle injury. Bupivacaine is not recommended for epidural use in cattle despite its prolonged duration of analgesia. In a study in goats, the patients were unable to stand for up to 11 hours after administration of bupivacaine 0.75% (1 mL per 4 kg body weight).[55]

Several other drugs have been used for epidural analgesia in cattle. Of particular interest are drugs such as α-2 agonists.[43] These drugs cause analgesia by stimulation of α-2 receptors in the spinal cord and inhibit norepinephrine and substance P release. These drugs may optimize analgesia with minimal motor nerve interference such that the patient may remain standing and stable throughout surgery. Chevalier and colleagues[56] showed that heifers having epidural xylazine administered before preparation for laparotomy had reduced distress in response to paravertebral anesthetic injection and surgical manipulations. Minimal to no postoperative benefit was found. Epidural administration of clonidine (2–3 μg/kg body weight), an α-2 agonist, was evaluated in bulls.[45] Both doses produced perineal analgesia for 192 minutes (2 μg/kg) and 311 minutes (3 μg/kg), but sedation was also dose dependent. No adverse cardiovascular effects were noted. In a study comparing epidural and intramuscular administration of detomidine (40 μg/kg body weight) in cattle, both routes of administration resulted in similar degrees of analgesia of the perineum and flank.[48] Use of α-2 agonists under emergency conditions is discouraged because the risk of profound cardiovascular instability or recumbency exceeds the benefits observed with the use of these drugs.

Opioids have been used in cattle but clinical results have been variable. Opioids act on μ, δ, and κ receptors, inhibit neurotransmitter release, and increase potassium influx into the neuron, thus hyperpolarizing the membrane.[2] Epidural administration of opioids, such as morphine (0.1 mg/kg) diluted in 20 mL of sterile saline, is used to provide analgesia for a prolonged period (approximately 12 hours) without interfering with motor function. Disadvantages of using opioids for epidural anesthesia are that the analgesia is not as potent as lidocaine and the maximum effect of a morphine epidural may not occur for 2 to 3 hours. Caudal epidural administration of morphine may be used to help alleviate pain in the perineal area and straining.[57] In our clinical experience in ruminants, morphine causes mild to moderate clinical analgesia.[47] Tramadol has been investigated as a complimentary drug for epidural use in cattle. Although the onset of analgesia was slower (14.1 minutes) than lidocaine (3.9 minutes), tramadol induced a prolonged period of analgesia (307 minutes) compared with lidocaine (69 minutes) and tramadol-lidocaine combination (174 minutes).[58]

Use of the NMDA receptor antagonist ketamine for epidural administration has shown promise in cattle. Ketamine noncompetitively binds to NMDA receptors and prevents response to adverse stimuli transmitted by C-fibers. Lee and colleagues[46] administered 5% ketamine by caudal epidural injection in volumes of 5, 10, or 20 mL. Cows having 5-mL injections had perineal analgesia for 17 minutes with no ataxia. Cows having 10-mL injections showed mild ataxia for 30 minutes, but had analgesia for 34 minutes. Cows with 20-mL injections had ataxia for 48 minutes, with 1 cow becoming recumbent. Analgesia lasted for 62 minutes. Heart rate, respiratory rate, rectal temperature, rumen motility, and mean arterial pressures did not change throughout the study.

CONTINUOUS CAUDAL EPIDURAL

Continuous caudal epidural anesthesia is used in cattle with chronic rectal and vaginal prolapse that experience continuous straining after the initial epidural. This procedure is performed by placing a catheter into the epidural space for intermittent administration of local anesthetic. A 17-gauge 5-cm spinal needle (Tuohy needle) with stylet in place is inserted into the epidural space at Co1 to Co2 with the bevel directed craniad. The stylet is removed and 2 mL of local anesthetic are injected to determine whether the needle is in the epidural space. A catheter is inserted into the needle and advanced cranially for 2 to 4 cm beyond the needle tip. The needle is then withdrawn while the catheter remains in place. An adapter is placed on the end of the catheter and the catheter secured to the skin on the dorsum. Local anesthetic solution may then be administered as needed.[58] This method of inducing continuous epidural anesthesia was used in a Brown Swiss cow suffering complex regional pain syndrome caused by severe, prolonged infections of a rear foot in which digit amputation failed to resolve clinical pain.[59] This cow received a mixture of methadone, ketamine, and bupivacaine continuously over a 17-day period.

ANESTHESIA OF THE FOOT

In many cases, intravenous regional anesthesia is the preferred technique for surgery of the foot. A tourniquet is placed proximal to the fetlock just before injection when the vein is maximally distended (**Fig. 8**). In the thoracic limb, intravenous regional analgesia can be performed using the dorsal metacarpal vein, the plantar metacarpal vein, and the radial vein (see **Fig. 9**). In the pelvic limb, the lateral saphenous vein or lateral plantar digital vein may be used for injection. Approximately 20 mL of local anesthetic are injected intravenously as close to the surgical site as possible using a 20-gauge 3.3-cm needle or 21-gauge butterfly catheter. It is only necessary to administer anesthetic into 1 vein to provide anesthesia to the area distal to the tourniquet. The tourniquet can be safely left in place for up to 1 hour to provide hemostasis during surgical procedures of the foot. Anesthesia of the foot occurs within 5 to 10 minutes. Once the surgical procedure is complete, the tourniquet is released.

In cases of severe cellulitis, local intravenous anesthesia can be difficult to perform. In these cases, a simple ring block or 4-point nerve block may also be performed. A ring block is a simple method for regional anesthesia distal to the injection sites. Using a 22-gauge 2.5-cm needle, a total of 10 to 15 mL of local anesthetic is injected at multiple sites around the limb adjacent to the superficial and deep digital flexor tendons and medially and laterally to the extensor tendons. The ring block should be performed at the junction of the proximal and middle metacarpus or metatarsus. Although a simple technique to perform, multiple injection sites increase the risk of infection. Problems achieving satisfactory or complete anesthesia of the digit may also be a concern when using a ring block. The 4-point nerve block anesthetizes the area from the pastern distally. A 20-gauge 3.8-cm needle is inserted into the dorsal aspect of the pastern, in the groove between the proximal phalanges, just distal to the fetlock. Five milliliters of local anesthetic injected deep and another 5 mL of local anesthetic are injected superficially. This injection is then repeated on the palmar or plantar aspect of the pastern, just distal to the dewclaws. Five milliliters of local anesthetic are then used to block the digital nerve on both the medial and lateral aspects of the fetlock, which are approximately 2 cm dorsal and proximal to the dewclaw. The 2 interdigital injections performed in the 4-point block may also be used for removal of an interdigital fibroma.[57]

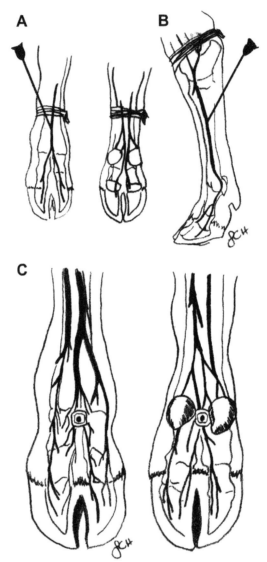

Fig. 8. Proper application of a tourniquet and placement of needle for intravenous administration of local anesthetic. (*A*) Plantar metacarpal vein. (*B*) Plantar metacarpal vein. (*C*) Radial vein.

ANESTHESIA OF THE EYE

Multiple techniques are available for anesthesia of the eye, eyelids, and orbit. Reasons for choosing 1 block rather than another should include the surgeon's comfort and skill at performing the blocks, the disease process present, and a knowledge of the risks associated with each block. Although the Peterson eye block is considered more technically challenging, it is associated with less risk of trauma to the orbit for penetration of the globe, hemorrhage, and damage to the optic nerve.

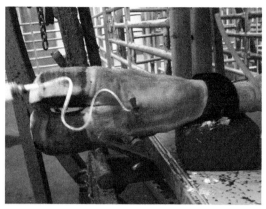

Fig. 9. Intravenous regional anesthesia of the foot. Lidocaine 2% HCl (20 mL) is infused into the dorsal common digital vein distal to a rubber tourniquet.

However, there is risk of neurologic signs or death because of cardiopulmonary arrest if lidocaine is injected into the optic nerve meninges or nasal turbinates. The 4-point block is technically less challenging to perform and seems to yield better anesthesia of the periocular tissues. Although there is risk of intrameningeal injection, the authors' clinical experience has shown it to be less of an issue than with the Peterson nerve block.

AURICULOPALPEBRAL NERVE BLOCK

Surgical manipulation of the eye is facilitated by nerve blockade of the eyelids. Auriculopalpebral nerve block can be placed to reduce upper eyelid movement before performing a Peterson or retrobulbar block. The auriculopalpebral nerve can be palpated as it crosses the zygomatic arch, roughly 5 to 6 cm behind the supraorbital process (**Fig. 10**). Inject 5 mL of 2% lidocaine HCl subcutaneously on the dorsal aspect of the zygomatic arch at this location.

PETERSON NERVE BLOCK

After performing a small local skin block over the intended site of puncture, a 3.8-cm 14-gauge needle is inserted through the skin as a cannula for introduction of an 18-gauge 9-cm needle for the nerve block. The cannula is inserted caudal to the junction of the supraorbital process and zygomatic arch and is introduced through the skin (**Fig. 11**). Then, the 18-gauge 9-cm needle is introduced through the cannula needle and is directed in a horizontal and slightly dorsal direction until the coronoid process is encountered. The needle is walked off the rostral aspect of the coronoid process and advanced in a ventromedial direction along the caudal aspect of the orbit until the needle encounters the bony plate encasing the foramen orbitorotundum. Once the needle is advanced to the foramen, it is advised that the needle be drawn back a few millimeters to reduce the risk of intrameningeal injection. After aspirating to ensure that the needle is not in the internal maxillary artery, 10 to 15 mL of lidocaine (2%) are deposited, with an additional 5 mL of lidocaine deposited as the needle is slowly withdrawn. Mydriasis indicates a successful block.

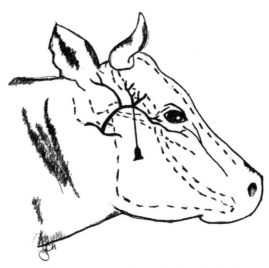

Fig. 10. Needle placement for desensitizing the auriculopalpebral nerve in cattle.

FOUR-POINT RETROBULBAR NERVE BLOCK

The 4-point retrobulbar block is technically easier and can be done more rapidly than the Peterson eye block. In this technique, an 18-gauge 9-cm needle is introduced through the skin on the dorsal, lateral, ventral, and medial aspects of the eye, at 12, 3, 6, and 9 o'clock positions, respectively. Introduction of the needle through the conjunctiva should be avoided to reduce the risk of ocular contamination. The needle is directed behind the globe using the bony orbit as a guide. When the needle is introduced into the retrobulbar sheath, the eye moves slightly with the tug of the needle. After this location is reached and aspiration is performed to ensure that the needle is not in a vessel, 5 to 10 mL of lidocaine (2%) are deposited at each site. Mydriasis indicates a successful block.

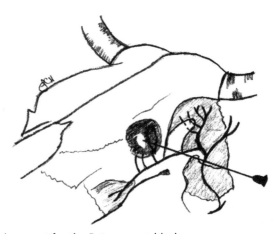

Fig. 11. Needle placement for the Peterson eye block.

RETROBULBAR BLOCK

An alternative to the 4-point retrobulbar block is the single retrobulbar block (**Fig. 12**). In this technique, the 9-cm 18-gauge needle is bent into a half circle. The needle is inserted immediately ventral to the dorsal orbital rim and directed such that the needle makes contact with the bone of the orbit. Then the needle is advanced as it is rotated ventrally in a progressive manner such that the needle remains in close proximity to the bone. After the needle is inserted to the caudal aspect of the eye, 20 mL of 2% lidocaine HCl are administered after aspiration to ensure that the needle is not positioned in a vessel or other fluid structure. Successful deposition of lidocaine causes mild proptosis of the globe.

RING BLOCK

Additional local anesthesia of the eyelids is recommended because the Peterson and retrobulbar blocks typically result in incomplete analgesia of the eyelids. Between 5 and 10 mL of lidocaine (2%) are infiltrated subcutaneously 2.5 cm from the eyelid margins as a ring block.

ANESTHESIA OF THE TEAT

Because most dairy cattle are accustomed to handling and restraint for milking, surgeries of the teat can often be performed with the animal standing and with minimal restraint. Because standing procedures are always preferred in order to prevent udder trauma, most surgical procedures of the teat are performed using local anesthesia.

INVERTED V BLOCK

The inverted V block is used primarily for specific lesions of the teat such as a teat laceration or wart. Using a 25-gauge 1.5-cm needle, approximately 5 mL of local anesthetic are injected into the skin and musculature dorsal to the surgical site in an inverted V pattern (**Fig. 13**).[39]

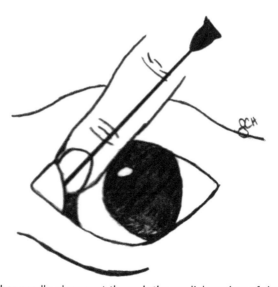

Fig. 12. Retrobulbar needle placement through the medial canthus of the eye in cattle.

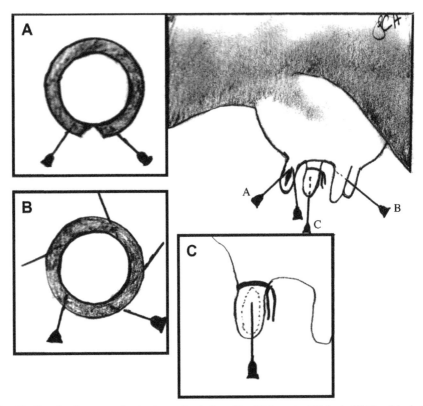

Fig. 13. Needle placement for teat anesthesia in cattle. (*A*) Inverted V block. (*B*) Ring block. (*C*) Placement of a tourniquet and teat cannula for infusion of local anesthetic into the teat cistern.

RING BLOCK

The ring block is a commonly used procedure for teat surgeries. Using a 25-gauge 1.5-cm needle, approximately 5 mL of local anesthetic are injected into the skin and musculature encircling the base of the teat (see **Fig. 13**).[39]

INFUSION OF THE TEAT CISTERN

The teat cistern may be infused with local anesthetic to assist in surgical conditions that only involve the mucous membranes (eg, removal of polyps). Before infusing the teat, the cistern should be milked out and the orifice thoroughly cleaned with alcohol. A tourniquet (rubber band) is then placed on the base of the teat with adequate tension to prevent leakage between the udder and teat cistern. A sterile teat cannula is introduced and approximately 10 mL of local anesthetic are infused to fill the teat (see **Fig. 13**). The teat cannula is removed, and the remaining anesthetic is milked out. Once the surgery is finished, the tourniquet is removed. The musculature and skin are not desensitized using this technique.

INTERNAL PUDENDAL NERVE BLOCK

The procedure for bilateral internal pudendal (pudic) nerve block was first described by Larson[60] to facilitate relaxation of the bull's penis without causing locomotor impairment. The internal pudendal nerve block can be used in the standing bull for penile relaxation and analgesia distal to the sigmoid flexure and examination of the penis. In the standing female, the internal pudendal nerve block can be used to relieve straining caused by chronic vaginal prolapse. This technique may also be used for surgical procedures of the penis such as repair of prolapses, removal of perianal tumors, removal of penile papillomas or warts, and other minor surgeries of the penis and prepuce.

This procedure involves desensitizing the internal pudendal nerve and the anastomotic branch of the middle hemorrhoidal nerve using an ischiorectal approach. The internal pudendal nerve consists of fibers originating from the ventral branches of the third and fourth sacral nerves (S_3 and S_4) and the pelvic splanchnic nerves. The skin at the ischiorectal fossa on either side of the spine is clipped, disinfected, and desensitized with approximately 2 mL of local anesthetic. A 14-gauge 1.25-cm needle is inserted through the desensitized skin at the ischiorectal fossa to serve as a cannula (**Fig. 14**). An 18-gauge 10-cm spinal needle is then directed through the cannula to the pudendal nerve. The operator's left hand is placed into the rectum to the level of the wrist and the fingers directed laterally and ventrally to identify the lesser sacrosciatic foramen. The lesser sciatic foramen is first identified by rectal palpation as a soft depression in the sacrosciatic ligament. The internal pudendal nerve can be readily identified lying on the ligament immediately cranial and dorsal to the foramen and approximately 1 finger's width dorsal to the pudendal artery passing through the foramen. The internal pudendal artery can be readily palpated a finger's width ventral to the nerve. The spinal needle is held in the operator's right hand and introduced through the cannula in the ischiorectal fossa. The spinal needle is directed medial to the sacrosciatic ligament and directed cranioventrally. The needle cannot be felt until it has been introduced approximately 5 to 7 cm, and it can then be repositioned to the nerve. Once at the pudendal nerve, 20 mL of local anesthetic are deposited at the nerve. The needle is then partially withdrawn and redirected 2 to 3 cm caudodorsally where an additional 10 mL of local anesthetic are deposited at the cranial aspect of the foramen to desensitize the muscular branches and the middle hemorrhoidal nerve. The needle is then removed and the sites of deposition are massaged to aid in dispersal of the local anesthetic. This procedure is then repeated on the opposite

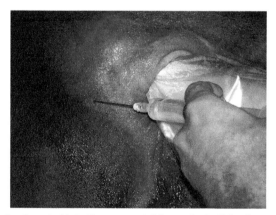

Fig. 14. Needle being inserted into the pararectal fossa of a bull for the purpose of blocking the pudendal nerve. Pudendal nerve block achieves paralysis of the retractor penis muscles and facilitates extension, manipulation, and surgery of the penis and prepuce.

side of the pelvis. Relaxation of the penis varies and may take as long as 30 to 40 minutes for full effect. The duration of the internal pudendal nerve block is from 2 to 4 hours.

ANESTHESIA FOR DEHORNING

The cornual nerve block is used for anesthesia for dehorning cattle. The horn and the skin around the base of the horn are innervated by the cornual branch of the lacrimal or zygomaticotemporal nerve, which is part of the ophthalmic division of the trigeminal nerve. The cornual nerve passes through the periorbital tissues dorsally and runs along the frontal crest to the base of the horns. Approximately 5 to 10 mL of a local anesthetic agent are deposited subcutaneously and superficially midway between the lateral canthus of the eye and the base of the horn along the zygomatic process (**Fig. 15**). Complete anesthesia may take 10 minutes. Larger cattle with well-developed horns require additional anesthetic infiltration along the caudal aspect of the horn, in the form of a partial ring block, to desensitize subcutaneous branches of the second cervical nerve.

NASAL ANESTHESIA

The infraorbital nerve block may be used for the repair of nasal lacerations and the placement of a nose ring. The infraorbital nerve is the continuation of the maxillary branch of the fifth cranial nerve after it enters the infraorbital canal. The infraorbital nerve has only sensory function and emerges on the face as a flat band through the infraorbital foramen where it is covered by the levator nasolabialis muscle. The infraorbital nerve is blocked as it emerges from the infraorbital canal. The nerve is difficult to palpate but is located rostral to the facial tuberosity on a line extending from the naso-maxillary notch to the second upper premolar. From 20 to 30 mL of local anesthetic agent are injected deep into the levator nasolabialis muscle with an 18-gauge 3.8-cm needle (**Fig. 16**). The injection should be repeated on the opposite side.

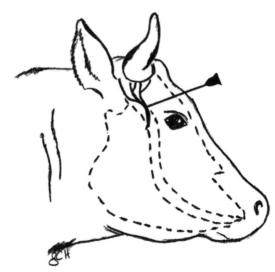

Fig. 15. Needle placement for desensitizing the cornual branch of the zygomaticotemporal nerve in cattle.

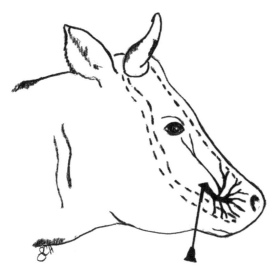

Fig. 16. Needle placement for desensitizing the infraorbital nerve in cattle.

ELECTROACUPUNCTURE AND ELECTROIMMOBILIZATION

Few scientific data are available for the use of acupuncture techniques in critical cases in cattle. Our clinical experience with acupuncture is limited to attempts to ameliorate chronic pain. Although we have observed profound short-term improvement in pain in cases of arthritis, myopathy, and a variety of injuries, we have not attempted to use acupuncture for surgery or management of critical cases. Kim and colleagues[61] evaluated the use of electroacupuncture for induction of analgesia for surgery in cattle. Cattle were assigned to (1) the dorsal acupoint (GV-20 and GV-5), (2) the lumbar acupoint (BL-21, BL-23, BL-24, and BL-25), (3) the combined dorsal and lumbar (BL-21, BL-23, BL-24, and GV-5), or (4) the control group. Analgesia was most profound after dorsal acupoint, followed by the combined group and then the lumbar group. The investigators stated that the dorsal acupoints cause recumbency and are only suitable for recumbent surgery in cattle, but that the combined or lumbar acupoints would be useful for standing surgery.

Electroimmobilization for surgical procedures is controversial. The ideal balance of control and inhibition of pain is difficult to achieve and monitor. In a study designed to examine the physiologic responses of heifers to spaying, flank ovariectomy was performed using electroimmobilization as the sole means of analgesia but administered by a veterinarian skilled in the use of the immobilizer.[62,63] Significant increases in serum cortisol were found compared with control heifers. Humane, effective use of electroacupuncture requires intensive training of the operator. Routine use of this technology is not recommended without special training.

REFERENCES

1. Coetzee JF. A review of pain assessment techniques and pharmacological approaches to pain relief after bovine castration: practical implications for cattle production within the United States. Appl Anim Behav Sci 2011;135:192–213.
2. George LW. Pain control in food animals. In: Steffey EP, editor. Recent Advances in anesthetic management of large domestic animals. International Veterinary

Information Service; 2003. p. 1–13. Available at: www.ivis.org Document No. A0615.1103. Accessed September 30, 2012.

3. Hewson CJ, Dohoo IR, Lemke KA, et al. Canadian veterinarians' use of analgesics in cattle, pigs, and horses in 2004 and 2005. Can Vet J 2007;48(2):155–64.

4. Fajt VR, Wagner SA, Norby B. Analgesic drug administration and attitudes about analgesia in cattle among bovine practitioners in the United States. J Am Vet Med Assoc 2011;238:755–67.

5. Laven RA, Huxley JN, Stafford KJ. Results of attitudes of dairy veterinarians in New Zealand regarding painful procedures and conditions in cattle. N Z Vet J 2009;57:215–20.

6. Huxley JN, Whay HR. Current attitudes of cattle practitioners to pain and the use of analgesics in cattle. Vet Rec 2006;159:662–8.

7. Broom DM. The evolution of pain. Vlaams Diergeneeskundig Tijdschrift 2000;69: 385–411.

8. Miranda C, Di Virgilio M, Selleri S, et al. Novel pathogenic mechanisms of congenital insensitivity to pain with anhidrosis genetic disorder unveiled by functional analysis of neurotrophic tyrosine receptor kinase type 1/nerve growth factor receptor mutations. J Biol Chem 2002;277:6455–62.

9. Craig AD. Pain mechanisms: labeled lines versus convergence in central processing. Annu Rev Neurosci 2003;26:1–30.

10. Woolf CJ. Pain: moving from symptom control toward mechanism-specific pharmacologic management. Ann Intern Med 2004;140:441–51.

11. Muir WW, Woolf CJ. Mechanisms of pain and their therapeutic implications. J Am Vet Med Assoc 2001;219(10):1346–56.

12. Woolf CJ, Slater MW. Neuronal plasticity: increasing the gain in pain. Science 2000;288:1765–9.

13. Carstens E, Mober GP. Recognizing pain and distress in laboratory animals. ILAR J 2000;41(2):62–71.

14. Scholz J, Woolf CJ. Can we conquer pain? Nat Neurosci 2002;5:1062–7.

15. Clark JD, Rager DR, Calpin JP. Animal well-being I. General considerations. Lab Anim Sci 1997;47(6):564–70.

16. Clark JD, Rager DR, Calpin JP. Animal well-being II. Stress and distress. Lab Anim Sci 1997;47(6):571–85.

17. Carr DB, Goudes LC. Acute pain. Lancet 1999;353:2051–8.

18. Desborough JP. The stress response to trauma and surgery. Br J Anaesth 2000; 85(1):109–17.

19. Weissman C. The metabolic response to stress: an overview and update. Anaesthesia 1999;73:308–27.

20. Chapman CR, Gavin J. Suffering: the contributions of persistent pain. Lancet 1999;353:2233–7.

21. Herskin MS, Munksgaard L, Ladewig J. Effects of acute stressors on nociception, adrenocortical responses and behavior of dairy cows. Physiol Behav 2004;83: 411–20.

22. Herskin MS, Kristensen AM, Munksgaard L. Behavioral responses of dairy cows toward novel stimuli presented in the home environment. Appl Anim Behav Sci 2004;89:27–40.

23. Herskin MS, Munksgaard L, Andersen JB. Effects of social isolation and restraint on adrenocortical responses and hypoalgesia in loose-housed dairy cows. J Anim Sci 2007;85:240–7.

24. Galindo F, Broom DM. Effects of lameness of dairy cows. J Appl Anim Welf Sci 2002;5(3):193–201.

25. Rushen J, Boissy A, Terlouw EM, et al. Opioid peptides and behavioral and physiological responses of dairy cows to social isolation in unfamiliar surroundings. J Anim Sci 1999;77(11):2918–24.
26. Otto KA, Short CE. Pharmaceutical control of pain in large animals. Appl Anim Behav Sci 1998;59:157–69.
27. Wittek T, Tischer K, Gieseler T, et al. Effect of preoperative administration of erythromycin or flunixin meglumine on postoperative abomasal emptying rate in dairy cows undergoing surgical correction of left displacement of the abomasum. J Am Vet Med Assoc 2008;232:418–23.
28. Guglielmini C, Giuliani A, Bernardini D, et al. Use of flunixin in cows with left abomasal displacement. Atti della Societa Italiana di Buiatria 2001;33: 269–73.
29. Walker KA, Duffield TF, Weary DM. Indentifying and preventing pain during and after surgery in farm animals. Appl Anim Behav Sci 2011;135:259–65.
30. Coetzee JF, KuKanich B, Mosher R, et al. Pharmacokinetics of intravenous and oral meloxicam in ruminant calves. Vet Ther 2009;10:E1–8.
31. Coetzee JF, Mosher RA, Kohake LE, et al. Pharmacokinetics of oral gabapentin alone or co-administered with meloxicam in ruminant beef calves. Vet J 2011; 190:98–102.
32. Coetzee JF, Gehring R, Tarus-Sang J, et al. Effect of sub-anesthetic xylazine and ketamine ("ketamine stun") administered to calves immediately prior to castration. Vet Anaesth Analg 2010;37:566–78.
33. Abrahamsen EJ. Chemical restraint in ruminants. Vet Clin North Am Food Anim Pract 2008;24:227–43.
34. Muir WW, Hubbell JA, Skarda R, et al. Local anesthesia in cattle, sheep, goats, and pigs. In: Muir WM, Hubbell JA, Skarda R, et al, editors. Handbook of veterinary anesthesia. 2nd edition. St Louis (MO): Mosby; 1995. p. 53–77.
35. Muir WW, Hubbell JA, Skarda R, et al. Local anesthetic drugs and techniques. In: Muir WM, Hubbell JA, Skarda R, et al, editors. Handbook of veterinary anesthesia. 2nd edition. St Louis (MO): Mosby; 1995. p. 39–52.
36. Rostami M, Vesal N. Comparison of lidocaine, lidocaine/epinephrine or bupivacaine for thoracolumbar paravertebral anaesthesia in fat-tailed sheep. Vet Anaesth Analg 2011;38:598–602.
37. Nelson ST. Skin lesions in cattle after use of lidokel-adrena. Norsk Veterinaertidsskrift (NVT) 2011;123:357–64.
38. Vesal N, Jahromi AR, Oryan A. Lidocaine containing high concentrations of a vasoconstrictor: is it safe for infiltration anesthesia? Comp Clin Pathol 2012; 21:1703–6.
39. Noordsy J, Ames N. Local and regional anesthesia. In: Noordsy J, Ames N, editors. Food animal surgery. 4th edition. Yardley (PA): Veterinary Learning Systems; 2006. p. 21–42.
40. Skarda R. Local and regional anesthesia in ruminants and swine. Vet Clin North Am Food Anim Pract 1996;12:579–626.
41. Nuss K, Eiberle BJ, Sauter-Louis C. Comparison of two methods of local anesthesia for laparotomy in cattle. Tierarztl Prax Ausg G Grosstiere Nutztiere 2012; 40(3):141–9 [in German].
42. Edwards B. Regional anaesthesia techniques in cattle. Practice 2001;23:142–9.
43. St-Jean G, Skarda RT, Muir WW, et al. Caudal epidural analgesia induced by xylazine administration in cows. Am J Vet Res 1990;51:1232–6.
44. Caron JP, LeBlanc PH. Caudal epidural analgesia in cattle using xylazine. Can J Vet Res 1989;53:486–9.

45. DeRossi R, Bucker GV, Varela JV. Perineal analgesic actions of epidural clonidine in cattle. Vet Anaesth Analg 2003;30:64–71.
46. Lee I, Yoshiuchi T, Yamagishi N, et al. Analgesic effect of caudal epidural ketamine in cattle. J Vet Sci 2003;4:261–4.
47. Fierheller EE, Caulkett NA, Bailey JV. A romifidine and morphine combination for epidural analgesia in the flank in cattle. Can Vet J 2004;45:917–23.
48. Prado ME, Streeter RN, Mandsager RE, et al. Pharmacologic effects of epidural versus intramuscular administration of detomidine in cattle. Am J Vet Res 1999; 60:1242–7.
49. Lin HC, Trachte EA, DeGraves FJ, et al. Evaluation of analgesia induced by epidural administration of medetomidine to cows. Am J Vet Res 1998;59:162–7.
50. Noordsy J, Ames N. Epidural anesthesia. In: Noordsy J, Ames N, editors. Food animal surgery. 4th edition. Yardley (PA): Veterinary Learning Systems; 2006. p. 43–55.
51. Araujo MA, Albuquerque VB, Deschk M, et al. Cardiopulmonary and analgesic effects of caudal epidurally administered ropivacaine in cattle. Vet Anaesth Analg 2012;39:409–13.
52. Meyer H, Starke A, Kehler W, et al. High caudal epidural anaesthesia with local anaesthetics or alpha-2 agonists in calves. J Vet Med A Physiol Pathol Clin Med 2007;54:384–9.
53. Offinger J, Meyer H, Fischer J, et al. Comparison of isoflurane inhalation anaesthesia, injection anaesthesia, and high volume caudal epidural anaesthesia for umbilical surgery in calves; metabolic, endocrine, and cardiopulmonary effects. Vet Anaesth Analg 2012;39:123–36.
54. Lewis CA, Constable PD, Huhn JC, et al. Sedation with xylazine and lumbosacral epidural administration of lidocaine and xylazine for umbilical surgery in calves. J Am Vet Med Assoc 1999;214:89–95.
55. Trim CM. Epidural analgesia with 0.75% bupivacaine for laparotomy in goats. J Am Vet Med Assoc 1989;194:1292–6.
56. Chevalier HM, Provost PJ, Karas AZ. Effect of caudal epidural xylazine on intraoperative distress and post-operative pain in Holstein heifers. Vet Anaesth Analg 2004;31:1–10.
57. Navarre C. Numbing - Nose to Tail. Proceedings from the 39th Annual Convention of AABP. 2006;39. p. 53–5.
58. Bigham AS, Habibian S, Ghasemian F, et al. Caudal epidural injection of lidocaine, tramadol, and lidocaine-tramadol for epidural anesthesia in cattle. J Vet Pharmacol Ther 2010;33:439–43.
59. Bergadano A, Moens Y, Schatzmann U. Continuous extradural analgesia in a cow with complex regional pain syndrome. Vet Anaesth Analg 2006;33:189–92.
60. Larson LL. The internal pudendal (pudic) nerve block. J Am Vet Med Assoc 1953; 123:18–27.
61. Kim DH, Cho SH, Song KH, et al. Electroacupuncture analgesia for surgery in cattle. Am J Chin Med 2004;32:131–40.
62. Petherick JC, McCosker K, Mayer DG, et al. Preliminary investigation of some physiological responses of Bos indicus heifers to surgical spaying. Aust Vet J 2011;89:131–7.
63. Anderson DE, Muir WW. Pain management in ruminants. Vet Clin North Am 2005; 21:19–31.

Assessment and Management of Pain in Small Ruminants and Camelids

Paul J. Plummer, DVM, PhD[a],*, Jennifer A. Schleining, DVM, MS[b]

KEYWORDS

- Sheep • Goat • Llama • Alpaca • Pain • Small ruminant • Analgesia

KEY POINTS

- Pain management of small ruminants has historically been discounted. We provide an evidence-based overview of the important aspect of pain control in these species.
- Economical options for pain management are available and efficacious.
- Many husbandry practices and postoperative case management can be improved with attention to pain management.

INTRODUCTION

Like other animal species, small ruminants and camelids experience pain after noxious stimuli. In some cases, the noxious stimuli may come in the form of a management procedure (eg, tail docking or castration). In other cases, the pain may be the direct or indirect result of a naturally occurring physiologic abnormality (eg, urethral obstruction or surgery for obstetrics, respectively). The prompt identification of pain in veterinary patients and the development of management plans to ameliorate the pain are of paramount importance to animal productivity and welfare. In cases in which the pain results from a management procedure, it is preferable for the veterinary practitioner to anticipate the pain and to develop and implement preemptive pain management strategies before conducting the procedure. The goal of this article is to summarize the current understanding of pain management in small ruminants and camelids. Toward that end, first, the methods used to evaluate pain in these species are reviewed and some management goals for pain control are outlined. A brief discussion of the predominant pharmacologic options follows, building into a discussion of multimodal therapeutic strategies that can be used. Some preemptive pain management

[a] College of Veterinary Medicine, Veterinary Diagnostic and Production Animal Medicine, 2426 Lloyd Veterinary Medical Center, Iowa State University, Ames, IA 50011, USA; [b] College of Veterinary Medicine, Veterinary Diagnostic and Production Animal Medicine, 2418 Lloyd Veterinary Medical Center, Iowa State University, Ames, IA 50011, USA
* Corresponding author.
E-mail address: pplummer@iastate.edu

Vet Clin Food Anim 29 (2013) 185–208
http://dx.doi.org/10.1016/j.cvfa.2012.11.004
0749-0720/13/$ – see front matter © 2013 Elsevier Inc. All rights reserved.

strategies for management procedures commonly performed in these species are discussed.

MANAGEMENT GOALS

Pain management strategies for small ruminants and camelids should be both clinically effective and economically feasible for the owner and adhere to the principles of the American Medicinal Drug Use Clarification Act (AMDUCA) and appropriate meat and milk withdrawal times. Because of the physiologic differences between ruminant species, pharmaceutical studies performed in large ruminants should be cautiously extrapolated to small and pseudoruminants. Therefore, the best practices for pain management in these smaller species should rely on scientific evidence, where available. Goals for managing pain should be centered on preemptive analgesia when possible (ie, preoperative administration of antiinflammatories or other pharmaceutical agents), interventions that provide a steady state of analgesia, and administration of medication that minimizes negative side effects. Arguably, one of the most difficult tasks in pain management is the recognition of pain in certain small ruminants, especially sheep and camelids, which tend to be stoic and do not readily show overt signs of discomfort. Subtle deviations of behavior, appetite, urination, or defecation from normal can be used to determine if a patient is experiencing pain. A good resource for pain recognition strategies in livestock is the Guidelines for Recognition and Assessment of Animal Pain resource published online by the Royal (Dick) School of Veterinary Studies, Edinburgh, Scotland.[1] Likewise, a challenge in interpreting pharmacologic data is the lack of published therapeutic concentrations for any of the available medications for use in small ruminants and camelids. Many of the therapeutic concentration ranges are extrapolated from companion animals or humans and may not reflect the concentration of drug required for analgesia in small ruminant species.

THERAPEUTIC DRUG OPTIONS

Generally, there are 3 primary classes of pharmaceutical agents routinely used to control pain in small ruminants and camelids. These classes are essentially the same as those used in other food-producing and fiber-producing species and have been discussed at length in other sections of this publication. In this section, the mechanism of action for these agents is reviewed and, when possible, the clinical usefulness of the agents in small ruminants and camelids is summarized. The use of all of these drugs in small ruminants is considered extralabel under AMDUCA and therefore requires the oversight of a licensed veterinarian and appropriate record keeping. One other significant difference between the broad classes of pharmaceutical agents is that some of these agents are considered controlled drugs that require Drug Enforcement Administration (DEA) registration and additional paperwork and drug security issues. This situation is especially true of the opioid class of compounds. Mobile veterinary practices should consult their local veterinary medical association, the state board of pharmacy, and the DEA regional office regarding the appropriate storage and transportation of these compounds.

α_2-Adrenergic Agonists

α_2-Adrenergic agonists are routinely used on small ruminants and camelids for both their sedative and analgesic properties. Examples of these drugs include xylazine, detomidine, and medetomidine. The analgesic potency of these compounds is generally considered to be similar to that of the opioids, given that they use the same effector mechanisms and are located on many of the same neurons of the brain as the μ-opioid receptor.[2] On binding to the α_2-adrenergic receptor in neurons of the brain, the drug induces signaling of the membrane-associated G-coupled proteins, which results in activation of potassium channels in the postsynaptic neuron. This process allows an influx of potassium into the cell, resulting in hyperpolarization and making cells unresponsive to stimulation.[2]

Ruminants and camelids are generally more sensitive to α_2-adrenergic agonist than other species like horses and small animals. Hence, appropriate dosing is important when designing a therapeutic regimen. For this reason, large animal preparations of xylazine (ie, 100 mg/mL) may not be appropriate for use in animals with a small body size. Many practitioners use 20 mg/mL xylazine and may even further dilute with sterile water as needed to a 1 to 2 mg/mL concentration when appropriate for the size of the animal being dosed. Similar dilution of other α_2-adrenergic agonists may be necessary. These drugs are eliminated from the plasma rapidly and have short elimination half-lives. For this reason, use of these drugs in an intramuscular (IM) or epidural manner may prolong the period of analgesia over that of intravenous (IV) dosing, albeit slower in onset than IV.[3]

Although there are limited data on the duration of analgesia, what data are available suggest that IM dosing of xylazine provides roughly 60 minutes of analgesic efficacy, with onset of action and the magnitude of effect being dose-dependent.[4] Xylazine does cause cardiovascular depression with a dose-dependent decrease in heart rate and cardiac output.[3] In pregnant animals, the drug also results in decreased heart rates of the fetuses. Xylazine has also been associated with decreased lung compliance, tachypnea, pulmonary edema, and hypoxia.[3] A transient hyperglycemia is often observed after use of xylazine in ruminants. This hyperglycemia results in increased urine output, and this class of drugs does have a propensity to induce a short-term diuresis. Although this side effect generally has minimal impact on the patient, it should be considered if the drug is being used to provide analgesia for a small ruminant that is experiencing an ongoing urethral obstruction. The analgesic effect and side effects of detomidine and medetomidine are similar to those described for xylazine.[3] Because of their short duration of potent analgesia, these compounds are most helpful in the management of acute and surgical pain in small ruminants and camelids. In some cases of chronic severe pain, a loading dose followed by continuous rate infusions (CRI) of these drugs is helpful; however, the analgesia is typically accompanied with a dose-dependent sedation. Given that the analgesic and sedative properties are both dose-dependent, high-dose analgesia typically results in profound sedation. The use of the epidural route in administering these drugs may lessen the sedation compared with other routes.

One benefit to the use of α_2-adrenergic agonist class is that their effects (including their side effects) can be rapidly reversed with the use of α_2-adrenergic antagonist such as tolazoline and yohimbine. When these antagonists are used, the analgesic properties of the drug are also reversed, potentially leaving the patient painful if alternate means of analgesia are not instituted. For this reason, multimodal analgesia protocols are encouraged when feasible and appropriate.

Nonsteroidal Antiinflammatory Drugs

The nonsteroidal antiinflammatory drug (NSAID) class of compounds provides analgesia indirectly by decreasing the inflammatory response to injury. Tissue damage generally results in the production of inflammatory mediators such as kinins and prostaglandins that activate primary afferent neurons and result in pain. By blocking the cyclooxygenase (COX) pathway, NSAIDs prevent the formation of prostaglandins and other signals.[5] Compared with the α_2-adrenergic agonist and the opioid classes of compounds, NSAIDs have several benefits. First, they do not result in sedation of the patient, a side effect of the other two drug classes. Second, they provide a longer duration of analgesia and a slower plasma half-life. They are generally considered most effective against pain of low to moderate intensity and originating from the somatic or integumentary systems. The general side effects of this class of drugs include gastrointestinal (GI) ulceration and nephropathy (especially in hypovolemic, dehydrated patients). Although these drugs may be helpful in the management of chronic pain, the clinician should consider these side effects in developing treatment regimens and should monitor for complications when long-term therapy is necessary. In patients who present with severe dehydration, fluid therapy to restore glomerular filtration rate may be warranted before the initiation of NSAID therapy, because of its propensity to cause nephropathies.

Flunixin Meglumine

Flunixin is generally administered as a parenteral formulation to ruminants and camelids. Although oral formulations exist for horses, their pharmacokinetics have not been determined in small ruminants and their use cannot be advocated. All commercially available formulations of flunixin as a single drug (ie, not mixed with an antimicrobial) are labeled for use by the IV route. Injection of these products by the IM route results in severe tissue damage, prolongs the drug withdrawal time, and can result in an anaerobic environment that predisposes to clostridial myositis. Because of these complications, the US Food and Drug Administration (FDA) has warned that they view the use of flunixin by a route of administration other than that labeled on the product as a violation of AMDUCA. Of the NSAIDs, flunixin is believed to have the most potent effects on relieving visceral pain. Although flunixin has a longer half-life than the opioid and α_2-adrenergic agonists, administration every 12 to 24 hours is generally recommended.

Phenylbutazone

Phenylbutazone is a potent NSAID, which is typically believed to provide better musculoskeletal pain control. It is available as both an oral and injectable product in the United States, with the oral product being most commonly used in small ruminants and camelids. The injectable product shares the side effects of tissue necrosis with flunixin and should be administered only IV. IM injection of phenylbutazone results in a significant local muscle necrosis and meat carcass defects and may predispose to clostridial myositis. Because of reports of an idiosyncratic serum-sickness–type hypersensitivity reaction in humans consuming milk contaminated with phenylbutazone, the use of this drug is prohibited in all female dairy cattle older than 20 months. Although not specified by the FDA, the use of this drug in commercial dairy goats or dairy sheep is likely not warranted and should be avoided.

Meloxicam

Although meloxicam has been heavily used in small animals, its usefulness in ruminants and camelids has only recently been appreciated. The product is available in the United States as an injectable product for small animals but is cost-prohibitive for use in large animals. Currently, the generic oral formulation of the compound is most widely used and validated in small ruminants and camelids. Comparative pharmacodynamics suggest that the oral formulation is highly bioavailable in sheep, goats, and camelids. Current cost for the generic tablets allows treatment of large animals at a reasonable cost of approximately US$0.20 per 45.35 kg (100 lb) of body weight. The tablets can be easily crushed and top-dressed onto grain, although such use is considered illegal under AMDUCA if a drug is used in an extralabel manner and compounded with feed. Because small ruminants tend to be more selective in their eating habits than cattle, the crushed tablets can also be mixed in molasses or water and drenched to the animals. Meloxicam also has the advantage of having a longer plasma half-life than that of flunixin or phenylbutazone and can be administered orally every 24 to 48 hours, maintaining plasma levels believed to provide sufficient analgesia.

Aspirin

Although aspirin has been on the market for a considerable period, it is not widely used in small ruminants or camelids. Well-designed studies of aspirin in cattle have failed to show significant benefits to its use, which has been associated with a short plasma elimination half-life.

Opioids

The opioid class of compounds is a broad group of drugs, all of which have been shown to bind to opioid receptors in the nervous system. These drugs are subclassified by their action as agonist, agonist-antagonist, or antagonist of one of several opioid receptors that have been identified. Like the α_2-adrenergic agonist, stimulation of the opioid receptors results in stimulation of the G-coupled protein pathways and the hyperpolarization of postsynaptic neurons. These compounds are generally believed to provide potent visceral analgesia.

Most opioids are considered controlled substances and are regulated by the DEA. They require special licenses to possess, order, and prescribe and must be stored in an approved manner. One important exception to this is nalbuphine, which is not a scheduled drug (in most states, except in Kentucky; check your local regulations before using) and has potential application in food animals as an analgesic therapy.

As a general class of drugs, the opioids can induce some degree of sedation, respiratory depression, decreased GI motility, and decreased appetite. In some cases, they can induce a hyperexcitable state that masks their sedative properties.[6] They do have potent analgesic activity, with some degree of variation in potency noticeable between the different specific compounds.

Morphine

Morphine is the prototypical opioid agonist. It is generally administered as an injectable product by either the IV, IM, or epidural routes. Morphine has a relatively short plasma elimination half-life and hence must be readministered frequently. In the United States, morphine is a scheduled drug and requires proper DEA licensing and record keeping. Compared with some of the other opioid products, it is generally less expensive; however, its analgesic potency is also less than many of the other opioids. The analgesic potency of morphine is similar to that of the α_2-adrenergic agonist.

Butorphanol

Butorphanol is a synthetic opioid, with both agonist and antagonist properties. Compared with morphine, it is 3 to 5 times more potent in its analgesic effects.[6] Butorphanol is considered to have fewer negative effects on the GI and respiratory system compared with morphine, but costs considerably more. In recent years, increased use of a combination of butorphanol, xylazine, and ketamine for restraint in small ruminants and camelids has shown potent analgesic effects. Butorphanol is a scheduled narcotic and requires DEA licensure and appropriate record keeping.

Nalbuphine

Nalbuphine is a lesser-known opioid agonist/antagonist, which in most (but not all) jurisdictions is not scheduled and hence does not require DEA licensure. It has a similar mechanism of action to butorphanol but is comparable with morphine in its analgesic efficacy, although some investigators dispute this. Nalbuphine is available at half the cost of butorphanol. It is supplied as an injectable product and can be substituted for butorphanol in many applications. No published studies have shown its use in small ruminants or camelids. However, clinical experience suggests that it performs equally well to butorphanol in these species.

Fentanyl

Fentanyl is a potent opioid analgesic, which is available as both an injectable and dermal patch formulation. Because of cost, the injectable formulation is rarely used in small ruminants or camelids; however, the dermal patch formulation can provide a good solution for moderately long potent analgesia. The patch can be applied to a clipped area of the skin in a portion of the body in which the animal is not likely to consume the patch. The patch can provide stable plasma concentrations for 2 to 3 days.[7]

Ketamine

In addition to the dissociative anesthetic effects of ketamine, it also has a potent analgesic effect at subanesthetic doses. Evidence suggests that the analgesia is more effective for somatic pain than for visceral pain.[8] Although it has a short plasma half-life, CRIs and epidural use of ketamine can be used in concert with other drugs to provide long-term analgesia, when necessary. Ketamine does not depress the respiratory system and stimulates the cardiovascular system. It is a scheduled drug and consequently requires DEA licensure and appropriate paperwork.

Lidocaine

Lidocaine is a local anesthetic, which blocks the depolarization of neurons and hence prevents the propagation of action potentials. It can also act as a systemic analgesic when administered as a CRI.[6] Consequently, lidocaine is used in two specific modalities for pain control in small ruminants and camelids. It is routinely used clinically to perform local nerve blocks and as a local anesthetic during management procedures required for production of these species. Second, it can be used as part of a multimodal analgesic protocol with either CRI or epidural administration. One downside to lidocaine injection for local anesthesia is that, in humans, it burns intensely at the site of injection because of the acidic pH of the commercial product. The burning sensation can be ameliorated by mixing 8.4% sodium bicarbonate with the lidocaine in a 1:10 dilution (ie, 1 mL of 8.4% sodium bicarbonate into 10 mL of lidocaine) (see article elsewhere in this issue). The lidocaine does not stay in solution long-term if the pH is neutralized, hence only the volume of lidocaine needed for a given procedure should be neutralized for immediate use within several hours. The addition of sodium bicarbonate to lidocaine has the added advantages of speeding the onset of action, prolonging the period of anesthesia/analgesia and enhancing the analgesia, and potentially decreasing the pain of the block (see article elsewhere in this issue).[9–12]

γ-Aminobutyric Acid Analogues

Gabapentin is a γ-aminobutyric acid analogue, which was initially developed to treat epilepsy in humans (see article elsewhere in this issue). It is also effective as an analgesic for chronic or neuropathic pain and is used for this function in human medicine. The drug binds to calcium voltage-gated channels and inhibits neuroexcitation. Initial studies in beef calves have shown synergism with NSAIDs (meloxicam) in relieving pain associated with an induced lameness model.[13] We have used the drug several times for treating chronic lameness in small ruminants with apparent success; however, no formal trials have been carried out.

ANALGESIC DRUG REGIMENS

Consult dosing **Tables 1–3** for dose information.

ORAL STRATEGIES

Oral medication has the benefit of ease of administration because most owners can administer an oral bolus, and most oral medications are relatively cost-effective. However, a disadvantage is that the rumen can inactivate certain medications, rendering them useless. This is an area in which the literature should be consulted for pharmaceutical studies for small ruminant species.

Morphine

Oral administration of morphine is not recommended because of inactivation by the rumen. In a study conducted in sheep, only one-third of the animals achieved good analgesia after oral administration.[14] Given the high variability, it does not make a good option for consistent pain control when administered orally.

Gabapentin

The use of gabapentin in small ruminants has not been described in the literature. However, anecdotally, it seems to offer analgesia to ruminants experiencing neuropathic pain, and the pharmacokinetics has recently been described in beef and dairy cattle.[13,15]

NSAIDS

Phenylbutazone

The use of phenylbutazone in food-producing species is not recommended for various reasons.[16] Phenylbutazone has been shown to be a carcinogenic in humans, as well as inducing blood dyscrasias (see article elsewhere in this issue). Because of these concerns, residues in meat and milk have a zero-tolerance level, meaning that residue detection is likely to come with a severe penalty. Supporting this situation is the fact that the elimination of phenylbutazone is extremely slow in ruminants.[17] In addition, flunixin meglumine is an approved nonsteroidal product for the treatment of pyrexia and as an antiinflammatory in major food-producing species (cattle and swine). This situation makes the use of phenylbutazone for the same indications illegal by the principles of AMDUCA. Therefore, even although there is scientific evidence to support the use of phenylbutazone in sheep and goats, because of regulatory guidelines, they are not covered here.

Meloxicam

The use of meloxicam as an analgesic is becoming more common. Its advantages include that it is generally considered to preferentially bind to the COX-2 isoenzyme (not confirmed in small ruminants), therefore theoretically decreasing the risk for harmful side effects common to nonpreferential NSAIDs, ease of administration, and cost-efficiency. Generic meloxicam is available in tablet form in 7.5-mg and 15-mg tablets

Table 1
Analgesic doses for llamas and alpacas

Drug	Dose	Route	Frequency	Comments	References
Opioids					
Morphine	0.1 mg/kg	PO		Not recommended	Abrahamsen 2009[22,a]
		IV, IM	Every 4 h		Grubb et al 2005[43]
Fentanyl	4 of the 75 ug/hr patches per adult llama	TD	Place new patch every 48 h		Abrahamsen 2009[22,a]
Butorphanol	0.05–0.1 mg/kg	IV, IM	Every 4–6 h		Abrahamsen 2009[22,a]
Tramadol	2.0 mg/kg	IV, IM	Every 2–3 h		Cox et al 2011[24]
NSAIDs					
Phenylbutazone	5.0 mg/kg	IV, PO	Every 24–48 h		Anderson 2002[59,a]
Meloxicam	1.0 mg/kg	PO	Every 3 d		Kreuder et al 2012[18]
	0.5 mg/kg	IV			Kreuder et al 2012[18]
Flunixin meglumine	1.1 mg/kg	IV	Every 8 h		Jensen 2003[60,a]
CRI Trifusion					
Butorphanol	0.05–0.1 mg/kg	IV or IM	Loading dose		Abrahamsen 2009[22,a]
	0.022 mg/kg/h	IV	CRI		Abrahamsen 2009[22,a]
Lidocaine	1.0 mg/kg	IV	Loading dose	Administer slowly	Abrahamsen 2009[22,a]
	3.0 mg/kg/h	IV	CRI		Abrahamsen 2009[22,a]
Ketamine	0.6 mg/kg/h	IV	CRI	No loading dose needed	Abrahamsen 2009[22,a]
OR					
Morphine	0.025 mg/kg/h	IV	CRI	No loading dose needed	Abrahamsen 2009[22,a]
Lidocaine	1.0 mg/kg	IV	Loading dose	Administer slowly	Abrahamsen 2009[22,a]
	3.0 mg/kg/h	IV	CRI		Abrahamsen 2009[22,a]
Ketamine	0.6 mg/kg/h	IV	CRI	No loading dose needed	Abrahamsen 2009[22,a]
Lidocaine	1 mL/22.67 kg (50 lb)	EP		Using 2% lidocaine	Anderson 2002[a]
Xylazine	0.1 mg/kg	EP			Anderson 2000[a]

Abbreviations: EP, epidural; PO, by mouth; TD, transdermal.
[a] Indicates published doses that are based on clinical experience.

Table 2
Analgesic doses for sheep

Drug	Dose	Route	Frequency	Comments	References
Opioids					
Morphine		PO		Not recommended	
	0.05–0.1 mg/kg	IV or SQ	Every 4–6 h		George 2003[14]
Fentanyl	0.2 mg/kg	TD			Ahern et al 2010[7]
		IV	Not recommended because of rapid clearance		Ahern et al 2010[7]
NSAIDs					
Phenylbutazone		IV, SQ, PO		Not recommended	
Meloxicam	0.5 mg/kg	IV	Every 12 h		Shukla et al 2007[19]
	2.0 mg/kg	PO	Loading dose		Stock 2012 [Personal communication]
	1.0 mg/kg	PO	Every 24 h after loading dose		Stock 2012 [Personal communication]
Flunixin meglumine	1.1 mg/kg	IV	Every 12–24 h		Cheng et al 1998[26], Welsh et al 1994[27]
Lidocaine	40 mg	IA			Shafford 2004[44]
	1 mL/50 kg	EP			Ivany and Muir 2004[33,a]
Bupivacaine	10 mg	IA			Shafford 2004[44]
	1–2 mg/kg	SQ			Hellyer et al 2007[61]

Abbreviations: EP, epidural; IA, intra-articular; PO, by mouth; SQ, subcutaneous.
[a] Indicates published doses that are based on clinical experience.

Table 3
Analgesic doses for goats

Drug	Dose	Route	Frequency	Comments	References
Opioids					
Morphine	0.05–0.1 mg/kg	PO		Not recommended	George 2003[14]
	0.1 mg/kg	IV or SQ	Every 4–6 h		Hendrickson et al 1996[36]
		EP			
Fentanyl		TD		Not supported by evidence-based medicine	Carroll et al 1999[25]
		IV	Not recommended because of rapid clearance		Carroll et al 1999[25]
NSAIDs					
Phenylbutazone		IV, SQ, PO		Not recommended	Shukla et al 2007[19]
Meloxicam	0.5 mg/kg	IV	Every 8 h		Ingvast-Larsson et al 2011[21]
	0.5 mg/kg	PO	Every 24 h		Ingvast-Larsson et al 2011[21]
	0.5 mg/kg	IM	Every 24 h		
Lidocaine	1 mL/50 kg	EP			Ivany and Muir 2004[33,a]
	1 mL/15 kg	EP			Van Meter 2010[34,a]
	1–2 mg/kg	SQ			Hellyer et al 2007[61]
	2.5 mg/kg	IV	Loading dose	Administer slowly!	Doherty et al 2007[29]
	0.1 mg/kg/min	IV	CRI after loading dose		Doherty et al 2007[29]

Abbreviations: EP, epidural; PO, by mouth; SQ, subcutaneous; TD, transdermal.
[a] Indicates published doses that are based on clinical experience.

and is extremely cost-effective. In llamas, a recent publication by our research group determined that oral dosing at 1.0 mg/kg maintains serum levels greater than 0.2 µg/mL for up to 72 hours. Oral administration of meloxicam in that study showed a high level of intestinal absorption, with 76% bioavailability. This finding suggests that oral dosing every 3 days is appropriate for analgesia in llamas. However, efficacy as an analgesic was not determined in that study.[18] A study examining the comparative pharmacokinetics of meloxicam between sheep and goats determined that meloxi-cam is metabolized at different rates between the 2 species, with goats metabolizing the drug faster than sheep.[19] The results of this study were not surprising, because it is known that goats have the ability to metabolize other drugs faster as a result of increased hepatic drug-metabolizing enzyme activity.[20] A single 0.5-mg/kg IV dose was used. The elimination half-life in sheep was determined to be 10.85 hours, whereas in goats, it was only 6.73 hours, but both species showed a similar small volume of distribution. That study extrapolated an effective concentration target of 0.73 µg/mL from previous published results in equines and concluded that meloxicam should be administered by the IV route every 12 hours in sheep and every 8 hours in goats to maintain levels considered to be analgesic. In a combined pharmacokinetic and efficacy study in goats in 2010,[21] oral administration was found to have high bioavailability (79%) and a half-life of nearly 11 hours. Based on these data, once-daily oral dosing at 0.5 to 1 mg/kg was recommended. In addition, in a small group of kids undergoing disbudding with cautery (n = 6), half received daily IM injections of meloxicam at 0.5 mg/kg and half received placebo. There was a significant increase in comfort level in the first 24 hours after disbudding in the meloxicam-treated group. Another recent study evaluated the oral bioavailability and pharmacokinetics of meloxicam in sheep. These investigators found a bioavailability of 72% in sheep. Based on their pharmacokinetics a reasonable dosing for oral meloxicam in sheep is a loading dose of 2 mg/kg followed by oral daily administration at 1 mg/kg (Stock ML, Coetzee JF, KuKanich B, Smith BI: Pharmacokinetics of intravenous and oral meloxicam in ruminant sheep, in press).

INJECTABLE STRATEGIES
IM

Butorphanol
Butorphanol as an IM injection provides a more sustained, yet lower peak concentra-tion of analgesia when compared with an IV bolus. However, when used concurrently with another form of analgesia (such as an NSAID), pain relief can be more efficacious than when butorphanol is used alone. In addition, the lower peak concentration reduces the risk of untoward side effects (ie, sedation).[22]

Flunixin meglumine
Although studies are available in sheep citing the use and efficacy of flunixin IM,[4,23] this constitutes an extralabel drug use, because the label indicates that the drug should be given IV. In addition, extensive muscle necrosis secondary to drug acidity and an extended withdrawal time support use of this product as labeled.

Tramadol
A pharmacokinetic study in llamas revealed that tramadol when given either IV or IM at 2.0 mg/kg produced levels consistent with analgesia in humans. However, the half-life when administered IV was only 2.1 hours and IM was only 2.5 hours. Bioavailability by either route was excellent. However, no known clinical data are available.[24]

IV

Morphine

Although morphine is ineffective when administered orally, it can be an effective pain control measure when used parenterally. The dose range varies greatly (0.05–0.1 mg/kg) and superior analgesia may not be evident until a 10-mg/kg dose is administered.[14]

Fentanyl

The injectable form of fentanyl is rapidly acting when given IV, but has a short duration of activity (~20 minutes) and therefore should be used as a constant-rate infusion to maintain analgesic levels. In a recent pharmacokinetic study in sheep, the half-life of IV-administered fentanyl was only 3 hours.[7] In goats, the half-life after an IV bolus of 2.5 µg/kg was even less, at 1.2 hours.[25] This finding suggests that the repeated dosing required and the economics of such preclude its clinical value.

Butorphanol

The use of butorphanol is common in camelid practice as both a sedative and an analgesic. Butorphanol can be used as an IV bolus or as an IM injection. When used together with an NSAID, analgesia may be more pronounced than when used alone.[22]

NSAIDs

Flunixin meglumine Flunixin has been in use for many years and is labeled for the treatment of pyrexia associated with respiratory disease and mastitis as well as treatment of endotoxemia-induced inflammation in cattle. However, its use extends to small ruminants, given the efficacy in cattle. A pharmacokinetic study in sheep undergoing a subcutaneous model of inflammation[26] showed that a single IV dose of flunixin administered at 1.1 mg/kg had good distribution into areas of inflammation, but had slow penetration and elimination from these areas. However, most notable was the dose at which significance was found. The investigators suggest that half the labeled dose of 2.2 mg/kg may be sufficient for analgesia in sheep. However, efficacy data were not presented in this study. Efficacy in sheep was shown in an in vivo pain model using a noxious stimulus on a distal limb.[27] In this study, IV flunixin used at 1.0 mg/kg attenuated hyperalgesia after the noxious stimulus.

Fentanyl No studies have been conducted on the use of fentanyl as a CRI in ruminant species. In dogs, the use of fentanyl as a constant-rate infusion has been described by Sano and colleagues.[28] After an IV loading dose of 10 µg/kg, fentanyl was administered IV at a rate of 10 µg/kg/h. Stable plasma levels were achieved at 3 and 4 hours of infusion, and fentanyl accumulation was not seen, as occurs in humans. However, the plasma concentration for analgesia was not studied, making clinical interpretation difficult.

Lidocaine When administered as a low-dose CRI, lidocaine has been shown to provide systemic analgesia. A loading dose of 2.5 mg/kg body weight followed by infusion at 0.1 mg/kg/min has been shown to decrease the isoflurane requirements in goats undergoing a nonsurgical noxious stimulus under general anesthesia.[29] Similar results have been observed in sheep undergoing orthopedic surgery with a combined CRI of ketamine and lidocaine (ketamine at 10 µg/kg/min and lidocaine at 20 µg/kg/min).[30] When used in a trifusion protocol in llamas and alpacas, a smaller loading dose of 1.0 mg/kg IV should be administered followed by a CRI dose of 3.0 mg/kg/h. Clinically, there has been good response to this protocol (see article by Abrahamsen elsewhere in this issue).

Ketamine CRIs of ketamine have been studied in goats and sheep, in which they were shown to decrease the isoflurane level required to maintain anesthesia while undergoing a nonsurgical noxious stimuli. The doses used in the study and shown to be effective were an IV loading dose of kg body weight followed by infusion/kg body weight followed by infusion at 50 μg/kg/min.[29] In sheep a CRI of lidocaine (20 microgram/kg/min) and ketamine (10 microgram/kg/min) was found to decrease the isofluorane requirement during orthopedic surgery.[30] As a component of the trifusion protocol in llamas and alpacas, ketamine is dosed at 0.6 mg/kg/h, with good clinical results. No loading dose was required using this protocol (see article by Abrahamsen elsewhere in this issue).

Morphine An opioid added to a trifusion CRI has clinically been shown to have increased analgesic properties in llamas and alpacas compared with when used alone. The CRI dose of morphine is 0.025 mg/kg/h. Negative side effects have not been observed following the trifusion protocol (see dosing table for llamas and alpacas).

Butorphanol Butorphanol can be substituted for morphine in the trifusion protocol for llamas and alpacas. However, analgesia may not be as potent with this substitution. A loading dose of 0.05 to 0.1 mg/kg IV is recommended followed by a CRI at 0.022 mg/kg/h (see dosing table for llamas and alpacas) (see article by Abrahamsen elsewhere in this issue).

Local Anesthesia

Perhaps one of the least used forms of pain control is local anesthesia. Local infiltration of lidocaine, bupivacaine, or mepivicaine preoperatively (ie, castration or tail docking) can greatly improve postoperative comfort and behavior. Lidocaine has long been the mainstay of local anesthesia, and especially in the case of goats, caution must be taken not to exceed a 10-mg/kg dose. However, other anesthetics may be used if it is anticipated that a longer duration of anesthesia is needed. A study comparing paravertebral anesthesia duration using lidocaine (180 mg) or bupivacaine (45 mg) in sheep concluded that bupivacaine resulted in a significantly longer duration of action (303 minutes) when compared with lidocaine alone (65 minutes) or to lidocaine with epinephrine (95 minutes).[31] Distal limb anesthesia, also known as the Bier block, is achieved in small ruminants, but with a modification to the technique used in large ruminants.

In regards to the use of local anesthesia (Bier block) for distal limb surgery or as a diagnostic aid in lameness detection in small ruminants, frustration has been encountered when attempting to use the dorsal digital vein or the palmar (plantar) digital veins as is common in large ruminants. Babalola and Oke[32] described the use of the Bier block in goats, in which the tourniquet was placed above the elbow in the forelimb and above the tarsus in the hind limb, allowing for use of the larger cephalic and recurrent tarsal veins, respectively. Lidocaine (2%) was infused into each vein at 3 to 4 mL per dwarf goat and resulted in total limb anesthesia for as long as the tourniquet was in place. No adverse effects were noted. This technique is preferred and could also be applied to other small ruminants.

The use of local anesthesia for the purposes of dehorning and disbudding is not only humane but also practical, because the animal is more compliant. Because of the differences in anatomy, the cornual nerve block in goats requires at least 2 injection sites per horn versus 1 site typical of cattle. In goats, the cornual nerve is a branch of the zygomaticotemporal nerve and lies midway between the lateral canthus of the eye and the lateral base of the horn. The horn base is also heavily innervated by the cornual branches of the infratrochlear nerve, which exits the orbit at approximately the medial canthus. Because of its extensive branching, this nerve is best blocked using a line block halfway between the medial canthus of the eye and the medial base horn to ensure all the branches are anesthetized (**Fig. 1**).[33]

Epidural

The application of epidural anesthetics is necessary in surgery of the caudal reproductive and GI tracts (eg, cervical lacerations, rectal prolapse) and in cases of reproductive emergencies. Analgesics can also be infused epidurally to alleviate pain in the hind limbs and caudal abdomen. The epidural space can be accessed at the lumbosacral space (cranial or high epidural) or at the sacrococcygeal or first coccygeal space (caudal or low epidural) (**Fig. 2**). Sheep with severely docked tails present a challenge in achieving a caudal epidural, and a cranial epidural may be the only option for access to the epidural space in these animals. The lumbosacral space can be accessed by palpating the space caudal to the dorsal vertebral process of the sixth lumbar vertebrae between the wings of the ilium. Usually an 18-gauge or 20-gauge, 3.8-cm (1.5-in) needle is sufficient. Llamas and animals with heavy body condition scores may require an 8.35-cm (3.25-in) spinal needle for the lumbosacral space. The needle should be advanced on midline in a perpendicular manner until a pop is felt. A drop of lidocaine placed in the hub of the needle should withdraw into the needle if in the epidural space. Injection should not have resistance. Some animals may react when the epidural space is entered. Injection should commence slowly over 60 to 90 seconds to prevent rapid cranial migration of the anesthetic or analgesic. It is also beneficial to keep the

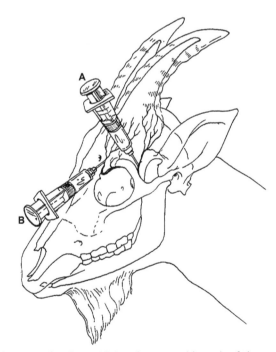

Fig. 1. Needle placement for desensitizing the cornual branch of the zygomaticotemporal (lacrimal) nerve (*A*) and cornual branch of the infratrochlear nerve (*B*) in the goat. (*From* Skarda RT. Techniques of local analgesia in ruminants and swine. Vet Clin North Am Food Anim Pract 1986;2:628; with permission.)

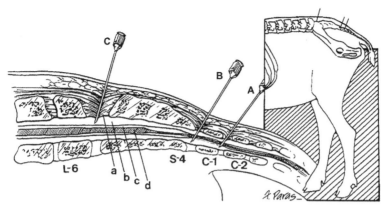

Fig. 2. Needle placement for caudal epidural analgesia (*A* and *B*) and anterior epidural analgesia (*C*) in the goat. (a) Interarcuate ligament. (b) Epidural space. (c) Subarachnoid space. (d) Spinal cord. C-1, first coccygeal vertebra; C-2, second coccygeal vertebra; L-6, sixth lumbar vertebra; S-4, fourth sacral vertebra. (*From* Skarda RT. Techniques of local analgesia in ruminants and swine. Vet Clin North Am Food Anim Pract 1986;2:638; with permission.)

head elevated. For caudal epidural, the tail should be pumped up and down to identify the cranialmost moveable space and the needle inserted at an approximate 45° angle. The hanging drop technique, in which a small amount of lidocaine is added to the needle hub after the needle is through the skin, is helpful. The lidocaine is aspirated into the needle when the epidural space is entered. In small ruminants, the dose of lidocaine ranges between 1 mL/50 kg[33] and 1 mL/15 kg[34] to achieve desensitization using either location. Although it is common practice to add xylazine to a lidocaine epidural in large ruminants to extend the duration of the epidural and as a method of sedation, caution should be used with this combination in goats, because they are especially sensitive to the effects of both xylazine and lidocaine.

In a study using bupivacaine (1 mL/4 kg) in a lumbosacral epidural block in goats, half the goats became recumbent immediately after the injection was completed because of loss of hind limb coordination. In addition, 30% of the goats had negative side effects involving the central nervous system after bupivacaine administration. Although the bupivacaine provided a longer duration of anesthesia than lidocaine, it was not consistent enough to warrant use clinically.[35] More recently, a comparison of lumbosacral application of saline, morphine, and bupivacaine was studied in goats undergoing right-sided abomasopexy.[36] In that study, it was concluded that morphine (0.1 mg/kg) was a useful postoperative analgesic and provided animals with increased levels of analgesia when compared with the saline group. Goats receiving bupivacaine were expectantly and unacceptably recumbent for significantly longer periods because of the blockade of motor nerves. These results were similar to a previous study using morphine at the same dose after orthopedic surgery of the stifle in goats.[37] In that study, goats receiving epidural morphine before anesthetic recovery had improved behavior scores and few side effects. The use of tramadol was outlined in a recent article investigating the use of lidocaine or tramadol in goats.[38] It was concluded that a combination of tramadol (1 mg/kg) and lidocaine (2.46 mg/kg) administered in the lumbosacral epidural space invoked skin desensitization in the perineal region that lasted longer than with lidocaine (2.86 mg/kg) alone. The group receiving tramadol alone (1 mg/kg) experienced the longest duration of effect, but the slowest onset of action. In addition, animals were found to be severely ataxic with lidocaine alone, moderately ataxic with the tramadol/lidocaine combination, and not ataxic with tramadol alone. However, no surgical stimulation was assessed in this study. These results were consistent with the same study design and dosages performed in lambs.[39] In alpacas undergoing castration, the use of lidocaine alone in the lumbosacral epidural space, IM xylazine plus lidocaine in the coccygeal space, or a combination of xylazine and lidocaine in the caudal epidural space failed to produce desensitization of the spermatic cord, even although skin sensation was lost.[40] This finding suggests that direct infiltration of a local anesthetic is required for complete anesthesia of the testicles and spermatic cords in this species. However, in llamas administered a caudal epidural using xylazine alone (0.17 mg/kg), lidocaine alone (0.22 mg/kg), or a combination of xylazine (0.17 mg/kg) and lidocaine (0.22 mg/kg), cutaneous sensation in the perineal area was eliminated in all groups. The combination group experienced significantly longer duration of activity (325 minutes) than with either group alone, and the groups receiving xylazine experienced varying degrees of sedation.[41]

TRANSDERMAL STRATEGIES
Fentanyl

Fentanyl in the transdermal delivery system can provide potent analgesia in a convenient delivery device. Patches are available in 1.2-mg, 2.5-mg, 5.0-mg, 7.5-mg, and 10.0-mg sizes. In sheep, a pharmacokinetic study described the placement of the appropriate-sized patch on the left antebrachium after removal of the wool with clippers and proper cleansing of the skin before undergoing tibial osteotomy and orthopedic plating.[7] The recommended dose in this study was 0.2 mg/kg. The concentration of fentanyl reached its maximum at 12 hours and maintained levels more than 0.5 ng/mL for 40 hours. Sheep in this study did not show any adverse effects from either the surgery or the fentanyl administration. This finding suggests that patches should be placed at least 12 hours before initiation of pain (such as surgery). This was a follow-up study to a previous publication by the same research group in which the analgesic properties of transdermal fentanyl were compared with intermittent IM injection of buprenorphine following the same surgical protocol.[42] This study showed that fentanyl was the superior analgesic from reduced pain scores in the fentanyl-treated group. In addition, the fentanyl-treated group required less preanesthetic sedation to achieve intubation. Contrary to the sheep studies, in goats, transdermal fentanyl was found to be unreliable enough in its absorption to warrant it for clinical use.[25] In that study, a single 5-mg patch was placed on the skin of the neck after clipping of the hair. The patch was left in place for 72 hours, during which consistent plasma levels were not achieved. The skin was not cleaned before application of the patch, and other factors in the study design could have confounded the results. However, the conclusions were consistent with the pharmacokinetics seen in dogs and humans. Another study conducted in healthy llamas[43] suggests that the use of 4 7.5-mg patches placed on the medial antebrachium results in steady serum concentrations without resulting in sedation. Skin-patch adherence is of utmost importance. It is critical that the hair/wool be clipped and the skin cleansed and dried thoroughly before applying the patch. Failure of adherence or inability of the fentanyl to be absorbed (eg, dirty skin, excessive hair) could result in suboptimal pain control by this method.

OTHER STRATEGIES
Intra-Articular

Intra-articular injection of a local anesthetic agent can be an effective means of controlling immediate postoperative pain in animals undergoing surgery of a joint.

However, repeated injections are not advisable given the risk for iatrogenic sepsis with repeated arthrocenteses. In sheep undergoing stifle arthrotomy, the use of intra-articular lidocaine preoperatively and intra-articular bupivacaine postoperatively significantly reduced postoperative pain for 3 to 7 hours compared with control animals that received no intra-articular therapies. All test animals also were treated with transdermal fentanyl and phenylbutazone perioperatively.[44] A study examining the use of intra-articular bupivacaine in goats undergoing stifle arthrotomy[45] found that use of bupivacaine preoperatively reduced the amount of anesthetic required, but that administration of intra-articular bupivacaine postoperatively had a short duration of effect. From this study, it is concluded that multimodal analgesia should be used perioperatively in goats undergoing stifle surgery.

PAIN MANAGEMENT IN SPECIFIC CONDITIONS
Tail Docking

Tail docking in wool-breed sheep is generally considered beneficial in decreasing the incidence of fecal soiling of the perineum and fly strike. For that reason, it is routinely performed in the basic management systems of sheep in the United States. For sheep breeds that do not have wool (hair breeds and some dairy sheep), the practitioner and flock manager should evaluate the need for docking, because it may not provide benefit. Docking is a noxious stimulus, and as such, preemptive analgesia is warranted in many cases. In developing a management plan for pain associated with tail docking, 3 issues should be addressed. (1) At what age should the procedure be performed? The answer to this question is not straightforward, and in many cases the management style of the operation should be considered. In many jurisdictions, animal welfare regulations suggest that tail docking should occur before a certain age because it is thought that docking at a young age is less painful.[46,47] In support of this assertion, Barrowman and colleagues[48] evaluated the behavior of lambs at different ages after castration/docking and concluded that there was "no apparent discomfort or pain in lambs docked before they were 48 hours old" using the rubber ring method. More recently, Kent and colleagues[49,50] evaluated the behavioral response and cortisol concentrations of lambs receiving 3 different types of docking (surgical resection, rubber ring alone, or rubber ring combined with Burdizzo) at 3 different ages (5 days, 21 days, and 42 days). In all cases, the lambs showed evidence of obvious pain; however, age (only looked at 42 days or less) was not a significant factor in terms of the cortisol levels or behavioral changes. (2) The practitioner must consider the method used to perform the tail dock. The most common methods used include hot docking iron, rubber ring banding, rubber ring banding followed by crushing with a Burdizzo, and surgical resection. Surgical resection under general anesthesia would be expected to provide excellent analgesia; however, routine use of this procedure as a management method is not feasible. In relation to the other methods of docking, hot docking iron has been shown to result in minimal differences in behavior and cortisol when compared with handled controls.[51] However, it does have an increased risk of postprocedure hemorrhage and an increased risk for the operator because of the hot iron. When directly compared, the use of the rubber ring method with the Burdizzo consistently results in less evidence of pain (cortisol and behavioral changes) than the rubber ring method alone.[49–54] Based on these results, the use of a bloodless castrator (Burdizzo type) after the application of a rubber band represents an easy and effective nonpharmaceutical means of decreasing the pain associated with tail docking. The procedure involves crushing the entire width of the tail for 3 seconds just above or below the level of the rubber band. In most cases, the rubber band then rolls into the groove made by the instrument. Ideally, the crushing surface of the bloodless castrator is honed to a thickness of 1 to 2 mm, but this is not mandatory. It is hypothesized that the crushing action of the bloodless castrator destroys the nerves of the tail distal to the site of the ring, preventing an afferent barrage of nervous tissue resulting from the developing ischemia of the tail.[51] (3) The third issue that must be considered by the practitioner is the administration of preemptive analgesics. The effect of 4 different ancillary analgesic approaches has been directly compared in a single study looking at 3 different methods of castration (hot docking iron, rubber ring alone, and rubber ring with Burdizzo).[51] In all cases, the administration of a local anesthetic ring block just proximal to the site of docking was most effective at decreasing behavioral response and minimizing cortisol spike.[51,52] Allowing appropriate time for the onset of local anesthesia is beneficial after injection, and the use of bicarbonate to buffer lidocaine (see earlier discussion of lidocaine) should be considered. Epidural blocks with local anesthetics or opioids have been evaluated but did not provide as much benefit as a local ring block.[51,55] At least 2 studies have evaluated the use of topically applied spray analgesics. The first study[51] looked at topical cold analgesic spray (Ralgex freeze spray: Seton Products Ltd, Tubiton House, OL) and found a reduction in cortisol levels but minimal impact of behavioral signs of pain. A second more recent study evaluated the use of Tri-Solfen, Bayer Animal Health, Australia, a topical analgesic marketed in Australia that includes lignocaine (lidocaine), bupivacaine, adrenalin, and cetrimide. This product was shown to alleviate wound pain and significantly decreased the behavioral signs of pain in animals treated with the spray compared with untreated controls.[56] Insufficient data are available to determine the benefit of using NSAIDs in the analgesic management plan for tail docks. If NSAIDs are used, selection of a product with a longer half-life and that is easy to administer, such as oral meloxicam, is preferable to injectable products with rapid elimination.

Castration

Similar to tail docking, the practitioner should consider 3 issues when planning castration of small ruminants and camelids. First, the practitioner should consider the appropriate age to conduct the procedure. For sheep and goats, castration of animals at the youngest age possible is generally encouraged, or in some cases required, to minimize the pain of the procedure if no ancillary analgesia is provided.[46,47] Although minimal data specifically testing this assertion are available, the research that has been conducted suggests that minimal differences exist in cortisol and behavior in animals castrated at 5, 21, and 42 days.[49,50] This study clearly showed that the animals do experience pain at all ages tested, hence analgesic therapy should be considered even although it may not be legally required. Ages more than 42 days have not been scientifically evaluated; however, in our opinion, these animals should always receive analgesic therapy. Castration of camelids is often delayed until the animals are mature, but the procedure is always performed with the addition of ancillary analgesia or full anesthesia. The second consideration in terms of pain management for castration is the method to be used to perform the procedure. The primary means of castration include rubber ring, rubber ring with Burdizzo, and surgical castration. As with tail docking, the evidence strongly suggests that use of the Burdizzo, in conjunction with rubber ring, is associated with a smaller cortisol spike and fewer behavioral changes than use of a rubber ring alone.[49–54] In camelids, surgical castration is the only viable method. The final consideration is the use of preemptive analgesic therapy. In the case of surgical castration of sheep and goats, local anesthesia with injection into the distal scrotum and testicular cords is beneficial. We prefer to perform a ring block around the distal scrotum (performed by holding the scrotum flat and placing a needle across the width of the scrotum one-third from the bottom and injecting lidocaine as removed, and then repeating this procedure on the back of the scrotum) using lidocaine buffered with bicarbonate. The testicular cords can then be palpated at the neck of the scrotum and a small volume of lidocaine injected directly into each cord as high as possible against the body wall. When using the rubber ring method of castration in sheep and goats, subcutaneous injection of local anesthetic at the site of ring placement has been shown to be beneficial.[51,52]

Disbudding

Disbudding is the management procedure used to prevent the growth of horns on young animals, predominantly dairy goats. The most common method of disbudding performed in the United States is the use of a hot iron similar to the method for disbudding dairy calves. Because of the rapid horn growth, it is recommended to perform disbudding early in life as soon as the horn bud can be identified (typically 2–6 days of age depending on breed and size of kids). Disbudding at this age allows for a significantly shortened procedure compared with that of kids with larger horns that develop by 1 to 2 weeks of age. Several options exist for analgesic management during disbudding. The use of local anesthetic nerve blocks, as described in the protocols section, allows for good anesthesia of the horn area. The technique requires injection in 4 sites (see **Fig. 1**) with a small volume of lidocaine. Use of bicarbonate to buffer the lidocaine decreases the objections of the kid to anesthesia placement. Care must be taken not to exceed the toxic dose of lidocaine, which can be very small for a young kid. In some cases, diluting the lidocaine from the standard 2% provided by the manufacturer to 1% with sterile saline may allow for more volume if needed. Alternatively, a ring block around the horn buds can be performed but requires more time and effort. Anecdotally, the use of oral meloxicam the night before disbudding or at the time of disbudding may provide some additional benefit. Results of a similar protocol in dairy calves (ie, appropriate dose crushed up and provided in milk by bottle at the regular bottle feeding 12 hours before disbudding) showed benefit (Coetzee, personal communication, 2012).

Dehorning

Dehorning is different than disbudding in that the procedure has been delayed until a time when the horn must be surgically removed. In these cases, local anesthesia and a good analgesic plan are necessary. Nerve blocks, as described earlier for disbudding, combined with sedation or general anesthesia should be considered. The procedure generally involves significant undermining of the skin and entering the sinus cavity, so appropriate postoperative analgesia should be provided.

Urethral Obstruction

The most important aspect of management in the small ruminant experiencing urinary obstruction is to restore urine outflow. This condition is painful and can be confused with colic by the inexperienced practitioner. However, pain management without recognizing the need for urinary continence can be catastrophic and result in loss of the patient. Appropriate pain management should be considered in conjunction with restoration of urine outflow. Caution should be exercised if xylazine is used as a sedative in a blocked animal, because xylazine is a diuretic and increases urine production. Flunixin used IV can offer pain relief to a recently unobstructed animal, and the animal may benefit from the antiinflammatory properties in an effort to decrease cystitis and inflammation associated with surgical correction. In our experience, as soon as the flow of urine is restored, in the absence of a necrotic bladder, straining is greatly diminished. In addition, animals generally are more comfortable postoperatively after a tube cystostomy than with a perineal urethrostomy. Although not routinely used at our hospital, epidural administration of an opioid could be beneficial if considerable discomfort is experienced postoperatively.

Cesarean Section

Emergency cesarean sections in small ruminants are often performed under sedation and not general anesthesia to allow the animal to remain standing and to minimize the risk of aspiration when 24 hours of fasting before surgery is not feasible. In such cases, complete local anesthesia of the surgical site should be achieved. This anesthesia can be achieved through several different methods or combinations of methods. In small ruminants, a lumbosacral epidural with lidocaine (0.4 mg/kg) often provides complete analgesia of the surgical site.[57] It results in complete, temporary (lasting up to 4 hours) paralysis of the pelvic limbs; however, recovery in small ruminants is generally good if the patient is placed on a nonslip surface. Alternatively, an epidural dose of an α_2 agonist or opioids might be combined with a local block using a local anesthetic with or without bicarbonate buffering. Local blocks can be performed in a manner similar to cattle with a line block, inverted L block, or paravertebral blocks.

Obstetrics

Obstetric manipulation of a fetus during dystocia can result in considerable pain for small ruminants and camelids. Use of a sacrococcygeal epidural with lidocaine (0.5 mg/kg) can provide rapid-onset and complete perineal anesthesia, which eases manipulation of the fetus and reduces pain for the patient. The addition of an α_2 agonist or opioids can be considered, as described earlier in the protocol section .

Lameness/Foot Rot

Management plans for controlling pain associated with lameness generally fall into 2 categories: acute pain associated with an acute injury or lesion or chronic pain associated with long-term arthritic or musculoskeletal abnormalities. In acute cases, the primary goal of the practitioner should be to determine the cause of the pain/lameness and address the underlying issue with appropriate therapy. Several options exist for ancillary management of acute pain in these cases. In some cases, administration of NSAIDs like oral meloxicam for 2 to 3 days can provide sufficient analgesia while the underlying issue is being addressed. If the pain results from lesions associated with 1 of the claws of the foot, a claw block similar to those used for lame dairy cattle can be fashioned out of wood and hoof adhesives to remove weight bearing from the affected claw. Application of these blocks often results in significant improvement in lameness. Regional limb blocks and ring blocks using local anesthetics can be performed for localization of lameness or short-term analgesia. If the severity of the case requires hospitalization, the use of fentanyl transdermal patches, epidural analgesic protocols, or CRIs of analgesics may provide more potent and sustainable analgesia. In cases in which the lameness is more chronic and associated with long-term changes of the musculoskeletal system, different approaches are necessary. Prolonged therapy with NSAIDs is possible and common; however, the owner should be warned of the potential side effects of long-term NSAID use, particularly GI ulceration and nephropathy. Anecdotally, some practitioners report success with intermittent injections of hyaluronic acid or polysulfated glycosaminoglycans marketed for equine patients. Early success with gabapentin (15 mg/kg every 24 hours) has been reported in a limited number of sheep and goats; however, little information is available regarding appropriate dosing and potential side effects in small ruminants, and practitioners should be cautious when using this drug in these species.

Rectal and Vaginal Prolapse

The pain associated with rectal and vaginal prolapses generally originates from edema or ischemia of the prolapsed tissue. In many cases, the continued sensation of the prolapse induces continued straining of the animal and exacerbates the prolapse and edema. Prevention of straining is best achieved through sacrococcygeal epidural anesthesia. Use of local anesthetics such as lidocaine or bupivacaine provides short-term analgesia, whereas combination epidural therapy including opioids, α_2 agonist, and local anesthetics as outlined earlier may provide longer-term relief. Several studies have evaluated the efficacy of a combination of xylazine and lidocaine (0.07 and 0.5 mg/kg, respectively) administered in the sacrococcygeal space, allowing for rapid anesthesia of the area to allow Buhner stitch placement while the xylazine provides analgesia for up to 36 hours.[58] In some cases, splash blocks with local anesthetics and installation of local anesthetics mixed with KY jelly into the distal rectum or vagina with a syringe and extension set may provide immediate analgesia and ease reduction of the prolapse.

SUMMARY

From both an animal welfare and a producer confidence perspective, it is incumbent on veterinary practitioners to make an effort to manage pain in small ruminants and camelids. In this article, a large variety of management options are outlined and specific examples are provided of how pain management protocols can be developed and used for routine procedures. On the most simple and least expensive end of the spectrum is the use of oral meloxicam, which can be administered every 1 to 2 days at a cost of less than $0.20 per 45.35 kg (100 lb) body weight. Therefore, with minimal effort, even the largest camelid can be treated for less than US$1 per day. In more severe or hospitalized cases, the use is outlined of multimodal CRIs or transdermal patches, which provide potent analgesia, but at a higher cost. Our goal is to provide a comprehensive, evidence-based review of the options for the practitioner to tailor a specific analgesic management plan for each case. No case is identical to another; hence, individualized pain management should be the goal.

REFERENCES

1. Kent JE, Molony V. Guidelines for the recognition and assessment of animal pain. Available at: http://www.link.vet.ed.ac.uk/animalpain/Default.htm. Accessed August 2, 2012.
2. Thurmon J, Tranquilli W, Benson GJ. Preanesthetics and anesthetic adjuncts. In: Thurmon J, Tranquilli W, Benson GJ, editors. Lumb and Jones' veterinary anesthesia. Philadelphia: Williams and Wilkins; 1996. p. 183–210.
3. Kastner SB. A2-agonists in sheep: a review. Vet Anaesth Analg 2006;33(2):79–96.
4. Grant C, Upton RN, Kuchel TR. Efficacy of intra-muscular analgesics for acute pain in sheep. Aust Vet J 1996;73(4):129–32.
5. Thurmon J, Tranquilli W, Benson GJ. Perioperative pain and distress. In: Thurmon J, Tranquilli W, Benson GJ, editors. Lumb and Jones' veterinary anesthesia. Philadelphia: Williams and Wilkins; 1996. p. 40–61.
6. Galatos AD. Anesthesia and analgesia in sheep and goats. Vet Clin North Am Food Anim Pract 2011;27(1):47–59.
7. Ahern BJ, Soma LR, Rudy JA, et al. Pharmacokinetics of fentanyl administered transdermally and intravenously in sheep. Am J Vet Res 2010;71(10):1127–32.

8. Lin HC. Dissociative anesthetics. In: Thurmon J, Tranquilli W, Benson GJ, editors. Lumb and Jones' veterinary anesthesia. Philadelphia: Williams and Wilkins; 1996. p. 241–96.

9. Curatolo M, Petersen-Felix S, Arendt-Nielsen L, et al. Adding sodium bicarbonate to lidocaine enhances the depth of epidural blockade. Anesth Analg 1998;86(2): 341–7.

10. Sinnott CJ, Garfield JM, Thalhammer JG, et al. Addition of sodium bicarbonate to lidocaine decreases the duration of peripheral nerve block in the rat. Anesthesiology 2000;93(4):1045–52.

11. Everest PH, Goossens H, Sibbons P, et al. Pathological changes in the rabbit ileal loop model caused by *Campylobacter jejuni* from human colitis. J Med Microbiol 1993;38(5):316–21.

12. McKay W, Morris R, Mushlin P. Sodium bicarbonate attenuates pain on skin infiltration with lidocaine, with or without epinephrine. Anesth Analg 1987;66(6):572–4.

13. Coetzee JF, Mosher RA, Kohake LE, et al. Pharmacokinetics of oral gabapentin alone or co-administered with meloxicam in ruminant beef calves. Vet J 2011; 190(1):98–102.

14. George L. Pain control in food animals. In: Steffey E, editor. Recent advances in anesthetic management of large domestic animals. Ithaca (NY): International Veterinary Information Services; 2003.

15. Malreddy PR, Coetzee JF, Kukanich B, et al. Pharmacokinetics and milk secretion of gabapentin and meloxicam co-administered orally in Holstein-Friesian cows. J Vet Pharmacol Ther. February 28, 2012. http://dx.doi.org/10.1111/j.1365-2885.2012.01384.x.

16. Davis JL, Smith GW, Baynes RE, et al. Update on drugs prohibited from extralabel use in food animals. J Am Vet Med Assoc 2009;235(5):528–34.

17. Lees P, Ayliffe T, Maitho TE, et al. Pharmacokinetics, metabolism and excretion of phenylbutazone in cattle following intravenous, intramuscular and oral administration. Res Vet Sci 1988;44(1):57–67.

18. Kreuder AJ, Coetzee JF, Wulf LW, et al. Bioavailability and pharmacokinetics of oral meloxicam in llamas. BMC Vet Res 2012;8(1):85.

19. Shukla M, Singh G, Sindhura BG, et al. Comparative plasma pharmacokinetics of meloxicam in sheep and goats following intravenous administration. Comp Biochem Physiol C Toxicol Pharmacol 2007;145(4):528–32.

20. el Sheikh HA, Ali BH, Homeida AM, et al. The activities of aminopyrine N-demethylase, aniline 4-hydroxylase and UDP-glucuronyltransferase in tissues of camels, desert sheep and Nubian goats. Gen Pharmacol 1988;19(5):713–7.

21. Ingvast-Larsson C, Hogberg M, Mengistu U, et al. Pharmacokinetics of meloxicam in adult goats and its analgesic effect in disbudded kids. J Vet Pharmacol Ther 2011;34(1):64–9.

22. Abrahamsen EJ. Chemical restraint, anesthesia, and analgesia for camelids. Vet Clin North Am Food Anim Pract 2009;25(2):455–94.

23. Fthenakis GC. Field evaluation of flunixin meglumine in the supportive treatment of ovine mastitis. J Vet Pharmacol Ther 2000;23(6):405–7.

24. Cox S, Martin-Jimenez T, van Amstel S, et al. Pharmacokinetics of intravenous and intramuscular tramadol in llamas. J Vet Pharmacol Ther 2011;34(3):259–64.

25. Carroll GL, Hooper RN, Boothe DM, et al. Pharmacokinetics of fentanyl after intravenous and transdermal administration in goats. Am J Vet Res 1999;60(8):986–91.

26. Cheng Z, McKeller Q, Nolan A. Pharmacokinetic studies of flunixin meglumine and phenylbutazone in plasma, exudate and transudate in sheep. J Vet Pharmacol Ther 1998;21(4):315–21.

27. Welsh EM, Nolan AM. Effects of non-steroidal anti-inflammatory drugs on the hyperalgesia to noxious mechanical stimulation induced by the application of a tourniquet to a forelimb of sheep. Res Vet Sci 1994;57(3):285–91.

28. Sano T, Nishimura R, Kanazawa H, et al. Pharmacokinetics of fentanyl after single intravenous injection and constant rate infusion in dogs. Vet Anaesth Analg 2006; 33(4):266–73.

29. Doherty T, Redua MA, Queiroz-Castro P, et al. Effect of intravenous lidocaine and ketamine on the minimum alveolar concentration of isoflurane in goats. Vet Anaesth Analg 2007;34(2):125–31.

30. Raske TG, Pelkey S, Wagner AE, et al. Effect of intravenous ketamine and lidocaine on isoflurane requirement in sheep undergoing orthopedic surgery. Lab Anim 2010;39(3):76–9.

31. Rostami M, Vesal N. Comparison of lidocaine, lidocaine/epinephrine or bupivacaine for thoracolumbar paravertebral anaesthesia in fat-tailed sheep. Vet Anaesth Analg 2011;38(6):598–602.

32. Babalola GO, Oke BO. Intravenous regional analgesia for surgery of the limbs in goats. Vet Q 1983;5(4):186–9.

33. Ivany J, Muir W. Farm animal anesthesia. In: Fubini S, Ducharme N, editors. Farm animal surgery. St Louis (MO): Saunders; 2004. p. 102–3.

34. Van Metre D. Small ruminant tips. In: 128th Annual Meeting of the Iowa Veterinary Medical Association. Ames, 2010.

35. Trim CM. Epidural analgesia with 0.75% bupivacaine for laparotomy in goats. J Am Vet Med Assoc 1989;194(9):1292–6.

36. Hendrickson DA, Kruse-Elliott KT, Broadstone RV. A comparison of epidural saline, morphine, and bupivacaine for pain relief after abdominal surgery in goats. Vet Surg 1996;25(1):83–7.

37. Pablo LS. Epidural morphine in goats after hindlimb orthopedic surgery. Vet Surg 1993;22(4):307–10.

38. Dehkordi SH, Bigham-Sadegh A, Gerami R. Evaluation of anti-nociceptive effect of epidural tramadol, tramadol-lidocaine and lidocaine in goats. Vet Anaesth Analg 2012;39(1):106–10.

39. Habibian S, Bigham AS, Aali E. Comparison of lidocaine, tramadol, and lidocaine-tramadol for epidural analgesia in lambs. Res Vet Sci 2011;91(3): 434–8.

40. Padula AM. Clinical evaluation of caudal epidural anaesthesia for the neutering of alpacas. Vet Rec 2005;156(19):616–7.

41. Grubb TL, Riebold TW, Huber MJ. Evaluation of lidocaine, xylazine, and a combination of lidocaine and xylazine for epidural analgesia in llamas. J Am Vet Med Assoc 1993;203(10):1441–4.

42. Ahern BJ, Soma LR, Boston RC, et al. Comparison of the analgesic properties of transdermally administered fentanyl and intramuscularly administered buprenorphine during and following experimental orthopedic surgery in sheep. Am J Vet Res 2009;70(3):418–22.

43. Grubb TL, Gold JR, Schlipf JW, et al. Assessment of serum concentrations and sedative effects of fentanyl after transdermal administration at three dosages in healthy llamas. Am J Vet Res 2005;66(5):907–9.

44. Shafford HL, Hellyer PW, Turner AS. Intra-articular lidocaine plus bupivacaine in sheep undergoing stifle arthrotomy. Vet Anaesth Analg 2004;31(1):20–6.

45. Krohm P, Levionnois O, Ganster M, et al. Antinociceptive activity of pre- versus post-operative intra-articular bupivacaine in goats undergoing stifle arthrotomy. Vet Anaesth Analg 2011;38(4):363–73.

46. Anonymous. Animal welfare (painful husbandry procedures) code of welfare. 2005. Available at: http://www.biosecurity.govt.nz/files/regs/animal-welfare/req/codes/painful-husbandry/painful-husbandry.pdf. Accessed August 20, 2012.

47. Anonymous. Code of recommendation for the welfare of livestock: sheep. 2007. Available at: http://www.defra.gov.uk/publications/files/pb5162-sheep-041028.pdf. Accessed August 20, 2012.

48. Barrowman J, Boaz T, Towers KG. Castration and docking of lambs: use of the rubber-ring ligature technique at different ages. Empire J Exp Agr 1954;22: 189–202.

49. Molony V, Kent JE, Robertson IS. Behavioural responses of lambs of three ages in the first three hours after three methods of castration and tail docking. Res Vet Sci 1993;55(2):236–45.

50. Kent JE, Molony V, Robertson IS. Changes in plasma cortisol concentration in lambs of three ages after three methods of castration and tail docking. Res Vet Sci 1993;55(2):246–51.

51. Graham MJ, Kent JE, Molony V. Effects of four analgesic treatments on the behavioural and cortisol responses of 3-week-old lambs to tail docking. Vet J 1997; 153(1):87–97.

52. Kent JE, Thrusfield MV, Molony V, et al. Randomised, controlled field trial of two new techniques for the castration and tail docking of lambs less than two days of age. Vet Rec 2004;154(7):193–200.

53. Kent JE, Jackson RE, Molony V, et al. Effects of acute pain reduction methods on the chronic inflammatory lesions and behaviour of lambs castrated and tail docked with rubber rings at less than two days of age. Vet J 2000;160(1):33–41.

54. Kent JE, Molony V, Robertson IS. Comparison of the Burdizzo and rubber ring methods for castrating and tail docking lambs. Vet Rec 1995;136(8):192–6.

55. Wood GN, Molony V, Fleetwood-Walker SM, et al. Effects of local anesthesia and intravenous naloxone on the changes in behaviour and plasma concentrations of cortisol produced by castration and tail docking with tight rubber rings in young lambs. Res Vet Sci 1991;51(2):193–9.

56. Lomax S, Dickson H, Sheil M, et al. Topical anaesthesia alleviates short-term pain of castration and tail docking in lambs. Aust Vet J 2010;88(3):67–74.

57. Aminkov BY, Hubenov HD. The effect of xylazine epidural anaesthesia on blood gas and acid-base parameters in rams. Br Vet J 1995;151(5):579–85.

58. Scott PR. The management and welfare of some common ovine obstetrical problems in the United Kingdom. Vet J 2005;170(1):33–40.

59. Anderson DE. Antibiotic usage in the llama and alpaca. Proceedings of the Camelid Medicine, Surgery, and Reproduction Conference. The Ohio State University, College of Veterinary Medicine. 2002:89–93.

60. Jenson J. Gastric ulceration in South American camelids. Veterinary Quarterly Review, Texas Cooperative Extension, Texas A&M University System. 2003;19:4–6.

61. Hellyer PW, Robertson SA, Fails AD. Pain and its management. In: Tranquilli WJ, Thurmon JC, Grimm KA, editors. Lumb & Jones' Veterinary Anesthesia and Analgesia. 4th edition. Blackwell Publishing: Ames, IA; 2007. p. 31–52.

Chemical Restraint and Injectable Anesthesia of Ruminants

Eric J. Abrahamsen, DVM

KEYWORDS

- Chemical restraint of ruminants (or ruminant chemical restraint)
- Injectable anesthesia of ruminants (or ruminant injectable anesthesia)
- Ketamine stun • CRI • TKX-Ru • Double drip • Ruminant triple drip

KEY POINTS

- The ketamine stun is basically the addition of a small dose of ketamine to any injectable chemical restraint technique.
- The ketamine stun technique provides enhanced patient cooperation when compared with more traditional injectable chemical restraint cocktails.
- The ketamine stun technique has been shown to reduce stress response to castration and dehorning in calves.
- Anesthesia should be considered for procedures requiring an extended period of immobility or a high level of systemic analgesia.
- Constant rate infusion techniques, such as double drip or ruminant triple drip, provide a more stable plane of injectable anesthesia than bolus administration techniques.

INTRODUCTION

This article covers techniques used to provide chemical restraint and injectable anesthesia of ruminant patients. Topics common to both of these subjects are covered in separate sections at the beginning of the article. Understanding the information contained in these sections will improve safety and efficacy when using the techniques presented in this article. This article is focused primarily on cattle. The author has not used all of the techniques presented in this article on every type of ruminant. Of the techniques that have been used, the dosing protocols provided have proven effective.

PREPROCEDURE CONSIDERATIONS
Physical Examination

Physical examination is not generally required when using chemical restraint in normal healthy ruminant patients. Because of the adverse side effects of some chemical

Conflict of interest: None.
Disclosure: None.
5160 Citadel, Kalamazoo, MI 49004, USA
E-mail address: abrahamsen@earthlink.net

Vet Clin Food Anim 29 (2013) 209–227
http://dx.doi.org/10.1016/j.cvfa.2012.11.005
0749-0720/13/$ – see front matter © 2013 Elsevier Inc. All rights reserved.

restraint cocktails, the cardiovascular status of potentially compromised patients should be evaluated when feasible before drug administration. Mucous membrane color and refill time provides a quick assessment of cardiovascular status. Turgidity and size of the median auricular artery can provide a useful estimate of arterial blood pressure and blood volume, respectively. Familiarizing yourself with the feel of the median auricular artery in normal patients will help in evaluating changes in turgidity and size in compromised patients.

When field anesthesia is contemplated, a brief physical examination should be performed when feasible to determine if patients are suitable candidates. It may also reduce liability should an anesthetic complication occur. The examination ideally includes an overall assessment of the patients' health status, auscultation of the cardiopulmonary systems, and evaluation of locomotor function. Cardiovascular status should more thoroughly evaluated in potentially compromised patients requiring field anesthesia.

Site Selection and Facility Requirements

A site that is quiet and free of distractions improves the response to chemical restraint. The sedation produced by alpha-2 adrenergic agonists (α_2) can be overridden by an elevated sympathetic tone in anxious or unruly patients. This point is especially true when a lower dose is administered, which is typically the case when using standing chemical restraint techniques in ruminants. A flat, even surface that provides good footing helps sedated patients maintain balance.

When recumbent chemical restraint or field anesthesia is contemplated, other factors must also be considered. A soft surface will reduce the chance of injury. The site selected should be free of hazards. Large ruminants are more difficult to physically control and require a somewhat larger safety zone. Ruminants tend to be very patient. They typically do not attempt to stand until they are awake and functional. Good footing is the primary requirement for achieving a good recovery. An open grassy area is generally ideal. A stall deeply bedded with shavings can be used, but the confined space increases the risk to the personnel involved and may interfere with the procedure. Proximity to water, electricity, and vehicle (how close are your emergency supplies) are also things to consider when selecting a site.

Patient Positioning and Airway Protection

Ruminants continue to produce a significant amount of saliva while sedated or anesthetized. The degree of protective laryngeal and eye reflexes retained will depend on the chemical restraint technique and drug doses selected. Milder levels of chemical restraint provide greater airway protection. When recumbency is produced, patients should be positioned so that saliva runs out of the mouth rather than pooling back near the larynx whenever possible. For patients in lateral recumbency, this can be accomplished simply by placing a pad under the head-neck junction so the opening of the mouth is below the level of the larynx.

Protecting the airway becomes much more challenging when patients are placed in dorsal recumbency. Smaller ruminants placed in dorsal recumbency will typically be under the influence of a potent chemical restraint protocol. The body of these patients should be elevated using foam pads or some other method with the head dependent and resting on the floor or surgery table surface. It is important that the head be supported rather than hanging in space to prevent excessive tension on neck structures. The head and neck are rotated to place the opening of the mouth below the larynx to facilitate saliva egress. The short, thick neck of many cattle breeds can make proper orientation difficult to achieve. When the head cannot be positioned to facilitate saliva egress or the procedure is expected to produce a significant amount of blood or other material that could enter the airway, patients should be intubated.

It is extremely difficult to position large ruminants in dorsal recumbency to facilitate saliva egress in a field setting. The degree of sedation used determines how these patients are managed. Larger ruminant patients are often cast and physically restrained in dorsal recumbency. Chemical restraint will reduce the level of distress in these patients. Lightly sedated patients are typically able to protect their airway but should be monitored for signs of respiratory distress. Heavy sedation markedly depresses the cough and swallow reflexes, increasing the risk of aspiration. Unfortunately, patients must be fairly obtunded to tolerate intubation. If you suspect that large ruminant patients will require more than light sedation to tolerate restraint in dorsal recumbency, injectable anesthesia with intubation may be a better choice.

Many practitioners carry a selection of long, small-animal endotracheal tubes and an AMBU bag (AMBU Inc, Glen Bernie, Maryland) for resuscitating newborn patients. The silicone endotracheal tubes used in larger ruminant patients are expensive (Cuffed Endotracheal Tube [Silicone], Smiths Medical/SurgiVet, St Paul, Minnesota). Practitioners planning to anesthetize larger ruminant patients in dorsal recumbency should add a small selection of larger endotracheal tubes to the equipment in their vehicle. A compromise might be to add 12-, 16-, and 22-mm endotracheal tubes, which will provide an adequate airway for a wide range of patient sizes. Patients more than 680 kg will experience increased work of breathing with a 22-mm endotracheal tube. Patients should be extubated with the cuff inflated in sternal recumbency to reduce the risk of aspiration.

Endotracheal Intubation

Smaller ruminants are intubated by direct visualization much like dogs or cats. Because of the small mouth opening and deep oral cavity, proper alignment is important to visualize the larynx. This technique is similar to looking through a long, narrow tube. A laryngoscope with an extra long blade aids the visualization of the larynx by allowing greater control of the base of the tongue (Wisconsin 11-, 14-, and 18-in laryngoscope blades, Anesthesia Medical Specialties, Beaumont, California). An assistant straddling the patient's back holds the patient in sternal recumbency. The assistant extends the head and neck up toward the individual doing the intubation and holds the jaws apart. The assistant's knees can be used to help control the patient's head/neck. The head should not be elevated until the intubation process is imminent to minimize pooling of saliva back around the larynx. A reduced level of jaw tone and the absence of a chewing or lingual response to this manipulation can be used to determine when intubation is appropriate. A stylet made from 0.125-in aluminum rod is used to facilitate intubation of small ruminants. The thin rod does not obstruct the view of the larynx. The ends of the stylet should be smoothed or rounded to minimize the risk of damaging the mucosal surfaces of the airway. The stylet is guided into the larynx first and the endotracheal tube passed over it into the airway. The stylet must be long enough so that it can be grasped above the endotracheal tube as it is advanced down the rod and into the trachea. With practice, the endotracheal tube can be positioned on the stylet and held in place with the hand guiding the stylet into the airway, making the process less cumbersome. In somewhat larger ruminants, the size of the oral cavity may be large enough to allow visualization of the larynx while the endotracheal tube is guided into the airway. The stylet is used to stiffen the endotracheal tube. Allowing the stylet to protrude slightly from the end of the endotracheal tube makes placement in the airway easier in these patients.

In large ruminants, the depth of the oral cavity and the size of the endotracheal tube make direct visualization difficult. Large ruminants are intubated by manually guiding the tube in the airway. The anesthetist carries the endotracheal tube into the mouth with one hand and then uses his or her fingers to guide the tube between the arytenoids as the other hand advances the tube. A speculum is required for this technique. The arm/hand size of the individual performing the intubation is the limiting factor in determining the patient size when this approach becomes appropriate. The oral cavity must be large enough to accommodate one's arm and the endotracheal tube. The lower limit for this technique is generally around 300 to 350 kg, unless the operator has an exceptionally small arm and hand. A somewhat undersized endotracheal tube can provide additional room for the operator's arm in marginally sized patients. The operator should wash his or her arms off afterward because ruminant saliva tends to irritate the skin of most people.

A flexible endoscope can be used to guide the endotracheal tube into the larynx. The endoscope serves as both a stylet and visualization device. This technique has proven useful when traditional methods cannot be used. The endoscope must be small enough to fit inside the endotracheal tube. Ruminants can be blindly intubated. With the head and neck extended, the endotracheal tube is gently advanced during inspiration. Repeated attempts will likely be required, and care must be exercised to minimize the risk of producing laryngeal trauma. This technique is not always successful and should not be counted on for routine intubation of ruminants.

Intravenous Catheters are Expensive and Time Consuming: Are They Really Necessary?

An intravenous (IV) catheter is not generally required for short-term chemical restraint but should always be used when patients are anesthetized. The jugular vein is the most commonly used site for IV catheter placement. The thicker skin of ruminants makes catheter placement more difficult, and accidental placement in the carotid artery has occurred. A 14-gauge 5.5-in catheter is used in most ruminant patients. An 18-gauge 2-in catheter is sufficient for lambs and kids. The catheter should be secured to the neck with a suture and/or bandage. The catheter should always be checked before anesthetic induction to ensure it is still functional.

The veins on the external surface of the ear are relatively large and accessible. The author frequently uses ear veins to deliver small-volume chemical restraint cocktails intravenously. A 25-gauge needle and good technique reduce the restraint required for this approach. Ear veins can also be used as an alternate site for venous catheter placement. An 18-, 20- or 22-gauge catheter should be used, depending of the vessel size, and secured with a combination of super glue and tape. A roll of gauze or 4 × 4 surgical sponges is placed inside the pinna to maintain its shape. Because of the increased level of stimulation produced by the catheter stylet, camelid patients are typically less than cooperative to ear catheterization unless chemically or medically obtunded. The cephalic vein can also be used as a site for venous catheter placement, much as it is in small animal patients. The smaller catheters will not provide the flow rate of the 14-gauge catheter but work well otherwise.

One injectable anesthesia approach practitioners may find useful is to administer the small volume of the IV recumbent ketamine stun via an ear vein and then place an IV catheter once patients are recumbent to deliver double drip or ruminant triple drip.

Oxygen Delivery, Muscle, and Nerve Protection

Oxygen supplementation is not generally required during short-term field anesthesia of normal healthy ruminant patients. Oxygen delivery, muscle, and nerve protection are covered in greater detail in *Current Veterinary Therapy*.[1]

A portable oxygen cylinder equipped with a pressure regulator, flowmeter, and appropriate tubing allows oxygen to be delivered via insufflation to patients requiring supplementation. The oxygen line can be attached to a port on the Ambu bag to deliver oxygen to newborn patients. Intermittently sealing the nares and mouth during insufflation can be used to provide some degree of positive pressure ventilation in the rare instance it is required. A 160-L/min demand valve (JDM-5041, JD Medical, Phoenix, Arizona) provides more effective positive pressure ventilation, especially in larger patients. There is no substitute for this equipment in the rare occasions it might be required, but justification of the expense and space required will vary from practice to practice. This equipment should be standard in all large animal clinics where anesthesia is regularly performed.

Fasting Before Anesthesia

Functioning ruminants should be starved before anesthesia. Starving reduces the volume of rumen contents, which reduces pressure on the diaphragm and the incidence of regurgitation. Ruminants properly starved are less likely to bloat during recumbency and anesthesia. Withholding food and water for 24 hours before surgery has been traditionally recommended. Experience with nonstarved emergency cases has shown proper technique to be the most important factor in reducing the risk of regurgitation during induction and intubation. Attempting to intubate patients with some degree of gag reflex present is more likely to result in regurgitation. A proper induction technique eliminates the gag reflex. Keeping patients in sternal recumbency with the head elevated reduces the risk of passive regurgitation during intubation. Withholding food for 12 to 18 hours (access to water is permitted) has proved effective in minimizing problems during intubation and anesthesia while not producing the adverse effects on rumen motility and acid base status associated with longer periods of starving. Some abdominal procedures benefit from a greater reduction of rumen volume, and a longer period of starving will be required in these cases.

Young animals have minimal energy stores. The risk of hypoglycemia in these patients increases with the duration of anesthesia. Nursing ruminants are typically anesthetized without starving to reduce the risk of hypoglycemia. Ruminants aged less than 2 months should be supplemented with dextrose during anesthesia. Adding 1.25% to 2.5% dextrose to the IV electrolyte solution (10 mL/kg/h) is generally sufficient to ensure blood glucose levels are adequately maintained in these patients. Generally, by 2 months of age, most healthy ruminant patients no longer require dextrose supplementation during shorter anesthetic procedures. Adding 1.25% dextrose to the IV fluids is cheap insurance against hypoglycemia in ruminant patients aged 2 to 4 months when a long period of anesthesia is anticipated. Elevated body temperature increases metabolism and increases the risk of hypoglycemia in younger patients. Patients aged up to 4 months should be supplemented with dextrose when the body temperature is significantly elevated.

Unless testing is preformed during anesthesia, hypoglycemia is typically not recognized until the recovery period. Hypoglycemia produces a stuporous state, and patients typically stall part way through the recovery process. Administration of dextrose has resulted in full recovery with no apparent adverse effects when this has occurred. As it is with most things medical, prevention is preferred to treatment. Protracted struggling during physical restraint of unruly young patients can produce substantial elevation of body temperature. Unruly patients should be sedated rather than battled.

Eye Protection

When ruminants are placed in lateral recumbency, care should be taken to ensure the lids of the down eye are closed. A towel or thin pad can be placed under the down eye to provide further protection. Ophthalmic ointment (bland or antibiotic) should be placed in the eyes to protect them during anesthesia. If the down eye ends up bathed in saliva or regurgitation, it should be rinsed out during recovery.

DRUGS USED IN RUMINANT CHEMICAL RESTRAINT AND ANESTHESIA
α_2

Xylazine is the most frequently used drug for sedation in large animals. Ruminants are 10 times more sensitive to xylazine than horses, whereas detomidine is dosed similarly in both species. Ruminants tend to lie down when dosed aggressively with α_2, whereas horses exhibit increasing levels of ataxia.

The initial demeanor of patients greatly influences the sedation produced by a given dose of an α_2. The sedative effect of α_2 can be overridden by elevated sympathetic tone. This results in 2 characteristic features of α_2 sedation. The sedative effect produced by lower doses of α_2 is not as stable. Calm, quiet patients require smaller doses, whereas anxious or unruly patients require larger doses. This sounds easy, but selecting the incorrect dose may result in working on your knees or getting kicked in them. The ideal dose can be difficult to predict, especially when recumbency is not desired. Experience makes the necessary adjustments easier, but even seasoned practitioners get surprised at times.

The α_2 can be administered IV, intramuscularly (IM), or subcutaneously (SQ) and produce a dose-dependent degree of sedation, muscle relaxation, and analgesia. IV administration of α_2 provides a faster onset and more intense level of chemical restraint and analgesia. The fairly rapid onset time can be used as an advantage, allowing multiple smaller IV doses of an α_2 to be administered in an attempt to titrate the effect to the desired level. IM administration results in a more gradual onset and provides a longer duration of less-intense chemical restraint and analgesia. IM administration is often used when patient cooperation does not allow IV administration or when extended duration is desired. The IM dose is traditionally twice the IV dose you would select for patients based on the desired level of effect and the patients' initial demeanor. SQ administration results in the most gradual onset, longest duration, and mildest peak effect. Administering the IV dose IM or SQ is a method used to produce a degree of sedation with a limited risk of recumbency.

The α_2 produce dose-dependent side effects, including decreases in gastrointestinal motility and cardiorespiratory function.[2] The α_2 should be avoided or used very cautiously in compromised patients and should be reversed on completion of the procedure. Even in normal healthy patients, when large doses of α_2 are administered (especially doses used to produce recumbency), reversal is advisable to minimize the risk of gastrointestinal complications. Xylazine has been reported to increase uterine tone in late gestation.[3]

In tractable ruminants, the response to xylazine is fairly predictable. Titrated administration (eg, initial conservative dose that is supplemented if necessary) minimizes the incidence of unintended recumbency. Extremely anxious or unruly patients require larger doses of xylazine to achieve adequate control. In these patients, the administration process often triggers even greater behavior problems, so they should be dosed fairly aggressively at the outset. IM administration is frequently the only option available in extremely anxious or unruly patients. A calm environment can also help to reduce the dose of xylazine required to calm patients. Restraint or interaction should be minimized whenever possible until xylazine has produced a reasonable degree of patient control.

Unless contraindicated, anxious or unruly patients should be sedated with xylazine 5 to 10 minutes before the anesthetic induction sequence. The dose of xylazine will depend on the demeanor of the patients. It could easily be argued that all healthy ruminant patients might benefit from a small dose of xylazine (0.0075–0.01 mg/kg IV or 0.015–0.02 mg/kg IM) 5 to 10 minutes before anesthetic induction because even the calmest of patients will experience some anxiety from the events surrounding anesthetic induction. The impact of anxiety on anesthetic induction is discussed in detail in *Current Veterinary Therapy*.[1]

α_2 Reversal

Yohimbine or tolazoline may be used to reverse the effects of α_2 at the end of a procedure to facilitate a quicker recovery and minimize the risks of gastrointestinal complications. IM administration of the reversal agent is preferred in all but emergency situations because it decreases the risk of central nervous system (CNS) excitement or cardiovascular complications. The shorter duration of action of reversal agents when administered IV can result in resedation in patients whereby the α_2 was administered IM, especially when larger doses were used. To reduce the risk of rough recovery, the reversal of α_2 should not be attempted until sufficient time has elapsed to allow any ketamine or tiletamine/zolazepam (Telazol) used to resolve (15 and 30 minutes after IV and 30 and 60 minutes after IM administration, respectfully). The amount of reversal agent used depends on the dose of the α_2 and duration since administration. The recommended emergency IV doses for yohimbine (0.125 mg/kg) and tolazoline (2 mg/kg) are typically used as the maximum IM dose and reduced to fit the circumstances. When dosed properly, the effects of reversal should start to become evident about 10 minutes following IM administration. Splitting the reversal dose (using both IV and IM routes) can produce a quicker recovery while minimizing the risk of resedation. The response to the small IV component will be fairly quick, so primary IM component should be administered first.

Benzodiazepines

Benzodiazepines (diazepam, midazolam) are centrally acting muscle relaxants with sedative effects. Benzodiazepines do not generally produce a beneficial calming effect when used alone in most species, but ruminants and camelids respond favorably. Benzodiazepines produce minimal cardiovascular or gastrointestinal effects at clinically used doses and provide viable options for producing mild sedation in compromised patients. Benzodiazepines can also be combined with other sedatives, allowing drugs with adverse side effects to be used in smaller doses. Diazepam can be administered IV or IM, but IM absorption is unpredictable. Midazolam is water soluble and can be administered IV, IM, or SQ. Midazolam is slightly more potent than diazepam, but the drugs are generally used interchangeably. Now that midazolam is available as a generic, the price differential is negligible.

Butorphanol

Butorphanol, an opioid agonist-antagonist, is an analgesic drug with sedative effects. Butorphanol does not generally produce a beneficial calming effect when used alone in most species, but ruminants and camelids respond favorably. Butorphanol produces minimal adverse cardiovascular effects at clinically used doses and provides a viable option for producing mild to moderate sedation in compromised patients. Butorphanol can also be combined with other sedatives, allowing drugs with adverse side effects to be used in smaller doses. Butorphanol can be administered IV, IM, or SQ.

Guaifenesin

Guaifenesin is a centrally acting muscle relaxant with mild to moderate sedative activity. At clinically used doses, it produces minimal cardiorespiratory effects. Guaifenesin is used in combination with ketamine and, in some cases xylazine, to produce anesthetic induction in food-animal patients. Guaifenesin-ketamine and guaifenesin-ketamine-xylazine combinations are also used in the IV maintenance of anesthesia in food-animal patients.

Guaifenesin concentrations of 10% have been shown to cause hemolysis in ruminant patients. Practices mixing guaifenesin from powder stock should prepare solutions of 5%. Premixed guaifenesin solution (5%) is now commercially available in 1-L bottles.

Muscle relaxation and ataxia limit the amount of guaifenesin that can be administered before the induction bolus in large patients. In horses, guaifenesin is typically preceded by xylazine, which also produces muscle relaxation and ataxia. The typically equine induction sequence delivers 40 to 50 mg/kg of guaifenesin. Anesthetic induction of small ruminants with double drip typically delivers 100 mg/kg. In larger cattle, the administration of double drip immediately preceding the induction bolus typically delivers 30 mg/kg.

Atropine

Premedication with atropine was commonly recommended in the early days of ruminant anesthesia to counter the profuse salivation of these patients. Atropine administration does not eliminate salivation in ruminant or camelid patients during anesthesia. Atropine tends to reduce the aqueous component of saliva, making it more difficult to clear from the mouth and oropharynx. Atropine also reduces gastrointestinal motility. Routine premedication with atropine is unnecessary and increases patient risk. Atropine (0.01–0.02 mg/kg IV) can be used to treat bradycardia or bradyarrhythmias.

Anesthetic Agents

Ketamine, tiletamine, and the ultrashort barbiturate thiopental are the injectable anesthetic agents used in large animal practice. Ketamine is by far the most common injectable anesthetic agent used in large animal practice. Sodium thiopental (sodium pentothal) is no longer generally used in large animal practice for induction or maintenance of anesthesia but remains the fastest option for restoring an anesthetized state when larger ruminant patients get too light during inhalation maintenance anesthesia. Thiopental (1.1 mg/kg IV) is also very useful in dulling the protective swallowing reflex present during ketamine-based injectable anesthesia. Tiletamine, a more potent and longer-lasting relative of ketamine, is available only in combination with the benzodiazepine zolazepam as Telazol. Because of the high cost of Telazol, it is primarily used in large animal practice for capturing intractable patients.[4,5]

Both ketamine and tiletamine draw on sympathetic nervous system reserve to augment cardiac output and blood pressure. This effect helps counter their direct negative inotropic and vasodilatory effects as well as the negative cardiovascular effects produced by xylazine. Cardiovascular function in normal healthy patients anesthetized with ketamine-based protocols is good to excellent. The author cannot emphasize enough the need for caution in dosing these seemingly safe drugs in compromised patients whereby sympathetic reserve may be severely limited.

CHEMICAL RESTRAINT TECHNIQUES

Physical restraint is generally required when working with food-animal patients. Adding a degree of chemical restraint can make many procedures more pleasant for both practitioners and patients. The enhanced level of patient cooperation improves efficiency, offsetting the modest additional cost of the drugs used.

Chemical restraint techniques used in ruminants range from mild sedation of standing patients to semianesthetized recumbency. When selecting a chemical restraint technique, you must first consider whether patients must remain standing or recumbent for optimal completion of the procedure. Patient cooperation and systemic analgesia are generally greater with techniques that reliably produce recumbency. Instances when either situation will facilitate successful completion of the procedure provide more latitude with regard to technique and doses.

Many of the drug combinations used to produce field anesthesia in ruminants are also used in chemical restraint. Drug doses are typically smaller when used in chemical restraint techniques, but the difference between these two applications is, at times, modest. The level of analgesia produced by chemical restraint varies with the technique and doses administered. Analgesia can approach surgical levels in some situations, but local anesthetic blockade should be used whenever feasible to reduce the risk of patient awareness and stress.

Unfortunately, things do not always go as planned. Should chemical restraint prove inadequate for the intended procedure, being prepared to convert to injectable anesthesia increases the likelihood of a successful outcome. An anesthetic bolus of IV ketamine may be sufficient for shorter situations. Infusion of double drip or ruminant triple drip provides a more stable plane of anesthesia when extended duration is required. Butorphanol (0.05–0.1 mg/kg IV or IM in small ruminants, 0.02–0.05 mg/kg IV or IM in larger ruminants) or morphine (0.05–0.1 mg/kg IV or IM) can be administered to augment the level of analgesia of chemical restraint techniques. The onset time for butorphanol and morphine is slow (peak effect is approximately 10 minutes after IV and 20 minutes after IM administration).

Xylazine

Xylazine sedation and its attendant analgesia are useful for facilitating short diagnostic or therapeutic procedures on less cooperative patients (**Table 1**). Although patients will generally tolerate mildly uncomfortable stimuli, standing xylazine sedation should not be counted on to provide significant analgesia. The duration of xylazine sedation and analgesia is dose dependent, generally lasting about 30 to 40 minutes following IV administration in standing or laterally recumbent patients. In dorsally recumbent patients, the duration of enhanced cooperation provided by IV xylazine may be as short as 20 minutes. The duration is typically doubled with IM administration, although intensity is commensurately reduced. Clinicians that have tried the ketamine stun technique tend to prefer it to pure xylazine chemical restraint.

Xylazine (0.05 mg/kg IV or 0.1 mg/kg IM) will result in recumbency in 50% of tractable cattle. Xylazine (0.1 mg/kg IV or 0.2 mg/kg IM) will result in recumbency is

Table 1 Dose range of xylazine expected to produce standing sedation with a low incidence of recumbency		
Patient Type	IV[a]	IM
Quiet dairy breeds	0.0075–0.01 mg/kg	0.015–0.02 mg/kg
Tractable cattle	0.01–0.02 mg/kg	0.02–0.04 mg/kg
Anxious cattle	0.02–0.03 mg/kg	0.04–0.06 mg/kg
Extremely anxious or unruly cattle	0.025–0.05 mg/kg	0.05–0.1 mg/kg

[a] Administering the IV dose IM further reduces the possibility of recumbency.

most tractable cattle. Anxious or unruly patients are more resistant, and somewhat higher doses of xylazine may be required to produce recumbency. Titrated administration (eg, initial conservative dose that is supplemented if necessary) minimizes the amount of xylazine administered and, therefore, the degree of adverse side effects produced. Physical methods can also be used to produce recumbency once patients are sufficiently sedated.

Detomidine

Although more expensive, detomidine can be used to produce sedation and systemic analgesia in ruminant patients (**Table 2**). Detomidine is a more potent α_2. Because of their increased sensitivity to xylazine, the dose relationship between xylazine and detomidine in ruminants does not reflect this difference.

Detomidine produces greater cardiorespiratory depression than xylazine and should not be used to produce recumbent sedation.

α_2 and Opioid

An opioid (butorphanol, morphine) can be administered to augment the level of systemic analgesia in ruminants sedated with an α_2. Butorphanol (0.05–0.1 mg/kg IV or IM in smaller ruminants, 0.02–0.05 mg/kg IV or IM in larger ruminants) or morphine (0.05–0.1 mg/kg IV or IM) can be administered with the initial dose of α_2 or added in situations when patient cooperation needs improvement. The α_2 dose can typically be reduced somewhat when used in conjunction with an opioid.

Ketamine Stun

The ketamine stun is basically the addition of a small dose of ketamine to any injectable chemical restraint technique. I initially developed the ketamine stun technique in the early 1990s to cover my limited cat handling abilities. My first exposure to camelid patients came when I left equine practice to teach at Ohio State. The recalcitrant behavior they frequently exhibited quickly led to experimentation with low-dose ketamine protocols to improve the level of patient cooperation during diagnostic and therapeutic procedures. Success was immediately evident, and the technique became wildly popular with the food-animal clinicians, residents, and students charged with the care of these patients.[6] Because of the success in camelid patients, the ketamine stun technique was adjusted for use in ruminants (less xylazine) and proved to be just as useful. Equine applications have proven more challenging. Dramatic improvement in cooperation evident a minute or two after the IV bolus of ketamine is administered in patients that were totally uncooperative under the prior detomidine-morphine sedation suggests the potential of this technique.[7] Unfortunately, the effective sedation-ketamine levels are not far removed from those that

Table 2		
Dose range of detomidine expected to produce standing sedation with a low incidence of recumbency		
Patient Type	**IV[a]**	**IM**
Tractable cattle	0.002–0.005 mg/kg	0.006–0.01 mg/kg
Anxious cattle	0.005–0.0075 mg/kg	0.01–0.015 mg/kg
Extremely anxious or unruly cattle	0.01–0.015 mg/kg	0.0015–0.02 mg/kg

Information regarding the use of detomidine in ruminants is limited. The dose ranges provided are estimates and should be adjusted based on experience.

[a] Administering the IV dose IM further reduces the possibility of recumbency.

produce instability in horses. The ketamine stun technique has been shown to reduce stress response to castration and dehorning in calves.[8,9]

I named this technique the ketamine stun (also known as ket stun) because of the stunned effect it produced in patients when administered at doses that produce recumbency. These patients seem to be awake but seem oblivious to the surroundings and the procedure being performed. The IV effect is quite brief (approximately 15 minutes), and patients typically stand and seem fairly normal at that time. I initially referred to this state as semianesthetized, but perhaps chemical hypnosis is more appropriate.

The α_2 possess potent sedative and analgesic effects. Opioids are typically thought of as analgesic drugs, but they possess CNS effects that, when combined with a tranquilizer or sedative, produce a greater level of mental depression. Ketamine is an N-methyl-D-aspartate receptor antagonist that possesses potent analgesic effects at subanesthetic doses. Ketamine was initially included in the stun technique for its analgesic properties but likely contributes to the mental aspects of the enhanced cooperation exhibited by patients under the influence of the ketamine stun technique. By combining drugs, one is able to use smaller doses of the individual components while still achieving the desired level of patient control. Dosing must be more conservative when using the ketamine stun technique in standing patients. This conservative dosing limits the degree of systemic analgesia relative to what can be achieved in recumbent patients but still provides improved patient cooperation when compared with more traditional methods of standing chemical restraint in both ruminants and horses.

In ruminants and camelid patients, I typically use a combination of xylazine, butorphanol, and ketamine. In equine patients, I generally use detomidine, morphine, and ketamine. Morphine is used to provide analgesic relief in food animal patients and is much cheaper than butorphanol. I have used morphine (0.05–0.06 mg/kg) in ruminant stuns. In standing adult cattle stuns, a similar level of cooperation is achieved with either opioid, but patients seem less obtunded when morphine is used. Some practitioners may find the obtunded appearance useful because it allows them to follow the decay over time in the level of chemical restraint. Deterioration in the level of patient cooperation can also be used to determine when supplemental drug administration may be required.

Ketamine stun techniques can be divided into 2 broad categories: standing and recumbent. The standing ketamine stun is used primarily in large ruminants and horses. The recumbent ketamine stun is used primarily in small ruminants, camelids, and foals. The level of effect achieved is determined by 3 variables: dose, route of administration, and initial demeanor of patients. The stun cocktail can be administered IV, IM, or SQ, depending on the systemic analgesia, patient cooperation, and duration desired (**Table 3**).

Aggressive dosing increases the level of systemic analgesia and patient cooperation but also increases the risk of instability, unintended recumbency, or the duration of intended recumbency. In patients that must remain standing, balance between the

Table 3	
Route of administration determines the relative impact of the ketamine stun technique	
Parameter	**Relative Ranking**
Intensity (analgesia/cooperation)	IV >> IM > SQ
Onset	IV >> IM > SQ
Duration of effect	SQ > IM >> IV

α_2 and ketamine is crucial. Greater levels of sedation require lower peak blood levels of ketamine to avoid producing a transient period of instability in equine patients and recumbency in ruminant and camelid patients. Obtaining maximum benefit from the ketamine stun technique requires pushing up against the limits of this balancing act. The rapid increase in blood levels produced by IV administration of ketamine presents the greatest challenge. Titrated administration of IV ketamine can be used to minimize the risk of untoward responses.

An endless number of permutations are possible when using the ketamine stun. Many years of experimentation in many different species have provided a great deal of insight into the potential of this technique but have not produced a definitive combination for all situations in each species. The following examples are provided as a guide, and practitioners are encouraged to experiment with adjustments in doses.

IV Recumbent Ketamine Stun

The IV recumbent ketamine stun was my first adaption for ruminants. It is intended for short procedures requiring a high level of systemic analgesia and/or patient cooperation. Numerous minor procedures (castrations, biopsies, flushing septic joints, casting fractures, and so forth) have been successfully completed in small ruminants using the IV recumbent ketamine stun.

A combination of xylazine (0.025–0.05 mg/kg), butorphanol (0.05–0.1 mg/kg), and ketamine (0.3–0.5 mg/kg) is administered IV. I generally use the upper end of the dose ranges unless contraindicated. The onset is approximately 1 minute. Patients gracefully become recumbent. Patients seem awake but seem oblivious to the surroundings and the procedure being performed. Mild random head or limb motion and vocalization are not unusual in patients under the influence of the ketamine stun. Purposeful movement or vocalization are signs of an inadequate ketamine stun level and additional drug should be administered. One-half of the initial ketamine dose should be administered IV and is often effective. If, after allowing 60 to 90 seconds for onset, this additional half dose of ketamine fails to produce the desired level of analgesia, a second half dose of ketamine along with one-half of the initial dose of xylazine should be administered IV. The level of systemic analgesia produced varies depending on the doses administered but tends to be fairly intense. Peak analgesia occurs at time of onset and decays over time. Surgical levels of analgesia have been achieved with this technique, but local anesthetic blockade should be used whenever feasible to reduce the risk of patient awareness and stress. Local anesthetic blockade also provides analgesia in the immediate postprocedure period. Having syringes preloaded with local anesthetic speeds the blockade process, which reduces its impact on the diminishing level of systemic analgesia. Duration of the stun effect is approximately 15 minutes, and patients are typically able to stand and walk immediately or shortly after this point.

The IV recumbent ketamine stun is designed for short procedures. One should plan ahead and work fast. Supplemental doses of ketamine or xylazine can be administered to extend the duration, but this technique is not intended for procedures that are expected to last significantly beyond the 15- to 25-minute range. The degree of extension is relative to the amount of supplemental drug administered.

An example of a somewhat more potent IV recumbent ketamine stun application in ruminants is a recent adaption developed by Dr David Anderson, DVM, MS, DACVS, Professor of Large Animal Surgery at Kansas State University College of Veterinary Medicine. He needed to do laparotomies on 100 ewes (60–75 kg), so efficiency was important. Safety was imperative because they needed to breed back 3 weeks after surgery. The ewes were held off water and feed overnight before surgery. Xylazine

(0.05 mg/kg IV), ketamine (1 mg/kg IV), and butorphanol (0.025 mg/kg IV) were administered as a combination (each ewe received 4 mg xylazine, 2 mg butorphanol, and 75 mg ketamine). Ewes were placed in dorsal recumbency (not intubated) and midline local anesthetic blockade performed. Surgery time was 15 to 20 minutes. When lifted off the table and rolled into sternal, 90% of the ewes stood and walked back to the pen. There was zero morbidity and mortality. David's summary defines the benefits of the ketamine stun technique: "Pretty awesome—totally conscious, aware and would watch you if you walked in front of them—but they did not have a care in the world, did not move a muscle." Movement occurred when a reduced dose of ketamine (50 mg IV) was tried.

IM or SQ Recumbent Ketamine Stun

Administering the upper end of the IV recumbent ketamine stun doses IM or SQ produces a longer, less intense form of chemical restraint. Local anesthetic blockade is required for painful procedures. A combination of butorphanol (0.025 mg/kg), xylazine (0.05 mg/kg), and ketamine (0.1 mg/kg) is administered IM or SQ. SQ administration provides a slightly longer duration of effect. This technique can also be used to improve cooperation in patients that have gone down before or during a surgical procedure.

The IM or SQ recumbent ketamine stun has been used at Kansas State to provide chemical restraint for umbilical hernia repair in calves. Onset time was approximately 3 to 10 minutes. The patients were obtunded enough to require (and tolerate) intubation when placed in dorsal recumbency. The duration of effect with SQ administration was approximately 45 minutes. Patients were typically ambulatory within 30 minutes following arousal.

IV Standing Ketamine Stun

Small doses of IV ketamine can markedly improve the level of cooperation in less cooperative standing patients. Dosing is more critical when the ketamine stun is administered IV in patients that must remain standing. I generally sedate the patient first with xylazine (0.02-0.0275 mg/kg IV depending on initial demeanor of patient) before slowly administering the ketamine (0.05–0.1 mg/kg IV). This practice allows me to reduce the dose of ketamine administered if I have any concerns regarding the level of sedation. An opioid (butorphanol 0.05–0.1 mg/kg IV or IM in smaller ruminants, 0.02–0.05 mg/kg IV or IM in larger ruminants, or morphine 0.05–0.1 mg/kg IV or IM) can be added to augment the level of systemic analgesia and patient control.

The following example demonstrates the value of this technique. A 725- to 775-kg Charolais bull was run into the chute for examination of a possible penile injury. He was extremely agitated and just kept banging around inside the chute despite being left alone. Examination was impossible, and patient injury was a valid concern. To calm him down, I administered 20 mg of IV xylazine (0.0275 mg/kg), which made him stand still when left alone, but he would not tolerate attempts at examination. I then administered 40 mg of IV ketamine (0.055 mg/kg). The ketamine made him extremely cooperative, but the chute hampered full examination. A decision was made to place him on the tilt table. He was very compliant during the tabling process and subsequent examination.

IM or SQ Standing Stun

The doses provided for the 5–10–20 technique were developed in range cattle. Dosages may need to be adjusted when using the IM/SQ standing ketamine stun in milder mannered cattle.

A combination of butorphanol (0.01 mg/kg), xylazine (0.02 mg/kg), and ketamine (0.04 mg/kg) is administered IM or SQ. In a 500-kg cow, this equates to butorphanol

(5 mg), xylazine (10 mg), and ketamine (20 mg). For a 680-kg patient, the doses are 7 mg butorphanol, 15 mg xylazine, and 25 mg ketamine. Morphine (25 mg for a 500-kg cow and 30 mg for a 680-kg cow) can be substituted for butorphanol. Patients will seem less obtunded, but the level of cooperation is similar to stuns using butorphanol. The level of systemic analgesia is limited, and local anesthetic blockade should be used to reduce the risk of patient awareness and stress.

The 5–10–20 standing ketamine stun technique is a modification developed in Kansas State University junior surgery laboratories where it was used to provide chemical restraint for standing cesarean deliveries in beef cattle. Patients received 5 mg of butorphanol, 10 mg of xylazine, and 20 mg of ketamine. Patient weights varied from 340 to 660 kg, but no adjustments were made in the combination administered. SQ administration is preferred to minimize the risk of recumbency; but in very unruly cows, IM administration provided better patient control. The onset is 5 to 10 minutes with SQ administration. The initial dose of 5–10–20 has not resulted in recumbency. Cows stood quietly during the cesarean deliveries (many were ill mannered before the ketamine stun). The duration of effect is approximately 60 to 90 minutes. Additional xylazine and ketamine can be administered SQ to extend the duration of chemical restraint. Recumbency has occasionally occurred with re-administration of 50% of all 3 components. The current recommendation for supplemental drug administration is 25% to 50% of the initial xylazine and ketamine doses, 0–2.5–5 and 0–5–10, respectively, depending on the degree of cooperation and the time required to complete the procedure.

A similar approach (10–20–40 technique) has been used successfully in adult bulls. Preputial surgery (with a local anesthetic block) is an example of the procedures performed using this technique.

IM Xylazine-Ketamine

A combination of xylazine (0.05–0.1 mg/kg IM) and ketamine (2 mg/kg IM) is administered. This combination can be useful for subduing combative patients. It will generally produce recumbency, although extremely unruly patients may not go down in a timely fashion without some physical assistance. The degree of chemical restraint and systemic analgesia achieved with this technique varies markedly. Patients typically tolerate physical manipulation and mildly painful procedures but respond to more intense levels of stimulation. Additional IV ketamine, double drip, or ruminant triple drip can be administered to enhance the level of patient cooperation and analgesia, if required. The reversal of xylazine should not be attempted until sufficient time has elapsed to allow the ketamine anesthesia to be resolved (30–40 minutes after IM and 15 to 20 minutes after IV administration).

IV Xylazine-Ketamine

Xylazine (0.025–0.03 mg/kg IV) is administered first. When marked sedation is evident or patients become recumbent, ketamine (1 mg/kg IV) is administered. The addition of the ketamine markedly augments the level of analgesia, although it varies somewhat from patient to patient. This combination may provide a brief period (5–10 minutes) of surgical analgesia. A half dose of ketamine IV can be used to extend the duration an additional 5 to 7 minutes.

Telazol-ketamine-xylazine

Ruminant Telazol-ketamine-xylazine (TKX-Ru) is a modification of porcine TKX (TKX-P). TKX-Ru is used for capturing intractable ruminant patients and large exotic hoof stock. TKX-Ru is created by reconstituting a 500-mg vial of Telazol with 250 mg of ketamine (2.5 mL) and 100 mg of large animal xylazine (1 mL). Because of the space occupied by the Telazol powder, the final volume is 4 mL. TKX-Ru is typically administered using a pole syringe or dart gun. The dosing protocol for TKX-Ru is still evolving. Current recommendations are 1.25 to 1.5 mL/110 to 115 kg for smaller ruminant patients and 1 mL/110 to 115 kg for larger ruminant patients. Patient should become recumbent and compliant approximately 5 (ideal) to 10 minutes following IM administration. An onset significantly less than 5 minutes indicates an excessive dose or accidental IV administration. If the onset has not occurred by 20 minutes, additional TKX-Ru (one-quarter to one-half of the original dose, depending on the urgency of the situation and health of the patient) can be administered. The degree and duration of chemical restraint and analgesia varies markedly from patient to patient. IV administration of double drip or ruminant triple drip can be used to enhance and/or extend the systemic analgesia and patient cooperation produced by TKX-Ru.

Patients are typically awake and sternal by 40 to 60 minutes after TKX-Ru administration. Because of the level of residual sedation, patients typically remain sternal for an additional 20 to 40 minutes (depending on demeanor and level of environmental stimulation) before attempting to stand. Recovery is generally smooth. Once patients are awake and sternal, xylazine can be reversed to speed the recovery process, although recovery quality may be reduced somewhat. Letting xylazine resolve on its own generally makes transporting unruly patients smoother.

TKX-Ru is fairly expensive. Leftover TKX-Ru can be frozen to preserve its function for up to 6 months.

INJECTABLE ANESTHESIA TECHNIQUES

Many diagnostic and therapeutic procedures in food-animal practice require physical and/or chemical restraint techniques. Anesthesia should be considered for procedures that require an extended period of immobility or high level of systemic analgesia. Certain aspects of anesthesia place patients at a greater risk than chemical restraint techniques. Knowledge and vigilance reduce the additional risks associated with anesthesia.

The choice of injectable (commonly referred to as *field* anesthesia) or inhalation maintenance (commonly referred to as *general* anesthesia) will depend on several factors, most prominent being the equipment available and the experience of the personnel involved. Injectable anesthesia has been traditionally considered proper only for shorter procedures, although its role is expanding in equine referral hospitals. When proper care is exercised, injectable anesthesia is safe and can be used effectively in both field and clinical settings.

Injectable anesthesia has been traditionally associated with IV or IM bolus administration of drugs. The level of patient cooperation and systemic analgesia decays over time when these methods are used, requiring a higher initial level of effect to achieve the desired duration. The risk of adverse side effects, such as cardiorespiratory depression, is greater during the initial stages of the anesthetic period when bolus administration techniques are used. Constant rate infusion (CRI) techniques, such as double drip or ruminant triple drip, are safer injectable anesthesia methods. Induction is more gradual with the double drip or ruminant triple drip. Continuous delivery also provides a more stable plane of anesthesia. The use of stock solutions with adjustments in delivery rate made to accommodate variations in patient size and/or alter the level of effect make CRI techniques easier to use.

Food animals tend to be patient during recovery from recumbent chemical restraint and anesthesia. They typically do not attempt to stand until they are awake and functional. Patient demeanor and the level of sensory stimulation (pain, environmental) influence the quality of recovery. Supplemental xylazine administration is rarely required but may be necessary in exceptionally unruly patients to prevent premature attempts to stand. Preemptive analgesic support should be used in painful procedures.

Ketamine Stun

The recumbent IV ketamine stun covered in the "Chemical Restraint Techniques" section typically produces a profound initial level of systemic analgesia. Brief periods of surgical analgesia have been produced in many patients but not consistently enough for the IV ketamine stun technique to be truly considered an injectable anesthetic technique.

IV Xylazine-Ketamine

IV xylazine and ketamine can be used to produce a short duration of injectable anesthesia in normal healthy ruminants. Because of the large dose of xylazine, this technique should not be used in compromised patients.

Xylazine (0.05 mg/kg IV) is administered first. When marked sedation is evident or patients become recumbent, ketamine (2 mg/kg IV) is administered. This combination provides approximately 15 minutes of anesthesia. Administering one-third to one-half of the original dose of each drug can be used to extend anesthesia, but recovery duration will increase with the number of supplemental doses administered because of the slower clearance of xylazine. Gradually reducing the xylazine component in the supplemental doses will reduce its adverse impact on cardiorespiratory function and recovery time. Extending anesthesia with boluses of IV xylazine-ketamine should be limited to cases that require only a few supplemental doses or in emergency situations in which other options are not available. Double drip or ruminant triple drip are the preferred methods for extending the duration of injectable anesthesia in ruminant patients.

IM Xylazine-Ketamine

IM administration of xylazine and ketamine can be used to produce an intermediate length of injectable anesthesia in normal healthy ruminants. Because of the large dose of xylazine, this technique should not be used in compromised patients.

A combination of xylazine (0.05–0.1 mg/kg IM) and ketamine (4 mg/kg IM) is administered. This combination will generally produce 30 to 40 minutes of recumbency. As with any bolus administration technique, analgesia will be highest at the outset and gradually diminish over time. A half dose of each drug can be administered IM to extend duration 15 to 20 minutes. A quarter dose of each drug can be administered IV to extend duration of anesthesia approximately 10 to 15 minutes.

Butorphanol-ketamine-xylazine

The butorphanol-ketamine-xylazine (BKX) technique was developed by Dr LaRue Johnson at Colorado State University. He prefers to call it XKB, but everyone else refers to it as BKX. A combination of xylazine, ketamine, and butorphanol is administered IM to produce an intermediate duration of injectable anesthesia in normal healthy ruminants. Because of the large dose of xylazine, this technique should not be used in compromised patients.

A stock solution can be created to provide numerous doses by adding 100 mg of large-animal xylazine (1 mL) and 10 mg of butorphanol (1 mL) to a 1000 mg bottle of ketamine (10 mg). Administer the mixture IM at a dose rate of 1 mL/20 kg. An alternative method is to draw up the individual components in a syringe as follows:

Butorphanol (0.0375 mg/kg)

Xylazine (0.375 mg/kg)

Ketamine (3.75 mg/kg)

Patients should become recumbent within 3 to 5 minutes, with a surgical plane of anesthesia lasting up to another 20 to 30 minutes. As with any bolus administration technique, analgesia will be highest at the outset and gradually diminish over time. For procedures requiring considerable surgical preparation, the effective period of analgesia can be extended by administering half of the initial BKX dose IV before the start of surgery. Expect approximately 25 to 35 minutes of working time when the additional dose is used. Patients tend to remain laterally recumbent much longer following the completion of the procedure when compared with the recumbent ketamine stun techniques.

Double Drip

Double drip is created by adding ketamine (1 mg/mL) to 5% guaifenesin. Double drip is the most commonly used method for inducing anesthesia to be maintained with inhalants in small ruminants. A CRI of double drip can be used to provide a stable plane of injectable anesthesia in ruminants. Because double drip does not contain xylazine, the level of analgesia provided is somewhat lower when compared with ruminant triple drip. The absence of xylazine's cardiovascular depressant effects makes double drip a better choice for injectable maintenance in compromised ruminant patients. Butorphanol (0.05–0.1 mg/kg IV or IM in smaller ruminants, 0.02–0.05 mg/kg IV or IM in larger ruminants) or morphine (0.05–0.1 mg/kg IV or IM) can be administered to augment the level of analgesia when double drip is used to maintain anesthesia.

Anesthetic induction is achieved by slowly administering double drip to effect. A syringe should be used to administer double drip in very small patients to reduce the risk of overdosing because this combination has a somewhat slow onset. Muscle relaxation and sedation typically produce recumbency well before patients are anesthetized. Anesthetic induction generally requires the administration of 1.7 to 2.2 mL/ kg. Anesthesia can be maintained by the continued infusion of double drip at a rate of 2.6 mL/kg/h without significant cardiorespiratory depression in normal healthy patients. In compromised patients, sympathetic nervous system reserve may be limited. Although double drip is the most benign method of injectable anesthesia, extra care must be exercised when using it in severely compromised patients whereby sympathetic reserve may be limited. Anesthetic depth and cardiorespiratory function should be closely monitored and supportive measures (IV fluids, dobutamine, oxygen, and so forth) implemented as required.

In large ruminants, double drip is generally used to soften up patients, but triple drip can also be used for this purpose. When early signs of sedation and muscle relaxation become evident, a combination of ketamine (1.5–2 mg/kg IV) and diazepam (0.06–0.1 mg/kg IV) is administered. This approach provides a more predictable and rapid drop, improving patient control and safety of the personnel involved in the induction process. Anesthesia can be maintained with continued infusion of either double drip or ruminant triple drip.

Ruminant Triple Drip

Ruminant triple drip (GKX-Ru) is created by adding ketamine (1 mg/mL) and xylazine (0.1 mg/mL) to 5% guaifenesin.[10,11] Equine triple drip contains a much higher concentration of xylazine (0.5 mg/mL). A CRI of GKX-Ru can be used to provide a stable plane of injectable anesthesia in normal healthy ruminants. Compromised ruminant patients should be maintained with double drip to eliminate the cardiovascular depressant effects of xylazine.

In small ruminants, anesthetic induction is achieved by slowly infusing GKX-Ru to effect. A syringe should be used to administer GKX-Ru in very small patients to reduce the risk of overdosing because this combination has a somewhat slow onset. Muscle relaxation and sedation typically produce recumbency well before patients are anesthetized. Anesthetic induction generally requires the administration of 1.0 to 1.5 mL/kg. Anesthesia can be maintained in normal healthy ruminants by continued infusion of GKX-Ru at a rate of 2.6 mL/kg/h without significant cardiorespiratory depression. Xylazine is cleared more slowly than ketamine. Because of this difference, postprocedure recumbency lengthens as the duration of GKX-Ru administration increases. Xylazine sedation can be reversed to speed the recovery process once patients are sternal and awake.

For large ruminants, refer to the previous "Double Drip" section.

Ketamine-diazepam

IV diazepam and ketamine can be used to produce a short duration of injectable anesthesia in normal healthy ruminants. Cardiovascular function is good to excellent following induction with this combination in normal healthy patients, and the absence of xylazine's cardiovascular depressant effects makes ketamine-diazepam (Ket-Val) a viable choice for injectable anesthesia of compromised patients. The same admonitions provided for double drip should be applied when using Ket-Val to anesthetize severely compromised patients. Titrated administration can be used to minimize the level of effect produced when administering boluses of Ket-Val. Butorphanol (0.05–0.1 mg/kg IV or IM in smaller ruminants and 0.02–0.05 mg/kg IV or IM in larger ruminants) or morphine (0.05–0.1 mg/kg IV or IM) can be administered to augment the level of analgesia when using Ket-Val to anesthetize ruminant patients.

In small ruminants, a mixture of equal volumes of ketamine (100 mg/mL) and diazepam (5 mg/mL) is administered IV at 1 mL/18 to 22 kg (which sounded better when it was 1 mL/40–50 lb). A single bolus of Ket-Val provides up to 15 to 20 minutes of surgical analgesia with patients remaining recumbent somewhat longer. As with any bolus administration technique, analgesia will be highest at the outset and gradually diminish over time. Administering smaller boluses (one-third to one-half of the original volume) can be used to extend anesthetic duration. Anesthesia can also be maintained with IV infusion of either double drip or ruminant triple drip, which will provide a more stable plane of anesthesia than intermittent boluses of Ket-Val.

For large ruminants, refer to the previous "Double Drip" section.

REFERENCES

1. Abrahamsen EJ. Inhalation anesthesia in ruminants. In: Anderson DE, Rings M, editors. Current veterinary therapy food animal practice. 5th edition. Saunders/Elsevier; 2009. p. 559–69.
2. Campbell KB, Klavano PA, Richardson P, et al. Hemodynamic effects of xylazine in the calf. Am J Vet Res 1979;40:1777–80.
3. LeBlanc MM, Hubbell JE, Smith HC. The effects of xylazine hydrochloride on intrauterine pressure in the cow and mare. Theriogenology 1984;21(5):681–90.
4. Abrahamsen EJ. Chemical restraint in ruminants. In: Anderson DE, Rings M, editors. Current veterinary therapy food animal practice. 5th edition. Saunders/Elsevier; 2009. p. 544–53.

5. Abrahamsen EJ. Telazol-based capture techniques for wild hoofstock. Proceedings of the American College of Veterinary Surgeons. Chicago (IL): 2011.

6. Abrahamsen EJ. Chemical restraint, anesthesia, and analgesia for camelids. Vet Clin North Am Food Anim Pract 2009;25(2):455–94.

7. Abrahamsen EJ. Standing chemical restraint techniques. Proceedings of the 2007 Western Veterinary Conference. Las Vegas.

8. Coetzee JF, Gehring R, Tarus-Sang J, et al. Effect of sub-anesthetic xylazine and ketamine ("ketamine stun") administered to calves immediately prior to castration. Vet Anaesth Analg 2010;37(6):566–78.

9. Baldridge SL, Coetzee JF, Dritz SS, et al. Pharmacokinetics and physiologic effects of intramuscularly administered xylazine hydrochloride-ketamine hydrochloride- butorphanol tartrate alone or in combination with orally administered sodium salicylate on biomarkers of pain in Holstein calves following castration and dehorning. Am J Vet Res 2011;72(10):1305–17.

10. Lin HC, Tyler JW, Welles EG, et al. Effects of anesthesia induced and maintained by continuous intravenous administration of guaifenesin, ketamine, and xylazine in spontaneously breathing sheep. Am J Vet Res 1993;54(11):1913–6.

11. Thurmon JC, Benson GJ, Tranquilli WJ, et al. Cardiovascular effects of intravenous infusion of guaifenesin, ketamine, and xylazine in Holstein calves. Vet Surg 1986;15:463.

The Economics of Pain Management

Heather P. Newton, BS,
Annette M. O'Connor, BVSc, MVSc, DVSc, FACVSc (Epidemiology)*

KEYWORDS

- Castration • Dehorning • Economics • Pain • Production

KEY POINTS

- There is little evidence that pain management is associated with increased production outcomes such as average daily gain, feed intake, or feed to gain.
- Most studies are too short to meaningfully assess production outcomes and few approaches to pain mitigation have been assessed multiple times.
- If assessing production outcomes is important, studies specially designed to assess this outcome are needed.
- Few studies have been conducted that assess the impact of cost-benefit on producers' motivation for adoption of pain mitigation.
- In the few studies conducted, it was common for producers to indicate that the cost of pain mitigation was a factor that affected its adoption.
- There are likely large regional differences in the cost of adopting pain mitigation so locally relevant studies will be important.

INTRODUCTION

The economics of pain management in livestock production encompasses an enormous number of issues including, but not limited to, trade implications, incentive programs, cost-benefit analysis, and consumer preferences. This article discusses two aspects of the question of the economics of pain management in cattle:

- What is the evidence that pain management for routine management procedures in cattle is associated with improved production?
- What is the evidence that producers consider that pain management must be economical?

The authors have nothing to disclose.
Department of Veterinary Diagnositic and Production Animal Medicine, Iowa State University College of Veterinary Medicine, 1600 South 16th Street, Ames, IA 50010, USA
* Corresponding author.
E-mail address: oconnor@iastate.edu

The rationale for evaluating these two aspects is to try to understand their role in the adoption of pain management practices. The working hypothesis is that if pain management was associated with greater gains in production than losses due to cost, this would remove a barrier to widespread adoption of pain management. However, that argument is predicated on the idea that gains versus costs have substantial bearing on the reason why producers do not use pain management. To evaluate the validity of this working hypothesis, the authors reviewed the publically available literature relevant to both topics.

The Scope

The scope of the review was limited to painful procedures that are part of routine bovine husbandry such as castration, dehorning, and tail docking. These topics were chosen because they are common livestock management procedures in beef and dairy herds. It is estimated that more than 16 million castrations were performed in the United States alone in 2011.[1] These procedures are considered to improve the safety of the producers, veterinarians, and other animals. The American Veterinary Medical Association considers castration and dehorning to be painful procedures and encourages the use of concurrent pain management techniques.[2]

Pain in Cattle Production due to Management Practices

Pain in cattle can be objectively or subjectively measured by factors including decreased movement, decreased interaction, reduced responsiveness, postural changes, increased heart rate, increased pupil size, altered respiration, serum cortisol response, and increased behavioral events like tail flicking and head shaking.[3–12] Several studies have also been suggested in that pain due to castration or dehorning in calves can adversely affect production parameters by decreasing average daily gain, daily feed intake, or feed efficiency.[4,5,11–15] If pain causes decreased production, it would be expected that mitigation of pain would decrease this loss, hence the rationale for assessing the impact of pain mitigation strategies on production parameters.

Use of Pain Management in North American Cattle Production

The use of pain mitigation for management procedures differs between countries and is reviewed elsewhere. In the United States, use of pain mitigation for procedures such as castration and dehorning is low.[16] There may be several reasons for slow adoption. One important factor is that in the United States there are no drugs approved by the Food and Drug Administration (FDA0 for the treatment of pain in livestock.[17] The FDA suggest that

> A major reason for the lack of approved food animal analgesics is that there are no validated methods for evaluating pain responses in food animals. For an analgesic to be FDA-approved, it has to undergo studies showing it is safe and effective. However, because no valid methods to measure food animal pain are available, the studies needed to show the analgesic actually controls pain are difficult to design.[18]

Consequently, veterinarians must use extralabel applications for pain management, which is a barrier to adoption.[16] Veterinarians and producers may also believe there is a dearth of evidence that pain medications have an appreciable effect on signs of pain in cattle.[16,19–23] Also, uncertainty about the cost-benefit balance may deter veterinarians from recommending (and producers from adopting) the use of pain medication during painful procedures in cattle.[24]

WHAT IS THE EVIDENCE THAT PAIN MITIGATION FOR ROUTINE MANAGEMENT PROCEDURES IN CATTLE IS ASSOCIATED WITH IMPROVED PRODUCTION?
The Review Question

"What is the magnitude of the effect on average daily gain, daily intake, and gain to feed ratio in cattle that received pain mitigation interventions compared with no treatment of painful management procedures?"

This format followed the PICO format recommended for systematic review by clearly identifying the relevant

- Population (cattle)
- Intervention (pain medication for painful procedures such as castration or dehorning)
- Comparator (no pain medication for painful procedures such as castration or dehorning)
- Outcome (magnitude of the effect on average daily gain, daily intake, and gain to feed ratio).

Relevant pain mitigation interventions were identified from a review of pain management in cattle[17] and included:

- Local anesthetics: lidocaine, bupivacaine
- Nonsteroidal antiinflammatory drugs: flunixin meglumine, phenylbutazone, salicylic acid derivatives, carprofen, meloxicam, ketoprofen
- Sedative analgesics: ketamine, xylazine, butorphanol, morphine.

The Literature Search

To identify primary research relevant to the review question, PubMed and CAB Abstracts were searched. The search terms used in PubMed are listed in **Fig. 1**. Analogous search terms were used in CAB Abstracts. All database searches were conducted in the last two weeks of May 2012. No language or date restrictions were imposed during the search. It was concluded that the performed search was comprehensive because all relevant articles identified in the bibliography of a review on the topic[17] were captured by the search.

Identifying Relevant Articles

Screening of the retrieved citations was conducted independently by one reviewer (HN) who was a DVM student working in a summer research program. The reviewer screened all retrieved citations or full text for inclusion based on the following eligibility criteria:

- Was the study conducted on cattle?
- Did the study involve a painful procedure or condition that was treated with a relevant pain medication in one group while assessing a parallel comparison group?
- Did the study describe primary research that compares at least one production outcome?

When the reviewer answered yes to all questions, the studies were included in the review.

Extracting Data from the Studies

Relevant data on the intervention and relevant outcomes were extracted by one reviewer (HN) for the following outcomes of interest: average daily gain, daily intake,

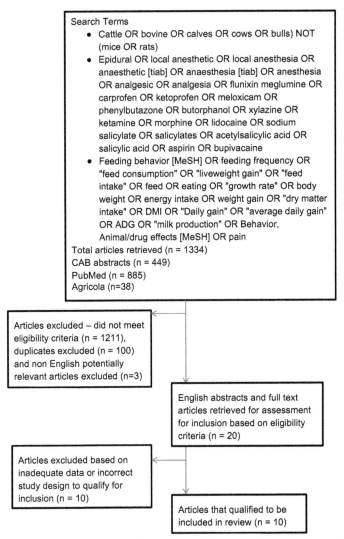

Search Terms
- Cattle OR bovine OR calves OR cows OR bulls) NOT (mice OR rats)
- Epidural OR local anesthetic OR local anesthesia OR anaesthetic [tiab] OR anaesthesia [tiab] OR anesthesia OR analgesic OR analgesia OR flunixin meglumine OR carprofen OR ketoprofen OR meloxicam OR phenylbutazone OR butorphanol OR xylazine OR ketamine OR morphine OR lidocaine OR sodium salicylate OR salicylates OR acetylsalicylic acid OR salicylic acid OR aspirin OR bupivacaine
- Feeding behavior [MeSH] OR feeding frequency OR "feed consumption" OR "liveweight gain" OR "feed intake" OR feed OR eating OR "growth rate" OR body weight OR energy intake OR weight gain OR "dry matter intake" OR DMI OR "Daily gain" OR "average daily gain" OR ADG OR "milk production" OR Behavior, Animal/drug effects [MeSH] OR pain

Total articles retrieved (n = 1334)
CAB abstracts (n = 449)
PubMed (n = 885)
Agricola (n=38)

Articles excluded – did not meet eligibility criteria (n = 1211), duplicates excluded (n = 100) and non English potentially relevant articles excluded (n=3)

English abstracts and full text articles retrieved for assessment for inclusion based on eligibility criteria (n = 20)

Articles excluded based on inadequate data or incorrect study design to qualify for inclusion (n = 10)

Articles that qualified to be included in review (n = 10)

Fig. 1. Flowchart of the search and identification of papers relevant to the review of the effect of pain medication on production parameters.

and gain to feed ratio. The outcomes of interest were continuous variables; therefore, for data analysis, group level means and SDs were required. Outcomes were reported as group means or pen-level means. When investigators reported only one SEM, this was interpreted as a pooled standard error across all treatment groups. Review Manager (RevMan) [Computer program]. Version 5.1; Copenhagen: The Nordic Cochrane Center, The Cochrane Collaboration, 2011. Software was used to back-calculate the SD for each treatment group based on the number of animals in each group and the pooled SEM. When multiple arm trials were conducted, the control arm was used for each active arm. This would lead to an overestimation of the sample size in the control arm and underestimation of the variation of the summary mean difference.

Meta-analysis Approach

Once extracted, the outcome data were entered into and analyzed using RevMan. Events of castration and dehorning were subdivided into outcomes of average daily gain, daily intake, and gain to feed ratio. Each outcome was divided into subcategories according to type of pain mitigation intervention (systemic, local, or caudal epidural pain medication). These data were used to create a summary mean difference when applicable and a forest plot for each outcome.

Forest Plots Show the Magnitude of Effect Across Studies

A forest plot is an approach to conveying the results of multiple studies on a single figure, to facilitate seeing each individual result and that of the combined body of work. On the left side of the forest plot are

- Column 1: Study identification
- Columns 2 to 4: mean and SD and the number enrolled in the medicated group
- Columns 5 and 6: mean and SD and the number enrolled in the comparison group
- Columns 7 and 8: the mean difference and 95% CI for the mean difference.

On the right side is a forest plot that contains a new line of data for each study:

- Each box in the forest plot represents the effect of pain management, the mean difference from each study
- The horizontal line through each box represents the 95% CI for the mean difference from each study
- The vertical line indicates where the mean difference is zero, which indicates no effect of pain management
- At the bottom of each forest plot is a diamond. The vertical points of the diamond represent the point estimate of the summary mean difference (ie, the weighted combination of the estimates from each study). The horizontal points of the diamond represent the boundaries of the 95% CI of the summary mean difference.

Assessing Statistical Significance

The authors assessed whether the association between pain mitigation interventions was statistically significant when all the controls were inactive products such as saline or placebo. The null hypothesis was that the overall mean difference was equal to zero. For all outcomes, it was expected that pain management would have a positive effect; therefore, the mean difference should be greater than zero if pain mitigation increased the production outcome. A subgroup analysis based on treatment type was conducted for all outcomes in which different interventions were used to assess the same outcome. Heterogeneity was assessed using the chi-square test for heterogeneity overall and within the subgroups. The null hypothesis was that heterogeneity was not present. If the P value for overall heterogeneity was greater than 0.1, the authors concluded the subgroups were not different. The authors also reported the I^2, which describes the percentage of variation across studies due to heterogeneity rather than chance.[25,26]

Assessing Biases in the Body of Work

To assess biases in the body of work, the outcomes reported were not subjective (ie, average daily gain was determined by measuring weight at given time intervals so that the impact of failure to blind on the risk of bias was considered minimal). Failure to randomize was considered important; however, its affect was most likely seen as publication bias. Suspicion of risk of publication bias was considered present if there was evidence that studies showing positive results were more likely to be published, whereas negative results were more likely to be excluded from the literature.[27] This was evaluated by looking at funnel plots created for each outcome.

RESULTS OF THE SEARCH

The results of the search are in **Fig. 1**. For several outcomes, relevant studies were retrieved in which the investigators did not report information in a manner that could be extracted. Tom and colleagues[28] reported that pain medication was not associated with changes in feed intake or milk production when tail docking was performed, but it was not possible to extract data from this article because only a *P* value was reported. Another study reported the effect of treating ulcera and foot conditions with pain medication and claw correction versus claw correction alone on spermiological and andrological data in bulls. Again, the authors were not able to extract data from this study to obtain an estimate of the effect for the same reason.[29] No studies reported on pain management for spaying or branding; therefore, these procedures were not considered.

The resulting literature included only information about pain management in castration and dehorning. A summary of the treatments used in each study is reported in **Tables 1** and **2**. Little evidence of publication bias was identified from the funnel plot analyses of the bodies of work contributing data to each outcome assessed, found in **Fig. 2**.

Effect of Pain Medication on Average Daily Gain After Dehorning

Two articles reported the effect of pain medication on average daily gain after dehorning.[5,13] The forest plot is presented in **Fig. 3**. To illustrate the different treatments, assessed subgroups were created according to treatment type:

- Systemic versus placebo (n = 1)[13]
- Multiple systemic and local versus single systemic and local (n = 1)[5]

Table 1
Summary of treatments studies analyzing outcome of pain management during dehorning on production parameters

Article	Procedure	Intervention	Control	Outcomes Observed
Baldridge et al,[13] 2011	Castration and dehorning	Xylazine, ketamine, butorphanol IM	Saline	Average daily gain
	Castration and dehorning	Xylazine, ketamine, butorphanol IM + sodium salicylate PO	Saline	Average daily gain
	Castration and dehorning	Sodium salicylate PO	Saline	Average daily gain
Duffield et al,[4] 2010	Dehorning	Ketamine + lidocaine	Saline + lidocaine	Feed intake
Faulkner and Weary,[5] 2000	Dehorning	Xylazine IM, lidocaine SC, ketoprofen PO	Xylazine IM, lidocaine SC	Average daily gain
Heinrich et al,[7] 2010	Dehorning	Meloxicam + lidocaine	Lidocaine	Feed intake
Milligan et al,[8] 2004	Dehorning	Ketoprofen + lidocaine	Saline + lidocaine	Feed intake

Table 2
Summary of treatment studies analyzing outcome of pain management during castration on production parameters

Article	Procedure	Intervention	Control	Outcomes Observed
Baldridge et al,[13] 2011	Castration and dehorning	Xylazine, ketamine, butorphanol IM	Saline	Average daily gain
	Castration and dehorning	Xylazine, ketamine, butorphanol IM + Sodium salicylate PO	Saline	Average daily gain
	Castration and dehorning	Sodium salicylate PO	Saline	Average daily gain
Coetzee et al,[15] 2012	Castration	Meloxicam PO	Placebo	Average daily gain, feed intake, Gain to feed ratio
Faulkner et al,[30] 1992	Castration	Butorphanol or xylazine IV	No treatment	Average daily gain, feed intake, Gain to feed ratio
Fisher et al,[14] 1996	Castration (burdizzo)	Local anesthetic	No treatment	Average daily gain, feed intake
	Castration (Surgical)	Local anesthetic	No treatment	Average daily gain, feed intake
Gonzalez et al,[6] 2010	Castration	Epidural xylazine, Flunixin megulmine IV	Saline	Average daily gain, feed intake
Pang et al,[9] 2006	Castration (Band)	Carprofen	Saline	Average daily gain, feed intake
	Castration (Burdizzo)	Carprofen	Saline	Average daily gain, feed intake
Ting et al,[11] 2003	Castration	Ketoprofen	Saline	Average daily gain, feed intake
	Castration	Lidocaine	Saline	Average daily gain, feed intake
	Castration	Combined xylazine HCl + lidocaine HCl caudal epidural	Saline	Average daily gain, feed intake
Ting et al,[12] 2003	Castration	Ketoprofen (3 mg/kg) at 0 min	Saline	Average daily gain, feed intake
	Castration	Ketoprofen (3 mg/kg) at 0 min	Saline	Average daily gain, feed intake
	Castration	Ketoprofen (1.5 mg/kg) at −20 and 0 min	Saline	Average daily gain, feed intake
	Castration	Ketoprofen (1.5 mg/kg) at −20 and 0 min	Saline	Average daily gain, feed intake
	Castration	Ketoprofen (1.5 mg/kg at −20 and 0 min; 3 mg/kg at 24 h)	Saline	Average daily gain, feed intake
	Castration	Ketoprofen (1.5 mg/kg at −20 and 0 min; 3 mg/kg at 24 h)	Saline	Average daily gain, feed intake

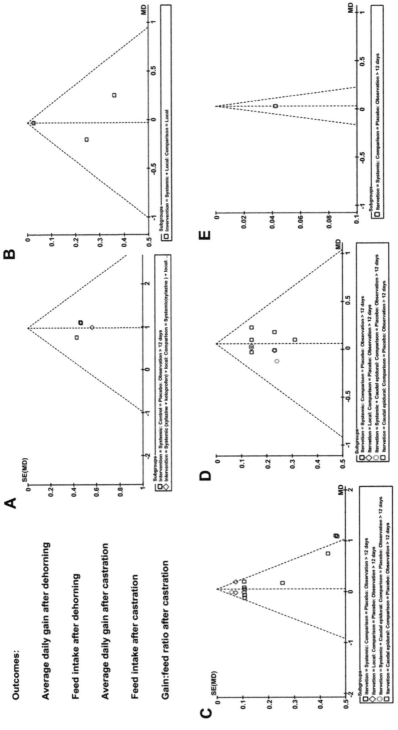

Fig. 2. Funnel plots for five continuous outcomes evaluated (*A–E*).

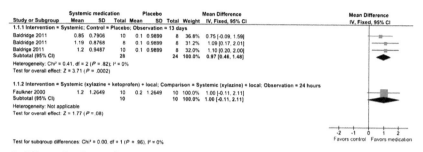

Study or Subgroup	Systemic medication			Placebo				Mean Difference		Mean Difference
	Mean	SD	Total	Mean	SD	Total	Weight	IV, Fixed, 95% CI		IV, Fixed, 95% CI
1.1.1 Intervention = Systemic; Control = Placebo; Observation = 13 days										
Baldridge 2011	0.85	0.7906	10	0.1	0.9899	8	36.8%	0.75 [-0.09, 1.59]		
Baldridge 2011	1.19	0.8768	8	0.1	0.9899	8	31.2%	1.09 [0.17, 2.01]		
Baldrige 2011	1.2	0.9487	10	0.1	0.9899	8	32.0%	1.10 [0.20, 2.00]		
Subtotal (95% CI)			28			24	100.0%	0.97 [0.46, 1.48]		
Heterogeneity: Chi² = 0.41, df = 2 (P = .82); I² = 0%										
Test for overall effect: Z = 3.71 (P = .0002)										
1.1.2 Intervention = Systemic (xylazine + ketoprofen) + local; Comparison = Systemic (xylazine) + local; Observation = 24 hours										
Faulkner 2000	1.2	1.2649	10	0.2	1.2649	10	100.0%	1.00 [-0.11, 2.11]		
Subtotal (95% CI)			10			10	100.0%	1.00 [-0.11, 2.11]		
Heterogeneity: Not applicable										
Test for overall effect: Z = 1.77 (P = .08)										
Test for subgroup differences: Chi² = 0.00, df = 1 (P = .96), I² = 0%										

Favors control   Favors medication

Fig. 3. Effect of pain medication on average daily gain after dehorning of calves.

The mean difference for systemic versus placebo was 0.97 kg (95% CI 0.46–1.48), suggesting a 1 kg greater daily gain in the medicated groups even in the short time frames studied. The mean difference for multiple systemic and local versus single systemic and local was 1.00 (95% CI −0.11–2.11), suggesting a 1 kg greater daily gain in the more highly medicated group. Of course, long-term impact was the important question, but no investigators conducted a study longer than longer than 13 days. A summary effect calculation would be invalid here because control groups were not the same.

Effect of Pain Medication on Daily Feed Intake After Dehorning

It was possible to extract data from three articles that reported the effect of pain medication on daily feed intake after dehorning.[4,7,8] The forest plot of the results is presented in **Fig. 4**. The intervention in all articles was the effect of systemic and local pain medications compared with local pain medication alone. However, the observation period for this outcome was very short—only 24 hours. For this outcome, it was expected that systemic and local pain medication would increase daily feed intake compared with local alone; therefore, a mean difference greater than zero would support this hypothesis. The overall mean difference was −0.03 (95% CI −0.09–0.02), suggesting no evidence of increased daily intake in the medicated groups. One surprising factor was the magnitude of the difference reported by Milligan and colleagues.[8] These investigators reported a mean difference of 0.03 kg (ie, 30 g) and an SEM difference of 0.02. Because these values were so small, these data are very heavily weighted in the meta-analysis. Given the time interval that these studies assess, it is not surprising that no effect was seen.

The Effect of Pain Medication on Average Daily Gain After Castration

This outcome was by far the most commonly reported. Eight articles reported the effect of pain medication on average daily gain after castration.[6,9,11–15,30] However, two of the eight articles reported relevant data that were in a format that could not be used in this analysis.[9,30] The forest plot of the results is presented in **Fig. 5**.

Study or Subgroup	Medication			Placebo				Mean Difference		Mean Difference
	Mean	SD	Total	Mean	SD	Total	Weight	IV, Fixed, 95% CI		IV, Fixed, 95% CI
Duffield 2010	1.8	1.3416	20	1.55	0.8944	20	0.6%	0.25 [-0.46, 0.96]		
Heinrich 2010	2.7	0.9859	30	2.9	0.9311	30	1.3%	-0.20 [-0.69, 0.29]		
Milligan 2004	0.09	0.0894	20	0.12	0.0894	20	98.1%	-0.03 [-0.09, 0.03]		
Total (95% CI)			70			70	100.0%	-0.03 [-0.09, 0.02]		
Heterogeneity: Chi² = 1.07, df = 2 (P = .58); I² = 0%										
Test for overall effect: Z = 1.09 (P = .28)										

Favors control   Favors medication

Fig. 4. Effect of pain medication on daily feed intake after dehorning in calves. Intervention = systemic + local; control = local; observation = 24 hours.

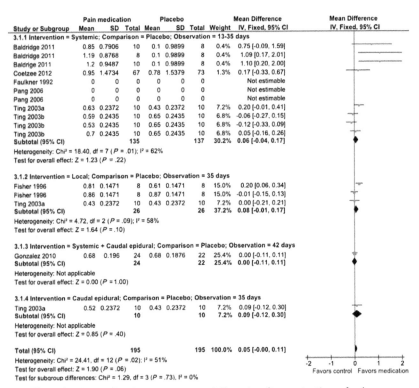

Fig. 5. Effect of pain medication on average daily gain after castration of calves.

To illustrate the different approaches assessed, these data were divided into subgroups by treatment type:

- Systemic versus placebo (n = 6)[9,11–13,15,30]
- Local versus placebo (n = 2)[11,14]
- Systemic plus caudal epidural versus placebo (n = 1)[6]
- Caudal epidural versus placebo (n = 1).[11]

Regardless of the type of pain management provided and duration of assessment, the magnitude of the effect was so small as to have little clinical relevance (summary mean difference = 0.05 kg and 95% CI = 0.00–0.11). It should be noted that the one study that did report a large effect is actually for animals that were both castrated and dehorned.[13] In addition, the funnel plot for this outcome suggests evidence of publication bias that would favor a positive result (ie, the smaller studies showed larger positive effects **Fig. 2**C).

The Effect of Pain Medication on Daily Feed Intake After Castration

Seven articles report the effect of pain medication on daily feed intake after castration.[6,9,11,12,14,15,30] Again, there was little evidence that pain medication had a meaningful effect on this outcome. The longest period of observation was 33 days[12] and likely not sufficient to document meaningful changes, especially in small studies. The forest plot of the results is presented in **Fig. 6**. Again, two of the seven articles reported relevant data that were in a format that could not be used in this analysis.[9,30]

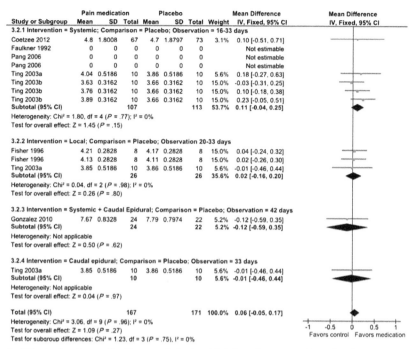

Study or Subgroup	Pain medication Mean	SD	Total	Placebo Mean	SD	Total	Weight	Mean Difference IV, Fixed, 95% CI
3.2.1 Intervention = Systemic; Comparison = Placebo; Observation = 16-33 days								
Coetzee 2012	4.8	1.8008	67	4.7	1.8797	73	3.1%	0.10 [-0.51, 0.71]
Faulkner 1992	0	0	0	0	0	0		Not estimable
Pang 2006	0	0	0	0	0	0		Not estimable
Pang 2006	0	0	0	0	0	0		Not estimable
Ting 2003a	4.04	0.5186	10	3.86	0.5186	10	5.6%	0.18 [-0.27, 0.63]
Ting 2003b	3.63	0.3162	10	3.66	0.3162	10	15.0%	-0.03 [-0.31, 0.25]
Ting 2003b	3.76	0.3162	10	3.66	0.3162	10	15.0%	0.10 [-0.18, 0.38]
Ting 2003b	3.89	0.3162	10	3.66	0.3162	10	15.0%	0.23 [-0.05, 0.51]
Subtotal (95% CI)			107			113	53.7%	0.11 [-0.04, 0.25]
Heterogeneity: Chi² = 1.80, df = 4 (P = .77); I² = 0%								
Test for overall effect: Z = 1.45 (P = .15)								
3.2.2 Intervention = Local; Comparison = Placebo; Observation 20-33 days								
Fisher 1996	4.21	0.2828	8	4.17	0.2828	8	15.0%	0.04 [-0.24, 0.32]
Fisher 1996	4.13	0.2828	8	4.11	0.2828	8	15.0%	0.02 [-0.26, 0.30]
Ting 2003a	3.85	0.5186	10	3.86	0.5186	10	5.6%	-0.01 [-0.46, 0.44]
Subtotal (95% CI)			26			26	35.6%	0.02 [-0.16, 0.20]
Heterogeneity: Chi² = 0.04, df = 2 (P = .98); I² = 0%								
Test for overall effect: Z = 0.26 (P = .80)								
3.2.3 Intervention = Systemic + Caudal Epidural; Comparison = Placebo; Observation = 42 days								
Gonzalez 2010	7.67	0.8328	24	7.79	0.7974	22	5.2%	-0.12 [-0.59, 0.35]
Subtotal (95% CI)			24			22	5.2%	-0.12 [-0.59, 0.35]
Heterogeneity: Not applicable								
Test for overall effect: Z = 0.50 (P = .62)								
3.2.4 Intervention = Caudal epidural; Comparison = Placebo; Observation = 33 days								
Ting 2003a	3.85	0.5186	10	3.86	0.5186	10	5.6%	-0.01 [-0.46, 0.44]
Subtotal (95% CI)			10			10	5.6%	-0.01 [-0.46, 0.44]
Heterogeneity: Not applicable								
Test for overall effect: Z = 0.04 (P = .97)								
Total (95% CI)			167			171	100.0%	0.06 [-0.05, 0.17]
Heterogeneity: Chi² = 3.06, df = 9 (P = .96); I² = 0%								
Test for overall effect: Z = 1.09 (P = .27)								
Test for subgroup differences: Chi² = 1.23, df = 3 (P = .75), I² = 0%								

Fig. 6. Effect of pain medication on daily feed intake after castration of calves.

To illustrate the different approaches assessed, these data were divided into subgroups by treatment type:

- Systemic versus placebo (n = 5)[9,11,12,15,30]
- Local versus placebo (n = 2)[11,14]
- Systemic plus caudal epidural versus placebo (n = 1)[6]
- Caudal epidural versus placebo (n = 1).[11]

All studies used an inactive control or no treatment and there was no evidence of heterogeneity among the subgroups (P = .75). The overall mean difference was 0.06 (95% CI −0.15–0.17) and was not statistically significant (P = .96).

The Effect of Pain Medication on Gain to Feed Ratio After Castration

Two articles reported the effect of pain medication on gain to feed ratio after castration.[15,30] The forest plot of the results is presented in **Fig. 7**. Both articles assessed systemic pain medication versus placebo and the observation period was 27 to 28 days. One article presented relevant data in a format that could not be used in this analysis.[30] The overall mean difference observed in this one study was 0.03 kg

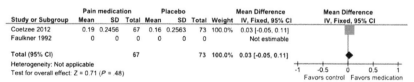

Study or Subgroup	Pain medication Mean	SD	Total	Placebo Mean	SD	Total	Weight	Mean Difference IV, Fixed, 95% CI
Coetzee 2012	0.19	0.2456	67	0.16	0.2563	73	100.0%	0.03 [-0.05, 0.11]
Faulkner 1992	0	0	0	0	0	0		Not estimable
Total (95% CI)			67			73	100.0%	0.03 [-0.05, 0.11]
Heterogeneity: Not applicable								
Test for overall effect: Z = 0.71 (P = .48)								

Fig. 7. Effect of pain medication on gain to feed ratio after castration of calves. Intervention = systemic; control = placebo; observation = 27–28 days.

gained per kg feed consumed (95% CI = −0.05–0.11) and was not statistically significant (P = .48).

CONCLUSION AND CRITIQUE OF THE EVIDENCE BASE

The body of work identified by the search does not support, and possibly refutes, the idea that pain medication has production benefits. With the exception of average daily gain after dehorning, the overall conclusion is that there is little to no evidence that the use of pain medication during painful procedures such as castration and dehorning results in an improvement in average daily gain, daily feed intake, or gain to feed ratio. For the one outcome that did seem to show an effect, the overall mean difference in average daily gain after dehorning implied that treated calves gained 1 kg more per day than control calves (see **Fig. 3**). Three studies from a single article found this outcome to be significant (0.97, 95% CI 0.46–1.48, P = .0002).[13] The other article analyzing this outcome reported a similar magnitude of effect, though the result was not statistically significant (1.00, 95% CI −0.11–2.11, P = .08).[5]

The body of work was likely never intended for this purpose. It seems most likely that most studies that reported production outcomes were designed to answer the question about behavioral or physiologic indicators of pain. This would explain the small sample sizes and the short duration. Eventually, if it is seen as critical to assess the question of whether pain management either increases production parameters or at least does not decrease it, studies purposefully designed for detecting meaningful differences in production outcomes will be needed. Such studies should be larger and, most important, of longer duration.

CRITIQUE OF THE REVIEW PROCESS

With respect to the execution of the review, the authors conducted a comprehensive electronic search; however, electronic citation databases were solely relied on and journals or conference proceedings were not manually searched for studies that may have been overlooked. This is a possible limitation in the search strategy. The authors did, however, verify that no relevant citations from the previous reviews were missed by the electronic search; therefore, the potential for bias is minimized.

Studies that failed to randomize were not excluded. Exclusion of nonrandomized studies would have further limited the information available to make meaningful conclusions because few studies explicitly reported randomization to group. Failure to blind was also not used as an exclusion criterion. The rationale for this was that the observed outcomes were objective and, therefore, most likely unaffected by blinding.

WHAT IS THE EVIDENCE THAT PRODUCERS CONSIDER THAT PAIN MANAGEMENT MUST BE ECONOMICAL?
Introduction

It is important to understand motivation among cattle producers to use or not use pain medication during painful procedures or conditions in cattle. The purpose of this literature analysis was to examine the question of whether economic factors influence this decision. The authors also included results from veterinary surgeons; however, the motivators of veterinarians to recommend the use of pain management are likely different from the motivators of producers to adopt its use.

The review question
What is the prevalence of producers who are motivated by or consider economic factors important when considering the use of pain management in cattle?

Identifying the literature
The electronic citation indexes PubMed and CAB Abstracts were searched. The search terms used in PubMed are provided in **Fig. 8**. Analogous search terms were used in CAB Abstracts. No language or date restrictions were imposed during the search. All database searches were conducted in the last 2 weeks of July 2012.

Identifying relevant articles
Screening of the retrieved citations was conducted independently by one reviewer (HN), a DVM student working in a summer research program. The reviewer screened all retrieved citations and full texts for inclusion based on the following eligibility criteria:

- Does the study describe a survey conducted among a population of cattle producers and veterinarians?
- Does the survey address economic motivation to use or neglect to use pain medication during painful procedures or conditions in cattle?

When the reviewer answered yes to each question, the studies were included in the review. Some retrieved surveys were eliminated because of failure to assess the question of economic motivation behind the use of pain medication in cattle[24,31–34]; however, other motivations may have been addressed.

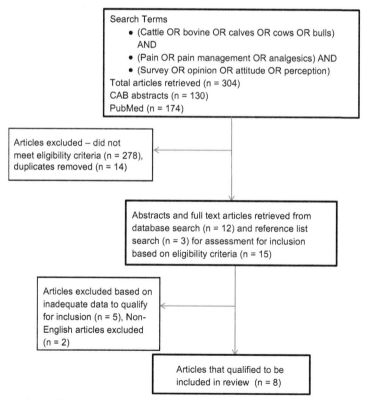

Fig. 8. Flowchart of the search and identification of surveys relevant to the question of motivation to use or neglect to use pain medication in cattle during painful procedures or conditions.

Extracting data from the studies
Once the full text for publications meeting the selection criteria (see previous discussion) were obtained, information about survey methods, demographic information about the population surveyed, as well as data regarding the motivation to use or not to use pain medication in cattle were extracted by one reviewer (HN).

SUMMARY OF DATA FROM THE STUDIES

The results of this literature search are summarized in **Fig. 8**. Data extracted from several surveys are summarized in **Tables 3** and **4**. Six of the eight relevant surveys had some respondents that expressed concern about the cost of analgesic use in cattle.[16,20,22,23,35,36] Two surveys found the results of this inquiry to be equivocal.[19,21] At the other end of the spectrum, one survey found that not a single producer surveyed was willing to pay the cost per animal to cover cornual nerve blocks.[20] Other deterrents of analgesic use included weight of calf,[16] time required for analgesic use,[22] absence of FDA-approved bovine analgesics,[16] governmental regulations,[23,36] and the perceived necessity of some pain to prevent excessive movement postsurgery.[23,36]

DISCUSSION
Responses from Producers

Surprisingly few studies were identified in which producers seemed to be explicitly asked if economics, cost-benefit, and so forth, were factors considered in the decision to adopt the use of pain medication.[20,22,35] These were conducted in Canada,[22] Italy,[20] and the United Kingdom.[35] In this survey of dairy producers and food-animal veterinarians in Ontario, no more than 25% of producers expressed concern about cost of either xylazine or lidocaine. In the survey of dairy producers in Italy, different results were obtained. None of the respondents were willing to pay enough per animal to cover the cost of a cornual nerve block. In the United Kingdom, though many cattle farmers were unwilling to cover the cost of analgesia in many procedures listed, 40% were willing to pay more than the cost of analgesia during surgical castration, and 24% were willing to pay more than the cost of analgesia during disbudding.

The question of cost is likely very different regionally and local surveys are likely needed. For example, in the United States and Canada, pain mitigation is entirely voluntary and also many producers perform the castration and dehorning procedures themselves. This obviously affects the economics of adoption of pain management. If the protocol for pain management, such as a cornual block, requires a veterinarian, the cost involved includes veterinary visits as well as medication and additional time. However, if the producer already uses a veterinarian for these procedures, the additional cost for pain medication will be substantially smaller. None of the surveys seemed to explicitly address this issue.

Responses from Veterinarians

Most relevant surveys identified were directed toward veterinarians in bovine practice.[16,19,21–23,36] A survey in the United States of American Association of Bovine Practitioners members,[19] as well as a survey of Canadian livestock practitioners,[21] revealed a lack of any strong opinion on whether the cost of pain management impedes its adoption. In the survey by Misch and colleagues[22] in Canada, 25% were concerned with the cost of xylazine, whereas only 4% were concerned with the cost of lidocaine. Almost 40% of veterinarians in a Scandinavian survey expressed recognition of clients' concern about the cost of analgesia.[23] In the United Kingdom, 65% of practitioners surveyed thought that the cost of analgesia was a major issue for producers.[36]

Table 3
Summary of surveys regarding veterinarians' opinions about the use of pain medication in cattle

Survey	Population	Selection Method	Average Age	Gender	Country	Type of Survey	Number of Surveys Sent	Number of Surveys Analyzed	Economic Reason for Choosing Whether to Use Pain Medication	Other Reasons for Choosing Not to Use Pain Medication
Coetzee et al,[16] 2010	AABP members; Members of Academy of Veterinary Consultants	Unclear	46	77% M 23% F	USA	Web-based survey	1,972	189	Four respondents: Cost of analgesia is an impediment to widespread use. Producers are resistant to incur the additional cost.	Adequate calf weight Four respondents: absence of FDA-approved analgesics
Fajt et al,[19] 2011	AABP members	All AABP members with email addresses listed	44	78% M 22% F	USA	Web-based survey	3,019	666	Concerns regarding drug costs seem to be equivocal	—

(continued on next page)

Table 3
(continued)

Survey	Population	Selection Method	Average Age	Gender	Country	Type of Survey	Number of Surveys Sent	Number of Surveys Analyzed	Economic Reason for Choosing Whether to Use Pain Medication	Other Reasons for Choosing Not to Use Pain Medication
Hewson et al,[21] 2007	Veterinarians in Canada listed by provincial licensing bodies as working in bovine, equine, and swine practice	Random	46	65% M 35% F	Canada	Paper questionnaire	1,431	586	Strong agreement (8/10) that long-acting and cost-effective analgesics for food animals are needed; No strong opinions about whether "owners are unwilling to pay for analgesia" (5/10 for beef vets; 3/10 for dairy vets); Neutral on whether "cost of analgesic drugs prohibits me from using them" (5/10).	—

Study	Population	Recruitment	Response rate	Country	Gender	Survey method	No. invited	No. responded	Results (cost)	Results (other)
Misch et al,[22] 2007	Dairy producers in Ontario that take part in Dairy Herd Improvement Program; Food-animal veterinarians in Ontario	Random	Not reported	Canada	Not reported	Paper questionnaire; Telephone questionnaire	Producers: 340 Veterinarians: 256	Producers: 207 Veterinarians: 65	Producers: 19% concerned with cost of xylazine, 23% concerned with cost of lidocaine. Veterinarians: 25% concerned with cost of xylazine, 4% concerned with cost of lidocaine	Producers: Time is most common concern in xylazine (18%) and lidocaine (22%) use. Veterinarians: Time is most common concern for xylazine (29%) and lidocaine (47%) use.
Thomsen et al,[23] 2010	Bovine practitioners in Scandinavian countries	All bovine vets on the mailing list of a pharmaceutical company (Boehringer Ingelheim)	Not reported	Denmark, Sweden, Norway	59% M 41% F	Paper questionnaire	1,164	352	37.8% Agree that farmers would like their cattle to be treated with analgesics, but the price is a major problem	21% Agree that some pain is necessary to prevent animal from being too active; 37.2% agree that EU legislation limits ability to use analgesics in cattle
Huxley and Whay,[35] 2007	Practicing cattle veterinary surgeons in the UK	All cattle vets on the mailing list of a UK pharmaceutical company	Not reported	Great Britain, Northern Ireland	Not reported	Paper questionnaire	2,391	616	36.3% agree the farmers are happy to pay the costs involved with giving analgesics to cattle 65.3% agree that farmers would like cattle to receive analgesia bust cost is a major issue	37.5% agree EU legislation limits ability to use analgesics in cattle 17.4% said some pain is necessary to stop the animal becoming to active Only 45.5% claimed to have adequate knowledge on the subject of pain in cattle

Table 4
Summary of surveys regarding producers' opinions about the use of pain medication in cattle

Survey	Population	Selection Method	Average Age	Gender	Country	Type of Survey	Number of Surveys Sent	Number of Surveys Analyzed	Economic Reason for Choosing Whether to Use Pain Medication	Other Reasons for Choosing Not to Use Pain Medication
Gottardo et al,[20] 2011	Dairy farmers that take part in Dairy Herd Improvement Program	Random	Not reported	Not reported	Italy	Paper questionnaire	1,500	639	Only 45% stated willingness to spend some money for analgesia. Within that group, none indicated they would spend enough per calf to cover cost of cornual nerve block	
Huxley and Whay,[24] 2006	Cattle farmers in the UK (survey of cattle practitioners conducted by these authors discussed in Whay et al)	Cattle farmers on the mailing list of a UK based pharmaceutical company (Pfizer Animal Health)	20–60+	92% M 18% F	Great Britain and Northern Ireland	Paper questionnaire	7,500	1,029	40% were prepared to pay more than the cost of analgesic therapy for surgical castration 24% were prepared to pay more than the cost of analgesic therapy for disbudding For several procedures listed, many farmers were not willing to cover cost of analgesia	62% agreed that farmers do not know enough about controlling pain in cattle 53% agreed that veterinary surgeons do not discuss controlling pain in cattle with farmers enough

| Misch et al,[22] 2007 | Dairy producers in Ontario that take part in Dairy Herd Improvement Program; Food-animal veterinarians in Ontario | Random | Not reported | Not reported | Canada | Paper questionnaire; Telephone questionnaire | Producers: 340 Veterinarians: 256 | Producers: 207 Veterinarians: 65 | Producers: 19% concerned with cost of xylazine, 23% concerned with cost of lidocaine Veterinarians: 25% concerned with cost of xylazine, 4% concerned with cost of lidocaine | Producers: time is most common concern in xylazine (18%) and lidocaine (22%) use. Veterinarians: time is most common concern for xylazine (29%) and lidocaine (47%) use. |

The authors think that, although interesting, a veterinarian's perspective of the economics of pain management is not entirely useful. Ultimately, it is the decision of the producer whether they are willing to pay for pain management and whether they think there are benefits to the added cost. This may result in discrepancies between the opinion of the producer and that of the veterinarian. For example, in the Canadian survey by Misch and colleagues,[22] 4% of veterinarians were concerned about the cost of lidocaine, whereas 23% of producers expressed this concern. It is also possible that veterinarians are unaware of the attitude of producers toward the cost of pain management in cattle.

Other Motivators

When considering why a veterinarian or producer would choose to use or not to use analgesics in cattle, factors other than cost may be of importance. In two surveys, for example, bovine practitioners held the opinion that some postsurgical pain is necessary and beneficial.[23,36] Time required for analgesic use was a concern for both practitioners and producers in a Canadian survey, though this could be considered a proxy for cost.[22] Governmental regulations also deterred some respondents from using analgesics in cattle. For example, a few AABP members expressed concern about the lack of FDA-approved cattle analgesics in the United States,[23] whereas Scandinavian and United Kingdom bovine practitioners expressed concern about preventive European Union regulations.[23,36] Inadequate knowledge of the subject may also be a major factor in this decision. In the survey by Whay and Huxley,[36] less than half of those practitioners surveyed (45.5%) claimed to have adequate knowledge on the subject of pain management in cattle. This is reflected in the United Kingdom survey by Whay and Huxley,[36] in which 62% of farmers agreed that they do not know enough about controlling pain in cattle and 53% agreed that veterinarians do not discuss the subject of pain management in cattle enough.[35] Either a lack of communication between veterinarian and producer, or inadequate education on the subject, may be important considerations.

SUMMARY

Future surveys on this issue of attitudes toward cost of pain management in cattle would be greatly beneficial. To increase analgesic use in cattle and thus improve animal welfare, it is essential that deterrents and motivators for their use among practitioners and producers are understood. The attitude on this subject among producers is particularly important because the final decision lies with them.

ACKNOWLEDGMENTS

The authors would like to acknowledge Dr Andrea Dinkelman of Iowa State University College of Veterinary Medicine for her assistance in constructing the literature search for research analyzing the effect of pain medication on production parameters.

REFERENCES

1. National Agriculture Statistics Service: Statistics of cattle, hogs, and sheep. Available at: http://www.nass.usda.gov/Publications/Ag_Statistics/2011/Chapter07.pdf. Accessed July 18, 2012.
2. AVMA policy: castration and dehorning of cattle. Available at: http://www.avma.org/issues/policy/animal_welfare/dehorning_cattle.asp. Accessed July 17, 2012.

3. Hudson C, Whay H, Huxley J. Recognition and management of pain in cattle. In Practice 2008;30:126–34.
4. Duffield TF, Heinrich A, Millman ST, et al. Reduction in pain response by combined use of local lidocaine anesthesia and systemic ketoprofen in dairy calves dehorned by heat cauterization. Can Vet J 2010;51(3):283–8.
5. Faulkner PM, Weary DM. Reducing pain after dehorning in dairy calves. J Dairy Sci 2000;83(9):2037–41.
6. Gonzalez LA, Schwartzkopf-Genswein KS, Caulkett NA, et al. Pain mitigation after band castration of beef calves and its effects on performance, behavior, *Escherichia coli*, and salivary cortisol. J Anim Sci 2010;88(2):802–10.
7. Heinrich A, Duffield TF, Lissemore KD, et al. The effect of meloxicam on behavior and pain sensitivity of dairy calves following cautery dehorning with a local anesthetic. J Dairy Sci 2010;93(6):2450–7.
8. Milligan BN, Duffield T, Lissemore K. The utility of ketoprofen for alleviating pain following dehorning in young dairy calves. Can Vet J 2004;45(2):140–3.
9. Pang WY, Earley B, Sweeney T, et al. Effect of carprofen administration during banding or burdizzo castration of bulls on plasma cortisol, in vitro interferon-gamma production, acute-phase proteins, feed intake, and growth. J Anim Sci 2006;84(2):351–9.
10. Stilwell G, Lima MS, Broom DM. Effects of nonsteroidal anti-inflammatory drugs on long-term pain in calves castrated by use of an external clamping technique following epidural anesthesia. Am J Vet Res 2008;69(6):744–50.
11. Ting ST, Earley B, Hughes JM, et al. Effect of ketoprofen, lidocaine local anesthesia, and combined xylazine and lidocaine caudal epidural anesthesia during castration of beef cattle on stress responses, immunity, growth, and behavior. J Anim Sci 2003;81(5):1281–93.
12. Ting ST, Earley B, Crowe MA. Effect of repeated ketoprofen administration during surgical castration of bulls on cortisol, immunological function, feed intake, growth, and behavior. J Anim Sci 2003;81(5):1253–64.
13. Baldridge SL, Coetzee JF, Dritz SS, et al. Pharmacokinetics and physiologic effects of intramuscularly administered xylazine hydrochloride-ketamine hydrochloride-butorphanol tartrate alone or in combination with orally administered sodium salicylate on biomarkers of pain in Holstein calves following castration and dehorning. Am J Vet Res 2011;72(10):1305–17.
14. Fisher AD, Crowe MA, Alonso de la Varga ME, et al. Effect of castration method and the provision of local anesthesia on plasma cortisol, scrotal circumference, growth, and feed intake of bull calves. J Anim Sci 1996;74(10):2336–43.
15. Coetzee JF, Edwards LN, Mosher RA, et al. Effect of oral meloxicam on health and performance of beef steers relative to bulls castrated on arrival at the feedlot. J Anim Sci 2012;90(3):1026–39.
16. Coetzee JF, Nutsch AL, Barbur LA, et al. A survey of castration methods and associated livestock management practices performed by bovine veterinarians in the United States. BMC Vet Res 2010;6:12.
17. Coetzee JF. A review of pain assessment techniques and pharmacological approaches to pain relief after bovine castration: practical implications for cattle production within the United States. Appl Anim Behav Sci 2011;135(3):192–213.
18. U.S. Food and Drug Administration. Pain measurement techniques for food-producing animals could lead to pain control drugs. Available at: http://www.fda.gov/downloads/AnimalVeterinary/ResourcesforYou/AnimalHealthLiteracy/UCM207088.pdf. Accessed July 26, 2012.

19. Fajt VR, Wagner SA, Norby B. Analgesic drug administration and attitudes about analgesia in cattle among bovine practitioners in the United States. J Am Vet Med Assoc 2011;238(6):755–67.
20. Gottardo F, Nalon E, Contiero B, et al. The dehorning of dairy calves: practices and opinions of 639 farmers. J Dairy Sci 2011;94(11):5724–34.
21. Hewson CJ, Dohoo IR, Lemke KA, et al. Canadian veterinarians' use of analgesics in cattle, pigs, and horses in 2004 and 2005. Can Vet J 2007;48(2):155–64.
22. Misch LJ, Duffield TF, Millman ST, et al. An investigation into the practices of dairy producers and veterinarians in dehorning dairy calves in Ontario. Can Vet J 2007; 48(12):1249–54.
23. Thomsen PT, Gidekull M, Herskin MS, et al. Scandinavian bovine practitioners' attitudes to the use of analgesics in cattle. Vet Rec 2010;167:256–8.
24. Huxley JN, Whay HR. Current attitudes of cattle practitioners to pain and the use of analgesics in cattle. Vet Rec 2006;159(20):662–8.
25. Higgins JP, Thompson SG. Quantifying heterogeneity in a meta-analysis. Stat Med 2002;21(11):1539–58.
26. Higgins JP, Thompson SG, Deeks JJ, et al. Measuring inconsistency in meta-analyses. BMJ 2003;327(7414):557–60.
27. Guyatt GH, Oxman AD, Montori V, et al. GRADE guidelines: 5. Rating the quality of evidence–publication bias. J Clin Epidemiol 2011;64(12):1277–82.
28. Tom EM, Duncan IJH, Widowski TM, et al. Effects of tail docking using a rubber ring with or without anesthetic on behavior and production of lactating cows. J Dairy Sci 2002;85(9):2257–65.
29. Babic NP, Radisic B, Lipar M, et al. Influence of lameness-caused stress, pain and inflammation on health and reproduction in Holstein-Frisian bulls. Veterinarska Stanica 2011;42(Suppl 1):3–6.
30. Faulkner DB, Eurell T, Tranquilli WJ, et al. Performance and health of weanling bulls after butorphanol and xylazine administration at castration. J Anim Sci 1992;70(10):2970–4.
31. Hoe FGH, Ruegg PL. Opinions and practices of Wisconsin dairy producers about biosecurity and animal well-being. J Dairy Sci 2006;89(6):2297–308.
32. Laven RA, Huxley JN, Whay HR, et al. Results of a survey of attitudes of dairy veterinarians in New Zealand regarding painful procedures and conditions in cattle. N Z Vet J 2009;57(4):215–20.
33. Phillips CJ, Wojciechowska J, Meng J, et al. Perceptions of the importance of different welfare issues in livestock production. Animal 2009;3(8):1152–66.
34. Raekallio M, Heinonen KM, Kuussaari J, et al. Pain alleviation in animals: attitudes and practices of Finnish veterinarians. Vet J 2003;165(2):131–5.
35. Huxley JN, Whay HR. Attitudes of UK veterinary surgeons and cattle farmers to pain and the use of analgesics in cattle. Cattle Pract 2007;15(2):189–93.
36. Whay HR, Huxley JN. Pain relief in cattle: a practitioners perspective. Cattle Pract 2005;13(2):81–5.

Index

Note: Page numbers of article titles are in **boldface** type.

A

Accelerometer(s)
  monitoring activity with
    in remote noninvasive assessment of pain and health status in cattle, 63–64
  in pain assessment in lame cattle, 140
Acepromazine
  extralabel use of, 30
α2-Adrenergic agonists
  for castration-related pain, 95–96
  in chemical restraint in ruminants, 214–215, 218
  effects on pain biomarkers in dehorning, 128
  in food animals
    in U.S., 21–22
  as injectable anesthesia in ruminants, 214–215
  for pain in small ruminants and camelids, 186–187
  reversal of
    in chemical restraint/injectable anesthesia in ruminants, 215
γ-Aminobutyric acid analogues
  for pain in small ruminants and camelids, 190–191
Analgesia/analgesic(s)
  for castration-related pain, 94–96
  for cattle
    in U.S.
      regulatory considerations for, **1–10**
        extralabel use of approved drugs, 8–9
        FOI Summary, 5–6
        identification of approved *vs.* unapproved drugs, 6
        introduction to, 1–2
        issues related to, 6–8
        new animal drug approval process, 2–5. *See also* New animal drug approval
          process, in U.S.
  in dehorned cattle
    assessment of, 117–121
    scientific studies, 106–116
    strategies for use
      effects on pain biomarkers, 121–129
  effects on pain biomarkers of castration-related pain, 88–91
  in food animals
    challenges associated with providing, 12–13
  opioid
    for castration-related pain, 94–95

Vet Clin Food Anim 29 (2013) 251–265
http://dx.doi.org/10.1016/S0749-0720(13)00009-1
0749-0720/13/$ – see front matter © 2013 Elsevier Inc. All rights reserved.

vetfood.theclinics.com

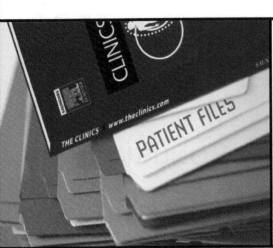

Printed and bound by CPI Group (UK) Ltd, Croydon, CR0 4YY

03/10/2024

01040440-0011